T0185935

Epilepsy Case Studies

William O. Tatum • Joseph I. Sirven
Gregory D. Cascino
Editors

Epilepsy Case Studies

Pearls for Patient Care

Second Edition

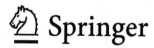 Springer

Editors
William O. Tatum
Mayo Clinic
Department of Neurology
Jacksonville, FL
USA

Joseph I. Sirven
Mayo Clinic
Department of Neurology
Jacksonville, FL
USA

Gregory D. Cascino
Mayo Clinic
Department of Neurology
Rochester, MN
USA

ISBN 978-3-030-59080-2   ISBN 978-3-030-59078-9   (eBook)
https://doi.org/10.1007/978-3-030-59078-9

This Springer imprint is published by the registered company Springer Nature Switzerland AG
The registered company address is: Gewerbestrasse 11, 6330 Cham, Switzerland

This book is dedicated to our patients and their families who have taught us so much about epilepsy and about life.

DKWILY

Foreword

What can we learn from the stories about a single patient with epilepsy? Consider the case of a young reporter who experienced "a month of madness" and was ultimately discovered to have anti-NMDA receptor encephalitis that uncovered the importance of autoimmune epilepsies. Consider genetics and rare diseases that have come to define populations with limited number of patients. Consider the impact from the unfortunate experience when a patient ultimately succumbs to epilepsy suddenly and unexpectedly is then impossible to "study" given ethical constraints and finality of the process. Consider the patient who has a rare disorder and epilepsy, experiences a rare side-effect, or becomes seizure-free with their ninth anti-seizure medication (ASM). Or when surgery becomes successful after failure of the same ASM usage. Consider the one case of Henry Molaison ("H.M."), who underwent bilateral temporal lobe surgery for drug-resistant epilepsy, and how this changed all subsequent surgeries from that time onward to avoid making a similar mistake.

The chapters in this book represent real people and real-life situations that had consequences both good and bad depending upon their individual situation. The intent of presenting these patients in a case-based format is designed to stimulate the same deductive reasoning on a personal level when we see patients in the clinic. The utility of neuroimaging and neurophysiology in the study of patients with epilepsy has become a staple with which the diagnosis and treatment of epilepsy has become inextricably intertwined. Therefore, the interpretation of these studies is essential for the neurologist and foundational for the epileptologist. Following the clinical scenario composed of a wide variety of epilepsy cases, questions are posed to organize the reader's thoughts in addressing the pertinent features of each case. Questions that include commonly asked ones such as, "How does this test help us with the diagnosis?" and "What is the relationship of the seizures to the patient's condition?" Other questions include, "How does this information help us to devise a treatment plan?" and "What do we know about the anticipated course and prognosis?" The questions raised in each section incorporate the clinical course and evaluation. They are addressed in a segment of the book that focuses on a discussion of the facts of the case. Where it is possible, these discussions rely upon the latest medical evidence to support the responses. At the end of each case, a few salient citations are referenced. Unlike a textbook, these cases include a few of the more pertinent articles that the reader can refer to obtain an overview of the topic and search for an expanded bibliography, if they so desire.

We learn from every patient. In the end, it is the individual report that "restores the human subject at the center of attention as the suffering, afflicted, fighting, human subject… only then do we have a 'who' as well as a 'what', a real person, a patient, in relation to a disease-in relation to the physical".* Our take-home messages are encapsulated in the form of clinical pearls. These "bullets" of information form the basis of our understanding of the case scenarios presented. Furthermore, they guide our decision-making in an approach to treatment for an individual patient. There is simply no written text that can replace the knowledge that is derived from hearing and seeing our patient and what they tell us. Additionally, our patients' case histories are the best tools to successfully guide us toward the correct approach to different clinical scenarios; the overuse of "tests" will never replace the clues that our patients give us. The field of epileptology encompasses some of the most dynamic and dramatic conditions that a neurologist will face. Little is more surprising in the field of medicine than the spontaneity and unpredictability of seizures. The second edition of *Case Studies in Epilepsy* will aid in selecting the approach to a clinically based problem list. Cases include the newly diagnosed to drug-resistant epilepsy, epilepsy from unknown causes to seizures caused by a brain tumor, infants and the elderly with epilepsy, diagnostic dilemmas, and treatment challenges. Novel associations involving genetics and autoimmunity are addressed. Surgical approaches in the uncontrolled person with epilepsy include non-medical treatment options, such as resective and laser surgery, neuromodulation, dietary control, alternative medicine, and investigational approaches. The cases in *Case Studies in Epilepsy* encompass a broad range and heterogeneous group of the epilepsies from those with genetic to structural-metabolic to those with unknown causes. Compiling these cases has been fun; we remember the people who taught us much about patient experiences and about the impact upon a full productive life. Today, even in the most highly regarded academic centers, professors from their subspecialties will be heard saying, "I remember the case of Mrs. Smith and will never forget it."

William O. Tatum IV

*O. Sacks The man who mistook his wife for a hat. Summit books. Simon & Schuster New York; 1999.

Acknowledgment

I would like to acknowledge my gratitude to my colleagues at the Mayo Clinic for both the opportunity to work alongside them and to learn from them. This multi-authored enterprise-wide work has been compiled by many outstanding clinicians, educators, and researchers, who freely and generously volunteered their precious time to contribute to this work, and serves as a testimony to their dedication to the field of epilepsy and to their colleagues. This book is about 50 people whose lives took a different course after they experienced seizures. The stigma and painful lack of predictability experienced by patients, friends, and families is something most of us will hopefully never know. The cases described in this book are presented in a didactic fashion, but lack the emotional content behind each case to limit the real impact that written text is too shallow to appreciate.

One of my first mentors taught me that patient care is the most noble aspect in the practice of neurology. Those who cannot work with people…teach or research sometimes in an effort to avoid patient care. What is missed is the humanity of suffering and the excitement of clinical success. We must always remember that it is people who are behind the symptoms of their illness and that treatment begins with the compassion displayed by a personal human touch. When we live our professional lives by the words of William and Charles Mayo, "The needs of the patient come first," we bring to light and acknowledge what is truly important for the focus in the practice of Medicine.

Mayo Clinic
Jacksonville, FL, USA

William O. Tatum IV

Contents

Contributors

Harry S. Abram, MD Department of Pediatric Neurology, Nemours Children's Specialty Care, Jacksonville, FL, USA

Rubina Bakerywala, MD Nemours Children's Specialty Care, Department of Neurology, Jacksonville, FL, USA

Karen Blackmon, PhD Mayo Clinic, Department of Psychology and Psychiatry , Jacksonville, FL, USA

Ben Brinkmann, PhD Mayo Clinic, Department of Neurology, Rochester, MN, USA

David B. Burkholder, MD Mayo Clinic, Department of Neurology, Rochester, MN, USA

Gregory D. Cascino, MD, FAAN, FANA, FACNS, FAES Mayo Clinic, Department of Neurology, Rochester, MN, USA

William P. Cheshire, MD Mayo Clinic, Department of Neurology, Jacksonville, FL, USA

Amy Z. Crepeau, MD Mayo Clinic, Department of Neurology, Phoenix, AZ, USA

Joseph F. Drazkowski, MD Mayo Clinic, Department of Neurology, Phoenix, AZ, USA

Cyrille Ferrier, MD University Medical Center Utrecht, Brain Center Rudolf Magnus, Department of Neurology and Neurosurgery, Utrecht, The Netherlands

Anteneh M. Feyissa, MD, MSc Mayo Clinic, Department of Neurology, Jacksonville, FL, USA

Anthony L. Fine, MD Mayo Clinic, Department of Neurology, Division of Child and Adolescent Neurology, Rochester, MN, USA

W. David Freeman, MD Mayo Clinic Florida, Departments of Critical Care Medicine, Neurology, and Neurosurgery, Jacksonville, FL, USA

Diogo M. Garcia, MD Mayo Clinic, Department of Neurosurgery, Jacksonville, FL, USA

Sanjeet S. Grewal, MD Mayo Clinic, Department of Neurosurgery, Jacksonville, FL, USA

Mayo Clinic, Department of Neurosurgery, Jacksonville, FL, USA

Vivek Gupta, MD Mayo Clinic, Department of Radiology, Division of Neuroradiology, Jacksonville, FL, USA

Matthew Hoerth, MD Mayo Clinic, Department of Neurology, Phoenix, AZ, USA

Mayo Clinic in Arizona, Epilepsy and Electroencephalography, Phoenix, AZ, USA

Brian N. Lundstrom, MD, PhD Mayo Clinic, Department of Neurology, Rochester, MN, USA

Erik H. Middlebrooks, MD Mayo Clinic Florida, Division of Neuroradiology, Jacksonville, FL, USA

Mayo Clinic, Department of Radiology, Jacksonville, FL, USA

Kai J. Miller, MD Mayo Clinic, Department of Neurosurgery, Rochester, MN, USA

University Medical Center Utrecht, Brain Center Rudolf Magnus, Department of Neurology and Neurosurgery, Utrecht, The Netherlands

Katherine Nickels, MD Mayo Clinic, Department of Neurology, Rochester, MN, USA

Katherine Noe, MD, PhD Mayo Clinic Arizona, Phoenix, AZ, USA

Anthony Ritaccio, MD, FAAN, FANA, FAES Mayo Clinic, Department of Neurology, Jacksonville, FL, USA

David Sabsevitz, PhD Mayo Clinic, Department of Psychology and Psychiatry, Jacksonville, FL, USA

Mayo Clinic, Department of Neurological Surgery, Jacksonville, FL, USA

Raj D. Sheth, MD, FAAN Mayo Clinic/Nemours Children's Health Systems, Department of Neurology, Jacksonville, FL, USA

Jason Siegel, MD Mayo Clinic Florida, Departments of Critical Care Medicine, Neurology, and Neurosurgery, Jacksonville, FL, USA

Joseph I. Sirven, MD Mayo Clinic, Department of Neurology, Jacksonville, FL, USA

Scott D. Spritzer, DO Mayo Clinic Health System, Department of Neurology, Eau Claire, WI, USA

Keith Starnes, MD Mayo Clinic, Department of Neurology, Rochester, MN, USA

William O. Tatum, DO, FAAN, FACNS, FAES Mayo Clinic, Department of Neurology, Jacksonville, FL, USA

Jamie J. Van Gompel, MD, FAANS Mayo Clinic, Department of Neurosurgery, Rochester, MN, USA

Mayo Clinic, Department of Neurologic Surgery, Rochester, MN, USA

Peter van Rijen, MD University Medical Center Utrecht, Brain Center Rudolf Magnus, Department of Neurology and Neurosurgery, Utrecht, The Netherlands

Prasanna G. Vibhute, MD Mayo Clinic, Department of Radiology, Division of Neuroradiology, Jacksonville, FL, USA

Robert E. Wharen, MD Mayo Clinic, Department of Neurosurgery, Jacksonville, FL, USA

Elaine Wirrell, MD Mayo Clinic, Department of Child and Adolescent Neurology and Epilepsy, Rochester, MN, USA

Lily C. Wong-Kisiel, MD Mayo Clinic, Department of Neurology, Rochester, MN, USA

Gregory A. Worrell, MD Mayo Clinic, Department of Neurology, Rochester, MN, USA

Epileptic Spasms

1

Elaine Wirrell

Case Presentation

A 7-week-old female presented with a 2-week history of recurrent, brief spells that consist of bilateral arm and leg flexion (left moreso than right). She also had head flexion to the left and leftward eye deviation. Each event lasted less than 1 s, but these occurred several times a day in clusters that lasted up to 10 min. Events were particularly prominent shortly after waking. She was diagnosed with a "seizure disorder" and started on topiramate by her local pediatric neurologist. The events persisted without a significant reduction in frequency, despite dose increases to 20 mg/kg/d.

She was the product of a healthy term pregnancy to a 31-year-old G1P0 mother. The delivery was a normal spontaneous vaginal delivery with a birth weight of 3600 grams. She was discharged from the hospital at 2 days of age and was well without incident until 7 weeks of age. Her previous family history was unremarkable.

The general examination was unremarkable. Her weight, height, and head circumference were all at the 25th percentile of growth for her age. A thorough examination of her skin was performed, including a normal evaluation with a Wood's lamp. There were no neurocutaneous lesions. She was alert and attentive at her neurological examination. Her cranial nerves were normal. Her motor examination demonstrated that she had mild hypotonia in her left upper arm and tended to use it less than her right arm. Sensory examination revealed that she had symmetrical withdrawal to stimulation. No pathological cerebellar functions or reflexes were evident. Interictal EEG (Fig. 1.1) and brain MRI (Fig. 1.2) were also subsequently obtained.

E. Wirrell (✉)
Mayo Clinic, Department of Child and Adolescent Neurology and Epilepsy,
Rochester, MN, USA
e-mail: Wirrell.Elaine@mayo.edu

© Springer Nature Switzerland AG 2021
W. O. Tatum et al. (eds.), *Epilepsy Case Studies*,
https://doi.org/10.1007/978-3-030-59078-9_1

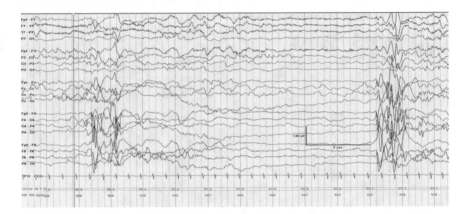

Fig. 1.1 Interictal EEG demonstrating right frontotemporal epileptiform discharges. Sensitivity 10 microvolts/mm, filter settings 1 and 70 Hz, display speed 30 mm/sec

Fig. 1.2 Coronal T1 MRI of the brain at 6 weeks of age. Note the hypointensity in the right frontotemporal region involving the insular cortex

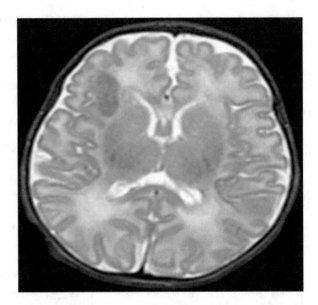

Clinical Questions

1. What specific type of spell is she presenting with clinically?
2. What is the most likely etiology for these events?
3. What does her neuroimaging and EEG demonstrate?
4. How do you classify dysplastic cortical malformations?
5. How should she be managed?

Discussion

1. She is presenting with epileptic spasms (ES), which have a focal component. Epileptic spasms are most seen commonly in the first year of life and characteristically occur in clusters, as in this child's case [1]. They are most commonly associated with West syndrome, though they may appear independent of a syndromic association. West syndrome is characterized by the triad of (a) spasms, (b) hypsarrhythmia on the EEG and (c) intellectual disability, and (d) most commonly present between 2 and 24 months of age. ES may also be associated with Ohtahara syndrome (early infantile epileptic encephalopathy), which frequently occurs with focal seizures. In Ohtahara syndrome, onset of spasms typically occurs at a younger age than West syndrome, often in the first 2 months of life. Most infants with Ohtahara syndrome will be found to have a structural brain abnormality; however, in approximately 10% of cases, a genetic etiology (particularly a mutation in *STXBP1*) is responsible. Children with Ohtahara syndrome are encephalopathic and show a burst-suppression pattern on EEG.

2. An underlying etiology can be identified in approximately 80% of cases; however, the etiologies are diverse. They include structural abnormalities of the brain that include, but are not limited to, prior injury, tuberous sclerosis, and malformations of cortical development. In addition, a genetic predisposition or chromosomal etiology (Trisomy 21, *CDKL5* mutation, *ARX* mutation, etc.) or metabolic disorders (mitochondrial cytopathies, pyridoxine dependency, etc.) may be involved.

3. The brain MRI scan that was done at 6 weeks of age showed a T2 hypointensity in the right anterior insular cortex. This is most likely due to a focal malformation of cortical development. In early infancy, focal cortical dysplasia is hypointense on T2. Due to ongoing myelination, such malformations can be very challenging to visualize between 4 and 24 months. After 2 years, focal cortical dysplasia can be detected by the more typical features of cortical thickening, blurring of the gray-white junction, abnormal gyral or sulcal patterns, or T2 hyperintensity.

4. Her interictal EEG pattern showed bursts of sharp waves rising from the right frontotemporal region. Ictal EEG later confirmed seizure onset that arose from the same area. Her EEG at this time was not consistent with hypsarrhythmia (note the absence of high voltage EEG).

   A clinicopathological classification system has been proposed, which divides these lesions into the following groups [2]:
   - FCD Type I: abnormal cortical layering that either compromise the radial migration and maturation of neurons (FCD Type Ia), the 6-layered tangential composition of the neocortex (FCD Type Ib), or both (Type Ic).
   - FCD Type II: a malformation that presents with disrupted cortical lamination and specific cytological abnormalities. FCD Type IIa has dysmorphic neurons without balloon cells, while FCD Type IIb has dysmorphic neurons with balloon cells.

- FCD Type III: cortical lamination abnormalities associated with a principal lesion: FCD Type IIIa (hippocampal sclerosis), FCD Type IIIb (tumor), FCD Type IIIc (vascular malformation), and FCD Type IIId (other lesion acquired early in life).
- FCD Types II and III may appear morphologically on the brain MRI. FCD Type I have histological features that may only be evident on histopathological examination and not the brain MRI. However, EEG may reveal focal or epileptiform abnormalities in FCD Type 1 that can reflect this MCD.

5. Epileptic spasms may occur independent of an association with either of the above epilepsy syndromes. Nevertheless ES are usually indicative of a severe epilepsy that is likely to be drug-resistant. Epileptic spasms can be challenging to treat. Despite the fact that her EEG does not yet show hypsarrhythmia, treatment should be initiated with vigabatrin, ACTH, or high-dose prednisolone. One recent study documented improved short-term outcome regarding spasm resolution with combination hormonal therapy with vigabatrin [3]; however follow-up after 18 months showed no difference in development between the two groups [4]. She was treated with vigabatrin 140 mg/kg/d and became seizure-free for 7 months. During that time, she also progressed developmentally in an age-appropriate manner. Unfortunately, her seizures recurred at 7 months. Despite addition of high-dose levetiracetam, focal seizures with left-sided motor symptoms occurred several times per day. She regressed in her development. She then underwent resection of the right frontal malformation of cortical development. Focal resections have been effective in patients with ES as it was in her case rendering her seizure free [5]. The pathology was consistent with FCD IIA (without balloon cells).

Pearls of Wisdom
1. Epileptic spasms are most common in infancy. They usually occur in clusters. Prompt diagnosis and effective therapy are crucial, as they are frequently associated with an epileptic encephalopathy with either failure of developmental progression or even regression.
2. Structural lesions may present with ES in infancy. They are frequently refractory to medical therapy.
3. The occurrence of focal ES with co-existent focal seizures or a focal abnormality on the neurological examination or EEG suggests the presence of a focal lesion.
4. Focal malformations of cortical development can be very challenging to visualize on MRI between 4 and 24 months due to the ongoing myelination process. Children with drug-resistant epilepsy should be considered for epilepsy surgery.
5. A referral for an epilepsy surgical center for assessment should be considered in a young child with drug-resistant seizures who has failed two anti-seizure medications due to a lack of efficacy. Such referral is urgent if there is evidence of developmental regression.

References

1. Shields DW. Infantile spasms: little seizures, big consequences. Epilepsy Curr. 2006;6(3):63–9.
2. Blumcke I, Thom M, Aronica E, Armstrong DD, Vinters HV, Palmini A, Jacques TS, et al. The clinico-pathological spectrum of focal cortical dysplasias: a consensus classification proposed by an ad hoc task force of the ILAE diagnostic methods commission. Epilepsia. 2011;52:158–74.
3. O'Callaghan FJ, Edwards SW, Alber FD, Hancock E, Johnson AL, et al. Safety and effectiveness of hormonal treatment versus hormonal treatment with vigabatrin for infantile spasms (ICISS): a randomised, multicentre, open-label trial. Lancet Neurol. 2017;16(1):33–42.
4. O'Callaghan FJK, Edwards SW, Alber FD, Cortina Borja M, Hancock E, et al. Vigabatrin with hormonal treatment versus hormonal treatment alone (ICISS) for infantile spasms: 18-month outcomes of an open-label, randomised controlled trial. Lancet Child Adolesc Health. 2018;2(10):715–25.
5. Moseley BD, Nickels K, Wirrell EC. Surgical outcomes for intractable epilepsy in children with epileptic spasms. J Child Neurol. 2012;27(6):713–20.

Neonatal Seizures and Metabolic Epilepsies

2

Anthony L. Fine and Lily C. Wong-Kisiel

Case

A 2-day-old girl was transferred for further evaluation of seizures. She was born at term to non-consanguineous parents with pregnancy complicated by group A beta-hemolytic streptococcus which was adequately treated with antibiotics. She was born via vaginal delivery, and Apgar scores were 8 and 9 at 1 and 5 min, respectively. There were no complications at delivery, and she appeared well on day of life 1 in the newborn nursery. On day of life 2, she began having stereotypic jerks of her upper extremities. On examination she was non-dysmorphic and noted to be diffusely hypotonic and hyporeflexic. She was noted to have quick, isolated jerks of her left and right upper extremities as well as frequent hiccups. She would have intermittent pauses in her breathing. She had depressed suck, rooting, and Moro reflexes. There were no abnormal skin findings, and she had no organomegaly.

She underwent evaluations including lumbar puncture, labs, EEG, and brain MRI and MR spectroscopy (MRS). The EEG recording showed a suppression-burst pattern with generalized burst activity alternating with generalized suppression, which lasted up to 10 s (Fig. 2.1). Generalized discharges were associated with body jerking, consistent with myoclonic seizures. The brain MRI showed hypoplasia of the corpus callosum and an immature sulcation pattern. The MRS showed an elevated glycine peak (Fig. 2.2). The serum glycine level was 2315 mmol/L (reference 232–740 mmol/L), CSF glycine was 370 umol/L (reference 5–38 umol/L), and the CSF/serum glycine ratio was 0.16 (reference < 0.03).

A. L. Fine (✉)
Mayo Clinic, Department of Neurology, Division of Child and Adolescent Neurology, Rochester, MN, USA
e-mail: fine.anthony@mayo.edu

L. C. Wong-Kisiel
Mayo Clinic, Department of Neurology, Rochester, MN, USA
e-mail: WongKisiel.Lily@mayo.edu

© Springer Nature Switzerland AG 2021
W. O. Tatum et al. (eds.), *Epilepsy Case Studies*,
https://doi.org/10.1007/978-3-030-59078-9_2

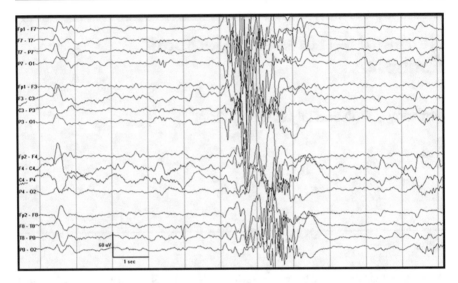

Fig. 2.1 EEG in bipolar montage demonstrating periods of EEG suppression and high amplitude generalized discharge (suppression-burst pattern)

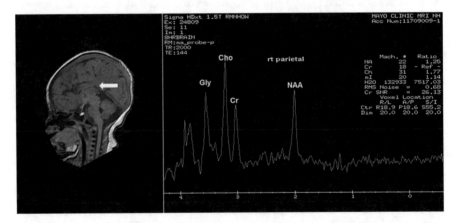

Fig. 2.2 Left panel: sagittal T1 brain MRI demonstrating hypoplastic corpus callosum (white arrow) and immature sulcation pattern. Right panel: MR spectroscopy with elevated glycine peak. *Cho* choline, *Cr* creatine, *Gly* glycine, *NAA* N-acetylaspartate

Questions

1. What is the differential diagnosis for a neonate with seizures and a suppression-burst pattern on EEG?
2. In what conditions can an elevated CSF-to-serum glycine ratio are seen, and what additional findings and/or studies can be helpful?

3. How would you classify this patient's seizures and epilepsy?
4. How would you treat this disorder?
5. What is the prognosis for this disorder?

Discussion

1. A neonate with seizures and a burst-suppression pattern on EEG suggests a severe encephalopathy, with a hypoxic-ischemic insult, metabolic, or epileptic encephalopathy being the most likely etiologies. The unremarkable pregnancy and birth history with an initially normal presentation would argue against hypoxic-ischemic encephalopathy. The presence of a burst-suppression pattern in a neonate also suggests an epileptic encephalopathy, with early infantile epileptic encephalopathy (a.k.a. Ohtahara syndrome) or early myoclonic epileptic encephalopathy (EME) potentially fitting with this patient's presentation. The clinical features (encephalopathy, myoclonic seizures, hiccups) and study/laboratory findings (suppression-burst pattern on EEG, elevated serum, and CSF glycine with elevated CSF-to-serum glycine ratio) are consistent with the diagnosis of nonketotic hyperglycinemia (NKH).

2. An elevated CSF-to-serum glycine ratio can be seen in several clinical scenarios. This can be seen in neonates with severe hypoxic-ischemic encephalopathy; however, additional findings in the history could include a difficult labor or delivery, low Apgar scores, acidosis, and a depressed newborn. In patients undergoing treatment with valproic acid, an elevated CSF-to-serum glycine ratio can be seen due to inhibition of the glycine cleavage system by valproic acid. This can be seen in metabolic disorders including NKH, pyridoxal 5'-phosphate oxidase (PNPO) deficiency, and organic acidurias. Pyridoxal 5'-phosphate oxidase deficiency most frequently will present as a neonatal epileptic encephalopathy. In addition to an elevated CSF glycine, testing would be notable for low CSF pyridoxal-5-phosphate. There may be a partial response to a trial of pyridoxine; however, treatment would be with pyridoxal 5-phosphate [1]. Elevated glycine levels can be seen in several organic acidurias, including propionic aciduria, methyl malonic aciduria, isovaleric aciduria, and multiple carboxylase deficiency; however, urine organic acid screen is typically normal in NKH and abnormal in these other disorders [2]. An elevated CSF-to-serum glycine is suggestive of NKH but is not confirmatory. Confirmatory testing could include assay of the glycine cleavage enzyme obtained with liver biopsy or by establishment of biallelic pathogenic variants in AMT, GLDC, or GCSH genes [3].

3. The description of the patient's seizures as quick jerks of the extremities associated with generalized discharges would be consistent with myoclonic seizures. The two epileptic encephalopathies to consider in this patient are early myoclonic encephalopathy (EME) and early infantile epileptic encephalopathy (EIEE). In EME, onset is frequently in the neonatal period and can be within the first hours of life with encephalopathy, frequent fragmentary myoclonus, and a suppression-burst pattern on EEG. The etiology for EME is most commonly a

metabolic disorder; however, genetic and structural etiologies have been reported. In EIEE/Ohtahara syndrome, onset is typically within the first 3 months of life and can be within the neonatal period. The presenting seizure type is tonic spasms, which can be generalized but more commonly are asymmetric and focal. NKH can be seen in association with two early onset epileptic encephalopathies, EME and EIEE. On EEG, a suppression-burst pattern will also be seen in Ohtahara syndrome. The most common etiology for Ohtahara is structural abnormalities due to an underlying genetic diagnosis; however this syndrome has been seen in metabolic disorders as well. Given the early onset myoclonus beginning shortly after birth and suppression-burst pattern on EEG, the epilepsy syndrome would be most in keeping with early myoclonic epilepsy secondary to NKH.

4. The treatment of NKH includes therapies aimed at reducing plasma glycine levels and NMDA excitatory signals. There is no cure for NKH, and disease course depends on the form of NKH. Treatment with sodium benzoate does not alter disease course but may improve seizure control [4]. Sodium benzoate conjugates glycine to hippurate which then can be excreted in the urine. Other therapies, including ketamine, dextromethorphan, and felbamate, which are NMDA-receptor antagonists, are used to potentially reduce glycine-induced excitotoxicity [5].

5. The prognosis for NKH is variable but tends to typically be poor. There are several forms including classic, transient, and atypical forms. The classic form of NKH is the neonatal form, with onset within hours to the first week of life, with lethargy, hypotonia, hiccups, and frequent myoclonic seizures. Apneas and respiratory failure can occur, which if untreated will result in coma and death. Survivors of classic NKH invariably have profound neurologic disability and drug-resistant epilepsy (a.k.a. intractable epilepsy), with evolution of burst-suppression pattern often to hypsarrhythmia and infantile spasms followed by Lennox-Gastaut syndrome. Death typically occurs within the first years of life [3, 4].

Transient NKH is a rare (and controversial) form, which has an identical initial presentation to the classic neonatal form and is felt to be due to immaturity of the glycine cleavage system. Children with transient NKH will have resolution of glycine elevations seen in serum and CSF over time and most frequently have normal neurodevelopment.

Atypical forms of NKH have heterogeneous age of onset and clinical presentations. In the late-onset form, seizures can be absent; however, other symptoms may include developmental delays, attention deficit disorder, ataxia, movement disorders, and spastic paraparesis. Some individuals will have normal cognition [3].

Our patient's clinical history of early onset myoclonic seizures with burst-suppression pattern on EEG, hypotonia, hiccups, and apneas and laboratory evaluations including elevated serum and CSF glycine levels and elevated CSF-to-serum glycine ratio would be most consistent with the neonatal form of NKH. She was initiated on sodium benzoate, ketamine, dextromethorphan, and topiramate. She was weaned off the ventilator on day of life 51 and discharged from the hospital at 2 months old. By 3 months of age, she developed infantile spasms. At 18 months, she had profound developmental delay and frequent hospitalizations for her drug-resistant seizures. She passed away at age 3 years due to respiratory failure and decompensation in the setting of illness.

Clinical Pearls

1. In a neonate with encephalopathy and seizures with an unremarkable perinatal course and without other features consistent with hypoxic-ischemic encephalopathy, additional etiologies such as an underlying metabolic or genetic disorder should be considered.
2. In a neonate with an epileptic encephalopathy with a suppression-burst pattern on electroencephalogram, diagnoses to consider include early myoclonic encephalopathy (EME) and early infantile epileptic encephalopathy/Ohtahara syndrome.
3. Nonketotic hyperglycinemia should be strongly considered as a possible diagnosis when findings are consistent with EME, and an evaluation of serum and CSF glycine should be performed.
4. In patients with NKH, the classic neonatal form has poor prognosis in terms of development, drug-resistant epilepsy, and death within a few years of diagnosis. In atypical forms, the disease course may be more attenuated with some individuals presenting with movement disorders and spastic paraparesis.
5. There is no curative therapy for NKH. Treatments are aimed at reducing excitotoxicity associated with excess levels of glycine, as well as, anti-seizure medications for seizure reduction.

References

1. Mills PB, Surtees RA, Champion MP, Beesley CE, Dalton N, Scambler PJ, et al. Neonatal epileptic encephalopathy caused by mutations in the PNPO gene encoding pyridox(am)ine 5'-phosphate oxidase. Hum Mol Genet. 2005;14(8):1077–86.
2. Kumps A, Duez P, Mardens Y. Metabolic, nutritional, iatrogenic, and artifactual sources of urinary organic acids: a comprehensive table. Clin Chem. 2002;48(5):708–17.
3. Dinopoulos A, Matsubara Y, Kure S. Atypical variants of nonketotic hyperglycinemia. Mol Genet Metab. 2005;86(1–2):61–9.
4. Swanson MA, Coughlin CR Jr, Scharer GH, Szerlong HJ, Bjoraker KJ, Spector EB, et al. Biochemical and molecular predictors for prognosis in nonketotic hyperglycinemia. Ann Neurol. 2015;78(4):606–18.
5. Bjoraker KJ, Swanson MA, Coughlin CR 2nd, Christodoulou J, Tan ES, Fergeson M, et al. Neurodevelopmental outcome and treatment efficacy of benzoate and dextromethorphan in siblings with attenuated nonketotic hyperglycinemia. J Pediatr. 2016;170:234–9.

Febrile Seizures

Harry S. Abram

Case Presentation

An 18-month-old girl presents to a local emergency room following a 20 min generalized tonic-clonic seizure. She has been an otherwise healthy child with age-appropriate developmental milestones. Upon assessment, in the emergency room, she has a temperature of 103° and an inflamed right tympanic membrane. She was initially irritable and uncooperative. Following ibuprofen, her temperature resolved, and within 60 min, she was cooperative, and she had a normal neurological examination.

Family history is notable for an older brother who had a similar event with a fever and a maternal aunt who developed epilepsy as a young adult. She has received all of her immunizations and has not been on any medications at home. The parents witnessed the seizure and were very frightened by it. Their fears concern further seizures, epilepsy, "brain damage," and death.

Clinical Questions

1. What are febrile seizures (FS), and how are they classified?
2. How should a child with febrile seizures be evaluated?
3. What is the reoccurrence risk of a second FS after the first? What is the risk of developing epilepsy in later childhood or adulthood? What is the risk of brain damage or death?
4. What are the treatment options?
5. What is the latest genetic research in FS?

H. S. Abram (✉)
Department of Pediatric Neurology, Nemours Children's Specialty Care,
Jacksonville, FL, USA
e-mail: harry.abram@nemours.org

© Springer Nature Switzerland AG 2021
W. O. Tatum et al. (eds.), *Epilepsy Case Studies*,
https://doi.org/10.1007/978-3-030-59078-9_3

Diagnostic Discussion

1. The International League Against Epilepsy (ILAE) defines a febrile seizure as "a seizure occurring in childhood after one month of age associated with a febrile illness not caused by an infection of the central nervous system, without previous neonatal seizures or a previous unprovoked seizure, and not meeting the criteria for other acute symptomatic seizures."

   This is considered a genetic age-limited seizure disorder in which seizures occur only with fever. This is the most common seizure type in early life, affecting 2–5% of all children. Peak incidence is between 18 and 24 months. FS are subdivided into two categories: simple and complex. Simple FS last for less than 15 min, are generalized and occur once in a 24-h period in a neurologically normal child. In contrast, complex FS are prolonged (>15 min), are focal, occur more than once in 24 h, or are in a neurologically abnormal child and risk factors for developing epilepsy (Table 3.1).

   Febrile status epilepticus, a subgroup of complex febrile seizures with seizures lasting more than 30 min, occurs in about 5% of cases. Seizure may consist of tonic or clonic movements which may be asymmetrical or have brief alterations of awareness.

2. Diagnostic evaluation of a child with a FS should be initially directed at determining the source of the fever. Meningitis should be considered in any febrile child. A lumbar puncture should be strongly considered in any child less than 12 months. The decision in older children should be based upon history and clinical examination, with attention to prior treatment with antibiotics and confirmation of appropriate immunizations. Typical meningeal signs such as stiff neck may not be reliably present under the age of 2 years. The overall risk of bacterial meningitis was 0.2% in children with an apparent first simple febrile seizure and 0.6% in children with complex febrile seizure [1]. Beware of an alternative diagnosis if the fever is less than 38.0 °C or if the child is over 5 years of age.

   An EEG is not indicated in a neurologically healthy child with a simple FS. There is no evidence to suggest that laboratory testing is of benefit in the evaluation of the child with a simple FS. These should be obtained only as indicated after appropriate history and careful physical examination. MRI and EEG

Table 3.1 Risk factors for febrile seizures to develop epilepsy

Reported risk factors for developing epilepsy
Complex febrile seizures
Prolonged
Recurrent
Focal features
Abnormal neurological status
1st degree relative with epilepsy

Table 3.2 Risk factors for recurrent febrile seizures

Reported risk factors for recurrent febrile seizures
Age <15 months
1st degree relative with febrile seizures or epilepsy
Low grade fever (<39 °C) at seizure onset
Short duration of fever prior to seizure (<1 h)
Daycare attendance
Complex febrile seizures
Developmental delay

are not typically indicated in simple FS but may be a consideration in children with complex FS [2].

3. After a single FS, the risk of a second is approximately one third, with the majority within 1 year (Table 3.2). This risk may range from approximately 5% up to 80% depending on the number of risk factors.

   The risk of developing subsequent epilepsy is only minimally greater than the risk to the general population, 5–7% versus 1%. However various risk factors have been noted to increase this risk: complex FS, onset younger than 12 months, a family history of epilepsy, abnormal neurological examination, or abnormal neuroimaging [3]. With multiple risk factors, the risk of developing epilepsy by the third decade is 17% versus 2.5% if there are no risk factors [4]. There is no evidence that the use of prophylactic anti-seizure medication with FS can prevent the later development of epilepsy. There currently is no evidence that simple FS cause structural damage to the brain or affect a child's cognition. There has never been a reported death from a simple FS.

   There has been a suggested link of FS to later development of temporal lobe epilepsy, but that exact role remains unclear. Some studies have suggested development of hippocampal sclerosis following a prolonged FS in young infants. Despite retrospective analyses demonstrating that as many as 35% of adults with temporal lobe epilepsy have a history of complex or prolonged febrile seizures in childhood, prospective outcome has been inconclusive and contradictory [5].

4. Despite the frequency of simple FS, long-term daily therapy with an anti-seizure medication is typically not warranted. Although there is evidence that both continuous anti-seizure therapy with phenobarbital, primidone, or valproic acid and intermittent therapy with oral diazepam are effective in reducing the risk of recurrence of further FS, the potential toxicities associated with antiepileptic drugs outweigh the relatively minor risks associated with simple FS [6]. In situations in which parental anxiety is high, seizures are prolonged or recurrent, there is a strong family history of epilepsy, or is there limited access to health care, intermittent use of a benzodiazepine at the onset of febrile illness may be effective in preventing recurrence. The prospective FEBSTAT (Consequences of Prolonged Febrile Seizure) demonstrated that the longer a seizure continues, the less likely they are to stop spontaneously [7]. The importance of pre-hospital treatment protocol with respiratory support and a rescue benzodiazepine is emphasized.

Although antipyretics may improve the comfort of the child, there is no data that this will prevent further febrile seizures [8]. This is useful to note for worried parents, who may blame themselves for not administering adequately antipyretics. A cool bath or washcloth is no longer recommended for febrile children as it may raise core body temperature.

5. Disorders involving voltage-gated ion channels have been of increasing noted in neurological disease. Greater than 300 mutations involving the gene controlling sodium channels (*SCN1A* and *SCN1B*) and *GABRG2* have been implicated in a broad spectrum of mild to very severe epileptic syndromes. These severe seizure disorders have many presentations and include FS, generalized epilepsy with FS plus (GEFS+), Dravet syndrome (severe myoclonic epilepsy of infancy), Doose syndrome (myoclonic-astatic epilepsy), Lennox-Gastaut syndrome, and vaccine-related encephalopathy. These disorders are important to recognize due to genetic implications and alteration in anti-seizure management (avoiding medications with sodium channel blocking properties) and family counseling.

Pearls of Wisdom
1. Though FS are frightening events for families, the crux of treatment is addressing the etiology of the febrile illness and counseling families of the benign nature and excellent prognosis of FS. Long-term anti-seizure medications are not typically recommended. Intermittent use of a benzodiazepine may be appropriate in certain clinical situations either as prophylaxis or as a rescue option.
2. Counsel parents of children who might be at an elevated risk for an initial febrile seizures as well as recurrent FS. Genetic factors are important. FS are 2–3 times more common in children whose parents or siblings experienced FS.
3. Epilepsy is uncommon following FS with the risk only being marginally greater than the normal population.
4. Follow updated published guidelines from the American Academy of Pediatrics for guidance regarding evaluation and management of simple febrile seizures [6, 7]. There are no published guidelines for complex FS. These should be evaluated and managed more cautiously with greater consideration for LP, EEG, and neuroimaging.
5. Consider molecular genetic testing in children who present with repetitive febrile seizures in the first year of life and proceed to develop intractable generalized epilepsy with neurological regression.

References

1. Najaf-Zadeh A, Dubos F. Risk of bacterial meningitis in young children with a first seizure in the context of fever: a systematic review and meta-analysis. PLoS ONE. 2013;8:e55270.
2. Subcommittee on Febrile Seizures. Febrile seizures: guideline for the neurodiagnostic evaluation of the child with a simple febrile seizure. Pediatrics. 2011;127(2):389–94.
3. Berg AT, Shinnar S, et al. Risk factors for a first febrile seizure: a matched case-control study. Epilepsia. 1995;36(4):334–41.
4. Annegers JF, Hauser WA, Shirts SB, et al. Factors prognostic of unprovoked seizures after febrile convulsions. N Engl J Med. 1987;316:493–8.
5. Tarkka R, Paakko E, Pyhtinen J, et al. Febrile seizures and mesial temporal sclerosis: no association in a long-term follow-up study. Neurology. 2003;60:215–8.
6. Steering Committee on Quality Improvement and Management, Subcommittee on Febrile Seizures. Febrile seizures: clinical practice guideline for the long-term management of the child with simple febrile seizures. Pediatrics. 2008;121(6):1281–6.
7. Seinfield S, Shinnar S, Sun S, FebStat, et al. Emergency management of febrile status epilepticus. Epilepsia. 2014;55:388–95.
8. Rosenbloom E, Finkelstein Y, Adams-Webber T, et al. Do antipyretics prevent the recurrence of febrile seizures in children? A systematic review of randomized controlled trials and meta-analysis. Eur J Paediatr Neurol. 2013;17:585.

Childhood Absence Epilepsy

4

Raj D. Sheth

Case Presentation

A 7-year-old girl presents with episodes of staring that were lasting a few seconds and recurring multiple times daily. Her symptoms were brought to the attention of her primary care physician when she was reported to suddenly stop walking in the middle of the intersection of a busy street. She appeared to abruptly freeze and was motionless until her parents noticed and returned to her to assist her safely across the remainder of the street. According to her parents, she had been an excellent student, although recently they had been receiving notes from her teachers that she was noticed to be periodically staring into space as though she was daydreaming to the point of failure to attend to her lesson instructions. The symptoms became alarming to her parents when she experienced an episode during the daytime that was associated with urinary incontinence during school. She had no other complaints and was developmentally and neurologically normal on examination. Laboratory studies were unremarkable, and she was referred for a routine EEG (Fig. 4.1).

Clinical Questions

1. Does this EEG support a particular clinical diagnosis?
2. What is the relationship between staring spells and epilepsy?
3. What is a *typical absence* seizure, and how does it differ from an *atypical absence* seizure?

R. D. Sheth (✉)
Mayo Clinic/Nemours Children's Health Systems, Department of Neurology, Jacksonville, FL, USA
e-mail: rsheth@nemours.org; Raj.sheth@nemours.org

© Springer Nature Switzerland AG 2021
W. O. Tatum et al. (eds.), *Epilepsy Case Studies*,
https://doi.org/10.1007/978-3-030-59078-9_4

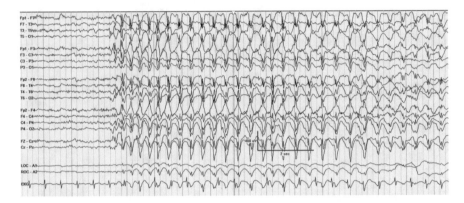

Fig. 4.1 EEG shows 3.5–4 Hz bi-synchronous and symmetrical anterior-predominant generalized spike-and-wave discharges lasting 5 s that was precipitated by hyperventilation

4. What are the anti-seizure medications that are used to treat childhood absence epilepsy (CAE)?
5. What is the anticipated clinical course and prognosis?

Diagnostic Discussion

1. The EEG shows a burst of 3–4 Hz anteriorly dominant generalized spike-and-wave discharges that in the context of a staring episode is diagnostic of absence seizures. The findings in this patient would be consistent with absence epilepsy and the childhood onset compatible with the epilepsy syndrome, childhood absence epilepsy [1].

   About 5–10% of all childhood epilepsies involves the presence of absence seizures. *Typical* absence seizures involve staring and impairment of consciousness that is associated with 3–4-Hz generalized spike-and-wave discharges on the EEG. The initial portion of the discharge may have a frequency of faster spike-and-wave and the terminal portion of the discharge a slower frequency. Impairment of consciousness may often be missed due to the subtlety of the clinical features and brevity of the attack. Special response testing methods may be required to demonstrate its presence. In addition to a blank stare, there are often other associated clinical manifestations, such as automatisms, eyelid myoclonia, and autonomic disturbances that may coexist. Absence seizures are often induced by hyperventilation.

2. The EEG is diagnostic of absence epilepsy and seizures that can be precipitated by hyperventilation. The discharges are frequently fragmented and last shorter periods of time during sleep. Differentiating absence seizures from focal seizures and episodic non-epileptic daydreaming is crucial to effective counseling and treatment. The EEG is important in addressing the mechanism to define the episode. Ictal recordings support childhood absence epilepsy when the 3 Hz

generalized spike-and-wave pattern is evident, focal epilepsy and focal seizures when focal or regional epileptiform discharges are captured, and non-epileptic staring spells when the EEG is devoid of epileptiform features entirely when the spells are recorded.

3. *Atypical* absence seizures are much less common than *typical* absence seizures. Atypical absence is seen in epileptic encephalopathies such as Lennox-Gastaut syndrome where it may be accompanied atonic and tonic seizures. Clinically, atypical absence is associated with developmental delay or intellectual disability whereas mental function in typical absence is normal. The EEG is useful in differentiation atypical absence from typical absence seizures by the presence of diffuse slow (<2.5 Hz) spike-and-wave on EEG (see EEG patterns elsewhere). In addition to this, the backgrounds compared to normal background frequencies seen in typical absence are slow and disorganized.

4. The most effective antiseizure medication used to treat absence epilepsy is ethosuximide and valproate [2]. However, a number of adverse events are associated with valproate treatment. Lamotrigine appears to have the best adverse event profile but is also less effective. Ethosuximide appears to have the best balance between efficacy and adverse effects. The most frequent adverse effect of ethosuximide is gastric irritation which can be controlled by taking medication with food [2]. Absence epilepsy is not effectively treated with phenytoin, gabapentin, and carbamazepine. Exacerbations of absence following the initiation of carbamazepine have been well documented. The mechanism is believed to be related to Na + channels medications activating absence seizures. Childhood absence epilepsy involves dysfunction of the thalamic relay neurons, thalamic reticular neurons, and cortical pyramidal neurons. Thalamic relay neurons activate cortical pyramidal neurons in either a tonic or in a burst mode. T-type calcium channels underlie the burst mode. Drugs, such as ethosuximide, are effective in controlling absence seizures by affecting the T-type calcium currents.

5. Epileptic syndromes that include typical absence in their spectrum include the genetic generalized epilepsies: childhood absence epilepsy, juvenile absence epilepsy, and juvenile myoclonic epilepsy. Myoclonic absence epilepsy also has absence seizures as a component of the generalized epilepsies. It is increasingly recognized, but while these syndromes are considered "benign," they can be associated with subtle language and other cognitive difficulties [3].

Pearls of Wisdom

1. Absence seizures can be detected in the clinical setting of the genetic generalized epilepsies when typical staring spells are provoked by hyperventilation. An EEG is diagnostic in over 90% of untreated patients with childhood absence epilepsy when the 3 Hz generalized spike-and-wave pattern is present.

2. Staring spells are very common in childhood and can be differentiated between absence seizure, focal impaired awareness seizures, and nonepileptic daydreaming by clinical and EEG means [4].

3. Effective treatment may be assessed by making sure that the EEG shows no prolonged bursts or clinical signs during the EEG findings of 3 Hz generalized spike-and-waves [5].
4. CAE is typically readily treatable with ethosuximide. Fifty percent of patients will have their absence seizures remit in early adolescence, while some develop other generalized seizure types such as myoclonus or generalized tonic-clonic seizures that require ongoing therapy.
5. Although the majority of patients respond to either first-line or a second-line antiseizure medication, there are patients that may be drug-resistant. In those patients, combining antiseizure medications such as valproate and ethosuximide may be effective. When medical treatment fails, consideration of rare metabolic encephalopathies such as glucose 1 deficiency should be considered. It is important to recognize this disorder since treatment with a ketogenic diet typically controls the epilepsy. Epilepsy gene mutations for SCL2A1 should be considered when patients with absence do not respond to treatment.

References

1. Berg AT, Shinnar S, Levy SR, Testa FM, Smith-Rapaport S, Beckerman B. How well can epilepsy syndromes be identified at diagnosis? A reassessment 2 years after initial diagnosis. Epilepsia. 2000;41:1269–75.
2. Glausser TA, et al. Ethosuximide, valproic acid, and lamotrigine in childhood absence epilepsy. N Engl J Med. 2010;362:790–9.
3. Jackson DC, Jones JE, Hermann BP. Language function in childhood idiopathic epilepsy. Brain. 2019;193:4–9.
4. Sheth RD. Absence epilepsy with focal clinical and electrographic seizures. Semin Pediatr Neurol. 2010;17:39–43.
5. French JA, Pedley TA. Initial management of epilepsy. N Engl J Med. 2008;359:166–76.

Lennox-Gastaut Syndrome

5

William O. Tatum and Raj D. Sheth

Case Presentation

A 36-year-old man with an intellectual disability disorder resided in a group home. His early history including birth, labor, delivery, and development was unavailable except for a hospitalization for the "shakes" when he was 1–2 years old. There was a history provided by his caretakers that he had received a series of "steroid shots when he was a child." The episodes eventually resolved though he remained cognitively impaired thereafter and never developed normally. He lost prior abilities of speech and fine motor skills and was unable to perform activities of daily living independent of supervision and assistance. He was diagnosed with a "seizure disorder" at 8 years of age and was maintained on two antiseizure medications (phenytoin and phenobarbital). Over time, several different types of seizure emerged. The most common type of seizure was a brief episode where he would suddenly "become stiff," lose consciousness, and fall to the ground. This frequently resulted in recurrent head injuries including contusions and lacerations, and with one fall, he fractured his right ankle leading to casting. He also experienced episodes involving a sudden onset of limp collapse where he would fall to the ground "like a sack of potatoes" resulting in injury. Falls were frequent, and "grand mal" seizures also occurred more infrequently. In addition, there were daily episodes of brief staring as well as "quick jerks" of his arms and legs at times where he would drop objects from his hands that he was holding. Further episodes of repetitive seizures and

W. O. Tatum (✉)
Mayo Clinic, Department of Neurology, Jacksonville, FL, USA
e-mail: tatum.william@mayo.edu

R. D. Sheth
Mayo Clinic/Nemours Children's Health Systems, Department of Neurology, Jacksonville, FL, USA
e-mail: rsheth@nemours.org; Raj.sheth@nemours.org

© Springer Nature Switzerland AG 2021
W. O. Tatum et al. (eds.), *Epilepsy Case Studies*,
https://doi.org/10.1007/978-3-030-59078-9_5

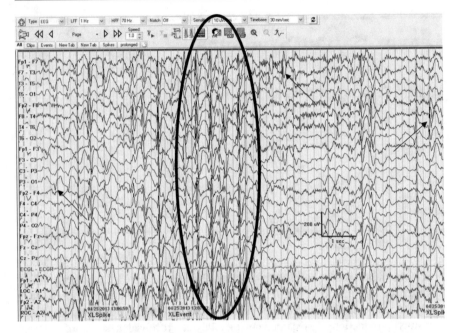

Fig. 5.1 24-channel EEG demonstrating bursts of 2-Hz slow spike-waves (oval) in seconds 5–6 in addition to multifocal spikes (arrows) and diffuse slowing of the posterior dominant rhythm. EEG parameters include anterior-posterior bipolar montage, sensitivity of 7 μv/mm, and filter settings of 1–70 Hz

prolonged convulsive events led to frequent visitation to the local hospital emergency department. He quickly proved drug-resistant to eight or nine antiseizure medications (ASM) and was taking phenytoin, phenobarbital, and levetiracetam at his group home. His group home managers were concerned that he was a liability for the home and wanted to have him "fixed" so that his seizures were controlled. He was referred for video-EEG monitoring (Fig. 5.1).

Clinical Questions

1. What is his diagnosis, and how did the EEG help to support his clinical diagnosis?
2. What are the common signs that suggest this condition?
3. What other conditions mimic this case presentation?
4. What is the best course of treatment?
5. What is the anticipated prognosis?

Diagnostic Discussion

1. The patient has the EEG features consistent with a clinical diagnosis of LGS. His EEG (Fig. 5.1) demonstrates slow generalized spike-and-slow waves which is one of the hallmark features of this drug-resistant epileptic encephalopathy [1].

EEG is one of the essential clues for a diagnosis of this well-known but devastating epilepsy syndrome, though other common features include diffuse slowing of the background activity, the presence of multifocal independent epileptiform discharges, and bursts of generalized paroxysmal fast activity [2].

2. Intellectual disability, the presence of multiple mixed seizure types, and characteristic EEG features are a triad that identifies LGS. Epileptic spasms and EEG demonstrating hypsarrhythmia (West syndrome) may precede LGS in about 40% of cases [3]. The early treatment of our patient with "steroid shots" likely reflects use of adrenocorticotropic hormone (ACTH) injections which are effective in majority of patients for cessation of spasms but not for preventing cognitive disability. The diagnosis of LGS is not particularly challenging compared with treatment. However, various EEG features and variable clinical phenotypes may occur that delay a definitive diagnosis [1]. The focus on treatment first includes measures to protect the patient from falls and injury optimizing patient safety. Protective head gear is often required due to the sudden unpredictability of drop attacks (a term used to identify tonic and atonic seizures often difficult to separate clinically). Discussion with family and caretakers should involve the expectation for poor seizure control, lack of reversible or surgical "cure," and the ongoing potential for injury despite treatment with one or more ASM.

3. LGS, like many epileptic encephalopathies, manifest uncontrolled seizures stemming from many different structural-metabolic etiologies [4]. LGS is considered a distinctive electroclinical syndrome based upon the following criteria:
   (a) Multiple mixed seizure types are present in LGS. These include tonic and atonic seizures (drop attacks) as the most common seizure type. However, tonic-clonic, myoclonic, atypical absence, and focal seizures may also occur.
   (b) The presence of an intellectual disability or evidence of cognitive impairment.
   (c) Slow spike-and-slow waves with or without GPFA present on the EEG [1, 2].
   The causes of LGS in many cases are unknown though symptomatic causes are common (i.e., tuberous sclerosis complex, hypoxic-ischemic encephalopathy, malformations of cortical development). Reversible etiologies of LGS such as hydrocephaly, endocrinopathies, inborn errors of metabolism, and drug-related causes in association with compromised mental function and seizures should be investigated and excluded initially to prevent ongoing physical and cognitive deterioration.

4. The best course of treatment is the use of broad-spectrum ASMs. ASMs that have proven useful in clinical trials include lamotrigine (LTG), topiramate (TPM), rufinamide (RUF), clobazam (CLB), and cannabidiol (CNB) [1]. Felbamate is useful, although its use is limited as a third-line ASM due to serious side effects, including aplastic anemia and hepatic failure. Valproate (VPA) is effective against multiple seizure types and may be helpful in combination with LTG or TPM. However, the combination of VPA with LTG may cause a higher risk of serious rash as an adverse event. RUF, CLB, and CNB are newer ASMs that may be useful in the treatment of LGS. Levetiracetam and zonisamide are broad-spectrum ASM that may also be considered with efficacy against myoclonus, focal, and GTC seizures. Dual ASM with the capability of utilizing

intravenous formulations are often used given the predisposition for frequent seizures and status epilepticus. The ketogenic diet and vagus nerve stimulator may also help with seizure reduction. Finally, corpus callosotomy is a palliative procedure reserved for those with disabling injurious drop attacks who experience repeat injury and in whom disability is significantly associated with uncontrolled seizures. Recently anterior nucleus of the thalamus deep brain stimulation has become available that may have a future treatment application in some carefully selected patients [5].

5. The clinical course for patients with LGS typically carries a poor prognosis [1–5]. It is important for the family to have reasonable expectations of seizure reduction despite use of ASM. They should understand that patients with LGS do not need to go to the emergency department with every seizure, but that injury, persistent seizures, cardiorespiratory compromise, and failure to recover after a seizure should rapid direct physician assessment. It is important for the family to be provided with supportive therapies including rescue medications (i.e., midazolam or diazepam nasal/oral/rectal preparations) in the case of serial or "cluster" seizures and prolonged seizure to limit repeat visits to the emergency department [1, 4]. Seizure counts to quantify the number of different seizure types are a helpful attempt to reflect the degree of change in seizure frequency. Disability due to epileptic seizures and comorbid intellectual disability disorders and behavioral disorders predispose the patient with LGS to multiple recurrent injuries and a sheltered supervised environment. Quality of life should balance the effect of intermittent seizures with the presence of constant side effects of treatment with multiple ASM.

Clinical Pearls

1. LGS often follows epileptic spasms associated with West's syndrome in early childhood and continues into adulthood. The classic clinical triad for patients with LGS is intellectual disability, drug- resistant mixed seizure types (especially tonic seizures), and slow spike-waves on the EEG to characterize the syndrome.

2. There is a limited expectation that patients with LGS will achieve seizure control. Therefore, the focus of treatment should be to attempt to balance seizure reduction with an effort to minimize side effects from ASMs to optimize an individual's quality of life.

3. Reversible structural lesions are seen infrequently in patients with LGS. Instead, diffuse injury or congenital malformations of the brain is oftentimes responsible for seizures and an underlying substrate for the patients with LGS. Intermittent exacerbation during periods of seizure control and alteration in mental status and behavior due to systemic or "toxic" effects from ASMs are common and require vigilance to resolve iatrogenic consequences that contribute to the appearance of clinical deterioration.

4. LTG and VPA or LTG and TPM are combinations that may be synergistic in the treatment of patients with the LGS. Vagus nerve stimulation may be a useful adjunct when ASM adverse effects are prominent to minimize the cumulative load of ASM. Vagus nerve stimulation may reduce seizures though is unlikely to result in seizure freedom. Corpus callosotomy should be considered for patients with disabling drop attacks in eligible candidates and is best performed at an experienced epilepsy center.

5. Safety includes safeguarding the home and protecting patients from dangerous objects that produce environmental risk, use of head gear during "at-risk" times where seizures could result in injury, and evaluation of significant medical issues requiring emergency care and emergency department visitation (e.g., serial seizures or status epilepticus). The overall prognosis for seizure control is poor, and the expectation for uncontrolled seizures is unfortunately anticipated to be lifelong.

References

1. Arzimanoglou A, French J, Blume WT, et al. Lennox-Gastaut syndrome: a consensus approach on diagnosis, assessment, management and trial methodology. Lancet Neurol. 2009;8:82–93.
2. Markand ON. Lennox–Gastaut syndrome (childhood epileptic encephalopathy). J Clin Neurophysiol. 2003;20(6):426–41.
3. Wheless JW. Managing severe epilepsy syndromes of early childhood. J Child Neurol. 2009;24(Suppl 8):S24–32.
4. Winesett SP, Tatum WO. Chapter 20: Encephalopathic generalized epilepsy and Lennox-Gastaut syndrome. In: Wyllie E, Gidal B, Goodkin H, Sirven J, Loddenkemper T, editors. Wyllie's treatment of epilepsy principles and practice. 6th ed. Philadelphia: Wolters Kluwer; 2015.
5. Douglass LM. Surgical options for patients with Lennox–Gastaut syndrome. Epilepsia. 2014;55:21–8.

Self-Limited Epilepsies in Childhood

6

Katherine Nickels

Clinical Case

A 7-year-old right-handed girl presented for a second opinion of focal epilepsy for the last year. She is a previously healthy girl without behavioral or academic disabilities, nor family history of epilepsy. She has one seizure type. All seizures arise from the first hour of sleep and are characterized by facial twitching on one side with excessive drooling. She retains awareness during the event and has minimal postictal symptoms. The events are all under 1 min in duration. Clinically, her healthcare providers felt her seizure in the setting of normal growth, and development was most consistent childhood epilepsy with centrotemporal spikes. However, her initial EEG demonstrated generalized spike-and-wave discharges that were maximal over the left hemisphere. Neuroimaging with MRI brain was normal.

She was subsequently given trials of three different anti-seizure medications, which were discontinued due to side effects or allergies. She then became seizure-free with the fourth antiseizure medication. Follow-up EEG demonstrated epileptiform discharges over the left central parietal region with spread to the right central region. There was increased activation during sleep, with the discharges occasionally occurring in runs. A third EEG demonstrated frequent epileptiform discharges independently over the bilateral central, bilateral temporal, and right central parietal regions. A broad field was noted with some of these discharges, with a more hemispheric distribution (Fig. 6.1a, b). However, the sleep recording was unsuccessful. Fortunately, she remained seizure-free, and her development and academic performance remained age-appropriate.

K. Nickels (✉)
Mayo Clinic, Department of Neurology, Rochester, MN, USA
e-mail: Nickels.Katherine@mayo.edu

© Springer Nature Switzerland AG 2021
W. O. Tatum et al. (eds.), *Epilepsy Case Studies*,
https://doi.org/10.1007/978-3-030-59078-9_6

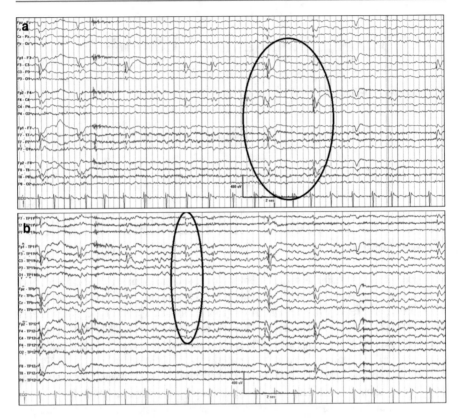

Fig. 6.1 (**a**) Awake EEG, bipolar montage, demonstrating age-appropriate posterior dominant rhythm with frequent multifocal potentially epileptiform discharges that were maximal over the bilateral centrotemporal regions. (**b**) Same EEG in a referential montage, highlighting the positivity over the frontal regions with negativity over the centrotemporal regions

Prolonged EEG was performed due to lack of sleep recorded on routine EEG, which demonstrated frequent to abundant bilateral centrotemporal epileptiform discharges with positivity over the frontal regions and negativity over the centrotemporal regions, as well as occasional multifocal epileptiform activity (Fig. 6.2a, b). During sleep, there was increased frequency and synchrony of discharges, demonstrating nearly continuous discharges occupying approximately 65% of sleep.

Clinical Questions

1. What electroclinical syndrome best fits this presentation, if any?
2. What syndromes must be excluded?
3. How should she be managed?
4. Are there preferred medications for this syndrome?
5. How will you counsel the family?

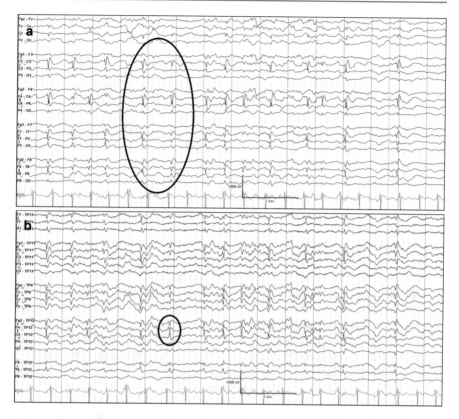

Fig. 6.2 (**a**) Sleep EEG, bipolar montage, demonstrating abundant activation of diffuse, synchronous, epileptiform discharges that were maximal over the bilateral centrotemporal regions. (**b**) Same EEG in a referential montage, highlighting continued positivity over the frontal regions with negativity over the centrotemporal regions

Discussion

1. Epilepsy syndrome classification is important to determine potential etiologies, preferred treatments, possible comorbidities, and expected outcomes. Epilepsies can be classified by seizure type (focal, generalized, unknown) and epilepsy type (focal, generalized, focal and generalized, unknown). The third level of classification is epilepsy electroclinical syndrome, which incorporates EEG findings, seizure types, age, and comorbidities. It is important to understand that not all epilepsies will be classified as a specific electroclinical syndrome [1].

   Based on her clinical presentation, the most likely syndrome for this child is childhood epilepsy with centrotemporal spikes, previously known as benign rolandic epilepsy or benign childhood epilepsy with centrotemporal spikes. Clinically, this epilepsy syndrome presents in otherwise healthy school-aged children (peak 8–9 years). A minority may have a history of febrile seizures.

The seizures are characterized by hemi-facial clonic movements, articulation difficulty, and hypersalivation. This may progress to clonic activity in the ipsilateral upper limb, ipsilateral hemi-clonic seizure, or bilateral tonic-clonic seizure [2].

The EEG in this syndrome would be expected to demonstrate high amplitude epileptiform discharges over the centrotemporal regions with increased activation during drowsiness and sleep. Furthermore, the morphology of the centrotemporal discharges demonstrates negativity over the centrotemporal electrodes and positivity anteriorly [2]. The patient's first EEG demonstrated generalized epileptiform discharges, and subsequent EEGs demonstrated epileptiform discharges over the bilateral centrotemporal regions but also parietal regions. However, generalized epileptiform discharges have been reported in children with typical clinical features of childhood epilepsy with centrotemporal spikes, although more typical features may be seen on subsequent EEGs [3]. Furthermore, focal epileptiform discharges can be present outside the centrotemporal region, including parietal region [2]. Therefore, the patient's EEG findings do not exclude childhood epilepsy with centrotemporal spikes.

2. The important differential diagnoses for childhood epilepsy with centrotemporal spikes that need to be excluded include focal epilepsy due to structural etiology, atypical childhood epilepsy with centrotemporal spikes, epileptic encephalopathy with continuous spike-and-wave during sleep (CSWS), and Landau-Kleffner (LKS) syndrome. Neuroimaging with brain MRI is important to perform if there are any atypical features. Our patient underwent brain MRI, which was normal.

Childhood epilepsy with centrotemporal spikes, atypical childhood epilepsy with centrotemporal spikes, LKS, and CSWS all demonstrate activation of epileptiform discharges during sleep, can have variable severity of seizures, may be associated with neurocognitive impairment, and are viewed by some as a spectrum. Children with atypical childhood epilepsy with centrotemporal spikes have an atypical evolution of their epilepsy, experiencing frequent seizures of multiple seizure types. When seizures are frequent, there may be cognitive and motor impairment. However, this is a self-limited epilepsy, and impairments resolve as seizures remit.

LKS and CSWS are self-limited epileptic encephalopathies. Both syndromes are self-limited and occur in children with previously normal development, with variable severity and frequency of seizures. LKS is associated with acquired aphasia, and there is a high risk of long-term language impairment, even after the EEG changes and seizures resolve. CSWS can also occur in children with prior neurologic deficits or neuroimaging abnormalities and is associated with global cognitive regression. Like LKS, neurologic impairments persist, even after remission of seizures and EEG abnormalities. Identification of LKS and CSWS through overnight sleep EEG is important in any child with a history of developmental regression because treatment of the EEG abnormalities can improve neurologic impairment. Furthermore, the EEG and developmental abnormalities can be exacerbated by some anti-seizure medications, including carbamazepine and oxcarbazepine previously used to treat our patient [2].

3. Childhood epilepsy with centrotemporal spikes is expected to be responsive to anti-seizure medication. Due to the self-limited nature of this epilepsy syndrome and the infrequency of seizures experienced by most children, some parents and physicians may opt not to initiate treatment in order to avoid potential side effects of anti-seizure medications. However, it is important to recognize that the frequent inter-ictal epileptiform discharges may be associated with cognitive and behavioral disabilities. Furthermore, daytime or frequent seizures can be detrimental physically, cognitively, and socially. Finally, there are rare reports of sudden unexpected death in epilepsy (SUDEP) in patients with this syndrome [4, 5]. Therefore, risks and benefits of treatment versus no treatment should be discussed and carefully weighed on an individual basis for each patient.

4. Currently, we lack level clear evidence of a preferred treatment for childhood epilepsy with centrotemporal spikes. Overall, this is a pharmaco-responsive syndrome. Therefore, most anti-seizure medications should be effective [4]. Similar to the treatment of any epilepsy in children, the goal should seizure freedom without medication side effects.

5. While the clinical presentation is most consistent with childhood epilepsy with centrotemporal spikes, there were some atypical features in the child's EEG, and her discharges were abundant, even while seizure-free. Furthermore, her sleep demonstrated a nearly continuous pattern of diffuse discharges, which can be seen in childhood epilepsy with centrotemporal spikes, but also in LKS and CSWS, and the child was treated with a medication that could potentially exacerbate these two syndromes. Therefore, the family was cautioned to watch for any signs or symptoms of cognitive or behavioral regression, and it was also suggested that her teachers also be alerted to this possibility. It was recommended that she continues her current medication regimen for now, given the abundance of epileptiform discharges and the patient's young age. However, her overall course was reassuring, and parents and providers were hopeful that she would continue to be consistent with this self-limited syndrome.

Pearls of Wisdom
1. Identification of epilepsy electroclinical syndrome, when possible, helps to provide guidance on potential etiologies, preferred treatments, and expected outcomes Childhood epilepsy with centrotemporal spikes is a self-limited epilepsy responsive to anti-seizure medication with characteristic clinical and EEG features. However, atypical features may occur.
2. Atypical features should not exclude classification into potential epilepsy electroclinical syndromes but often warrant additional evaluation, as well as more cautious counseling of expected outcomes. Additional childhood-onset epilepsy syndromes share clinical and EEG features with childhood epilepsy with centrotemporal spikes. Excluding these potential diagnoses is essential to providing preferred treatments and advising families on expected outcomes.

3. Activation of frequent epileptiform discharges during sleep can be seen in childhood epilepsy with centrotemporal spikes but can also represent epileptic encephalopathies, including LKS and CSWS. Therefore, a careful developmental history, including inquiring about developmental plateau or regression, should be obtained.

4. Although the seizures are infrequent and long-term seizure outcome is expected to be good in childhood epilepsy with centrotemporal spikes, epilepsy comorbidities and SUDEP can occur. Risks and benefits of treatment versus no treatment should be discussed and carefully weighed on an individual basis for each patient. All epilepsy syndromes can be associated with comorbidities and should not be considered "benign."

5. Epilepsy syndromes that are self-limited and responsive to antiseizure medication can still be associated with cognitive and behavioral impairment. Therefore, the term "benign" is no longer applied.

References

1. Scheffer IE, Berkovic S, Capovilla G, Connolly MB, et al. ILAE classification of the epilepsies: position paper of the ILAE Commission for Classification and Terminology. Epilepsia. 2017;58(4):512–21.
2. Epilepsydiagnosis.org. Accessed 12 Dec 2019.
3. Vargas R, Beltran L, Lizama R, Reyes Valenzuela G, Caraballo R. Benign rolandic epilepsy and generalized paroxysms: a study of 13 patients. Seizure. 2018;57:27–31.
4. Shields WD, Snead OC III. Benign epilepsy with centrotemporal spikes. Epilepsia. 2009;50(Suppl. 8):10–5.
5. Doumlele K, Frieman D, Buchhalter J, Donner EJ, Louik J, et al. Sudden unexpected death in epilepsy among patients with benign childhood epilepsy with centrotemporal spikes. JAMA Neurol. 2017;74(6):645–9.

Genetics and Epilepsy

7

Anthony L. Fine

Case

A 3-year-old female presents to a local emergency department for evaluation following a 5 min convulsion. At daycare, the child was playing when she was seen to have an abrupt pause in activity, turned her head to the left, and was staring to the left. Her arms then came up with her left arm flexed and right arm extended to the side for a few seconds before she had jerking of her entire body.

She was the full-term product of non-consanguineous parents following a spontaneous vaginal delivery. Pregnancy was complicated by identification of a renal tumor in mother during pregnancy. Her mother had a history of learning disorders and epilepsy and passed away when the child was 6 months old following nephrectomy for a renal tumor. The child has been living with her aunt who reports that the patient has had some speech delay, as well as hyperactive behavior.

On examination, the child is tired and wants to be held. She is noted to be using her right side less than the left and will preferentially reach for a toy or her stuffed animal with her left hand. Physical examination, including a brief skin examination, was notable for multiple hyperpigmented birthmarks scattered over her trunk and extremities. A systolic ejection murmur was heard on auscultation. A head CT was performed in the ER (Fig. 7.1), in addition to an echocardiogram given the murmur on examination (Fig. 7.2).

A. L. Fine (✉)
Mayo Clinic, Department of Neurology, Division of Child and Adolescent Neurology, Rochester, MN, USA
e-mail: fine.anthony@mayo.edu

© Springer Nature Switzerland AG 2021
W. O. Tatum et al. (eds.), *Epilepsy Case Studies*,
https://doi.org/10.1007/978-3-030-59078-9_7

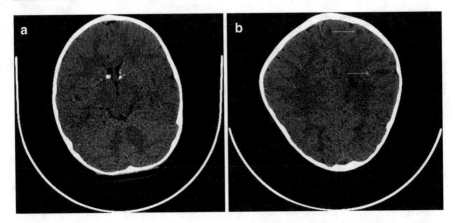

Fig. 7.1 (a) Axial computed tomography scan demonstrating several subependymal calcifications (dashed arrows). (b) Axial head CT with subcortical hypodensities (white arrows)

Fig. 7.2 Transthoracic echocardiogram with an apical four-chamber view showing multiple cardiac tumors (arrows)

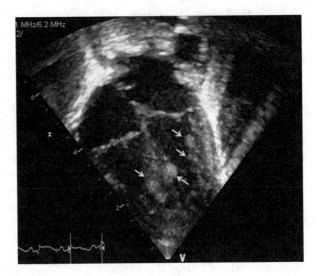

Clinical Questions

1. What diagnosis does this patient have?
2. What is the etiology for this patient's seizures?
3. What additional testing would you recommend?
4. How would you classify this patient's seizures?
5. What treatment implications can this diagnosis have?

Discussion

1. This child likely has tuberous sclerosis complex (TSC). In individuals with TSC, over 85–95% will present as children with seizures [1]. Children with TSC can have multiple seizure types, including both focal and generalized seizures. One of the most commonly seen seizure semiology in infants with TSC is epileptic spasms. The other features which suggest a diagnosis of tuberous sclerosis include the cardiac murmur (likely from a cardiac rhabdomyoma), multiple hyperpigmented macules, and cortical tubers on head CT. Additionally, the history of the child's mother having a renal tumor is suggestive of the multiorgan system involvement seen in TSC. Associated comorbidities in tuberous sclerosis complex include autism spectrum disorder, developmental delays, cognitive and learning disabilities, and mood and behavior disorders (depression, anxiety, ADHD, etc.) [2]. The degree to which an individual is affected can be quite variable given the variable expressivity seen in TSC, even among affected family members.

2. The etiology is genetic-structural. TSC is caused by mutations in TSC1 located on chromosome 9q34 and TSC2 located on 16p13.3, encoding hamartin and tuberin, respectively. These proteins function as regulators of the mTOR (mammalian target of rapamycin) pathway. Up to 25% of individuals with TSC will not have an identifiable gene mutation [1]. TSC exhibits complete penetrance with variable expressivity. Therefore, individuals can have a variable degree of symptom severity, and age of presentation and presenting symptoms can be variable. Seizures are most likely to arise from a cortical tuber. These cortical malformations are highly epileptogenic. On histopathology, these lesions correspond to focal cortical dysplasia (FCD) type IIb.

3. The child should undergo a thorough skin examination. It would be recommended that a brain MRI be performed to fully evaluate for cortical tubers, white matter radial migration abnormalities, subependymal nodules, and subependymal giant cell astrocytoma (SEGA). Repeat imaging with MRI should be performed every 1–3 years in patients under the age of 25 years for monitoring for new or growing SEGA. The child should undergo baseline ophthalmologic examination, and if lesions are present or other vision concerns, they should continue to undergo annual eye exams. Additional testing, as suggested by the child's murmur, would be an echocardiogram looking for evidence of a cardiac rhabdomyoma. A baseline electrocardiogram should be obtained to evaluate for conduction defects. In asymptomatic children, repeat echocardiography should be performed every 1–3 years until regression of cardiac rhabdomyoma is seen. Repeat electrocardiography should be performed every 3–5 years for evaluation of cardiac conduction defects. Abdominal imaging with MRI is also recommended to evaluate for the presence of renal cysts and angiomyolipomas. Subsequent surveillance would include repeat abdominal imaging every 1–3 years. Further evaluation of renal function should include blood tests for glomerular filtration rate. Additional testing, which should start at age 18 years in females and in symptomatic males, would include baseline pulmonary

function studies and high-resolution chest CT evaluating for lymphangiomyomatosis (LAM). If lung cysts are seen, then monitoring with repeat chest CT every 1–3 years would be recommended, otherwise, repeat imaging every 5–10 years. Given the child's history of developmental delays, baseline neuropsychometric testing would be recommended [3].

4. The seizure described is a focal impaired awareness seizure with evolution to bilateral convulsive seizure (secondary generalization). The child has head turn and eye deviation to the left with left arm flexion and right arm extension, which can be called a Figure 4 or fencer's pose. From the features described, this seizure likely is arising from the left frontal region and could be consistent with a seizure from the supplementary motor area (SMA).

5. Due to the variable presentation and severity of symptoms in TSC, the treatments can also be quite variable. Anti-seizure medications can include both those with focal and generalized seizure indications depending on the clinical scenario. Some individuals have refractory epilepsy and Lennox-Gastaut syndrome and require multiple daily medications. In some individuals with refractory epilepsy, surgical therapies are indicated. If supportive neuroimaging and electroencephalographic studies can identify a "dominant" tuber, then focal surgical resection can be helpful if reducing seizure frequency [4]. Additional treatment options can include the use of mTOR inhibitors such as everolimus and sirolimus which can reduce the size of both brain and renal lesions [5]. In epileptic spasms secondary to TSC, vigabatrin is the recommended treatment [6].

This child was initiated on oxcarbazepine for treatment of focal seizures. Her seizures have been relatively well controlled with intermittent breakthrough seizures occurring in the setting of illness and missed medication dosages. She was found to have a cardiac rhabdomyoma, which was clinically followed with serial echocardiograms and has demonstrated expected involution. On follow-up imaging, she was found to have a non-obstructing subependymal giant cell astrocytoma which has been stable on serial MRI studies. She is currently in the second grade and has an individual education plan (IEP) for help with math and reading and extra time for classroom assignments. She has been given a diagnosis of attention deficit hyperactivity disorder (ADHD), which has been treated with methylphenidate.

Key Points/Clinical Pearls
1. A child presenting with new onset seizures should undergo detailed physical examination including skin examination with a Wood's lamp. Additionally, family history is important and can be suggestive of an inherited disorder.
2. The identification of the underlying etiology is critical to informing additional diagnostic and treatment decisions.
3. Given the variable expressivity in TSC, patients can present with any number of findings. Seizures are the most common presenting complaint. Epilepsy severity can range from mild to severe.

4. In TSC, additional investigations for multiorgan system involvement vary by age and presenting symptoms. In children, additional evaluation should include a cardiac echocardiogram as well as abdominal imaging. In teens and adults, chest imaging is recommended.

5. Treatment of TSC depends upon epilepsy type and severity. In children with epileptic spasms, vigabatrin is the maintenance antiseizure medication of choice. In those with a highly epileptogenic tuber, focal resection can reduce seizure frequency. The use of mTOR inhibitors (sirolimus and everolimus) can reduce the size of both brain and renal lesions.

References

1. Northrup H, Krueger DA, International Tuberous Sclerosis Complex Consensus G. Tuberous sclerosis complex diagnostic criteria update: recommendations of the 2012 International Tuberous Sclerosis Complex Consensus Conference. Pediatr Neurol. 2013;49(4):243–54.
2. Curatolo P, Moavero R, de Vries PJ. Neurological and neuropsychiatric aspects of tuberous sclerosis complex. Lancet Neurol. 2015;14(7):733–45.
3. Krueger DA, Northrup H, International Tuberous Sclerosis Complex Consensus G. Tuberous sclerosis complex surveillance and management: recommendations of the 2012 International Tuberous Sclerosis Complex Consensus Conference. Pediatr Neurol. 2013;49(4):255–65.
4. Jansen FE, van Huffelen AC, Algra A, van Nieuwenhuizen O. Epilepsy surgery in tuberous sclerosis: a systematic review. Epilepsia. 2007;48(8):1477–84.
5. Krueger DA, Wilfong AA, Holland-Bouley K, Anderson AE, Agricola K, Tudor C, et al. Everolimus treatment of refractory epilepsy in tuberous sclerosis complex. Ann Neurol. 2013;74(5):679–87.
6. van der Poest Clement EA, Sahin M, Peters JM. Vigabatrin for epileptic spasms and tonic seizures in tuberous sclerosis complex. J Child Neurol. 2018;33(8):519–24.

Epileptic Encephalopaties and Developmental Disorders

8

Keith Starnes and Raj D. Sheth

Case Presentation

A typical developing 6-year-old right-handed boy presented to clinic for concerns of developmental regression. He had a history of a single febrile seizure at 9 months and a focal seizure at 3 years, with the latter characterized by slurred speech and drooling that occurred during wakefulness. He had an EEG and was diagnosed with childhood epilepsy with centrotemporal spikes. His parents were counseled that this would likely be self-limited, and no treatment was started.

About a year later, he abruptly began having similar focal seizures about 3–4 times per month. Some of these were also associated with right-sided facial twitching. He was started on oxcarbazepine, but there was no improvement in focal seizures over the next year. The seizures began to occur mostly at night. He had an overnight EEG which demonstrated ESES, with spike-wave index (SWI) 95%. He was diagnosed with CSWS and started on valproic acid. He began to have frequent, brief, head-drop seizures. He was more lethargic and developed subacute language and behavioral regression.

Over the next 4 months, several therapies were used. Clobazam was added to valproic acid without much success. He was started on oral steroids, which appeared to improve symptoms for redundant 2–3 weeks. He received pulse-dose intravenous steroids, which also conferred only temporary benefit. He started biweekly intravenous immunoglobulin. Following failure of these treatment regimens, he was transitioned to a ketogenic diet. Despite these efforts, his seizures worsened, occurring

K. Starnes (✉)
Mayo Clinic, Department of Neurology, Rochester, MN, USA
e-mail: starnes.donnie@mayo.edu

R. D. Sheth
Mayo Clinic/Nemours Children's Health Systems, Department of Neurology,
Jacksonville, FL, USA
e-mail: rsheth@nemours.org; Raj.sheth@nemours.org

© Springer Nature Switzerland AG 2021
W. O. Tatum et al. (eds.), *Epilepsy Case Studies*,
https://doi.org/10.1007/978-3-030-59078-9_8

up to 300 times a day. His neurocognitive abilities also deteriorated, with persistent dysarthria, loss of spontaneous speech, inability to follow commands, and slowed processing speed. He also began to hold his right hand in a fist and preferred using his left hand for most tasks. He was unable to swallow, necessitating gastrostomy tube placement. His behavior was increasingly aggressive, and he was unable to attend school. Epilepsy pre-surgical phase II evaluation with intracranial grid placement over the left perirolandic region was contemplated.

He was admitted for overnight EEG monitoring. Exceedingly frequent seizures with left centrotemporal onset and rapid secondary bisynchrony were recorded, with clinical manifestations of head dropping, negative myoclonia of the right hand and behavioral arrest. Hundreds of seizures were recorded within 24 h. His spike frequency during wakefulness was approximately 2–3 per min, but his SWI in sleep was 100% (Fig. 8.1). His MRI was non-lesional. Laboratory evaluations with serum

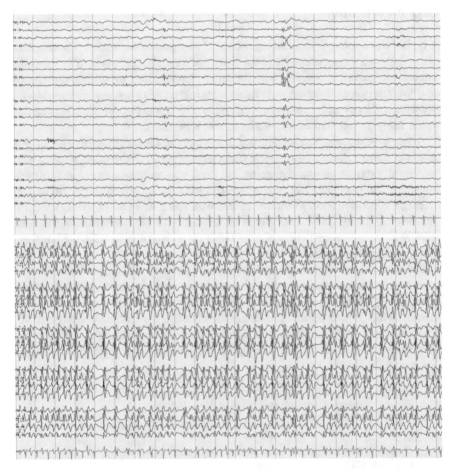

Fig. 8.1 Comparison of representative samples of awake (top) and asleep (bottom) EEG segments at presentation. During sleep, there was continuous activation of spike-wave discharges with rapid secondary bilateral synchrony

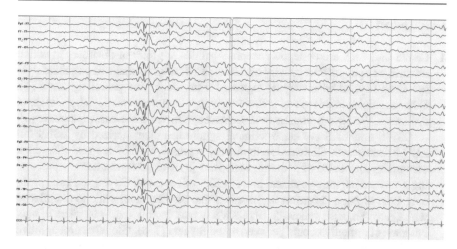

Fig. 8.2 Sleep sample recorded after 6 months of sulthiame treatment, showing markedly reduced activation of epileptiform discharges

and CSF testing for genetic, metabolic, and autoimmune conditions were negative. Clobazam was converted to nocturnal diazepam at 0.5 mg/kg, and topiramate was added.

There was little initial improvement, but seizures began to decrease after 2 weeks. Two weeks later, he was started on sulthiame, a carbonic anhydrase inhibitor, and his drop seizures abated completely concurrent with an improvement in encephalopathy. Within a month, he was speaking in sentences again, began to eat by mouth, and was more interactive with his environment. His right hand coordination improved dramatically. In 3 months, he was climbing trees, learning to play piano, writing all of his numbers and letters with his right hand, and spelling out words. His facial twitching seizures stopped after 4 months, and he was seizure-free for more than 6 months at last follow-up. At age 7, he still had difficulty with reading. His behavior had improved, though he remained impulsive and continued to be home-schooled. His SWI improved to 20% (Fig. 8.2). All treatments besides sulthiame and nocturnal diazepam were discontinued.

Clinical Questions

1. What are the ages of presentation and clinical features of CSWS and LKS?
2. What factors predispose children to developing ESES?
3. How does EEG assist in diagnosing and following CSWS and LKS?
4. What treatment options exist for CSWS and LKS?
5. What is the neurocognitive outcome for treated CSWS and LKS?

Discussion

1. CSWS and LKS are epileptic encephalopathies, a group of disorders in which seizures or epileptiform activity contribute to developmental and cognitive dysfunctions beyond what may be expected from underlying pathology alone [1]. Other examples in this group include early myoclonic encephalopathy, Ohtahara syndrome, West syndrome, Lennox-Gastaut syndrome, and Dravet syndrome [2].

   CSWS and LKS are electroclinical syndromes characterized by ESES (an EEG pattern) with clinical developmental regression. They are rare disorders, comprising 0.2–0.4% of pediatric epilepsies [3]. Seizures are often the presenting symptom but may be absent in up to 20% of cases [4]. CSWS and LKS probably exist along a spectrum of disorders that also includes childhood epilepsy with centrotemporal spikes [5, 6]. CSWS occurs in children 1–14 years of age, but most commonly occurs between 4 and 8 years [7, 8]. Global neurocognitive problems develop, with worsening deficiencies in expressive language, behavior, attention, and sometimes motor control (often unilateral). Autistic-like behavioral features can develop [9]. Seizures tend to be frequent and difficult to control. Multiple seizure types can occur [7, 8].

   In LKS, onset is between 3 and 8 years of age and most common at 4–5 years [7]. Receptive language is primarily affected, with acquired auditory progressing over weeks to months. Seizures are usually infrequent, nocturnal, and easily controlled [10].

2. One-third to one-half of children with CSWS or LKS have underlying prenatal or perinatal abnormalities [4, 10, 11]. Predisposing factors include cortical dysplasia, vascular insults, tuberous sclerosis, and abnormal myelination. Lesions to the thalami seem to be particularly associated with development of ESES [12, 13]. Genetic and metabolic factors have been implicated in some cases, with GRIN2A most commonly linked to the disorder [14]. However, ESES commonly occurs in normally developing children without identifiable predisposing factors.

3. ESES is an EEG pattern defined by significant activation of epileptiform discharges in non-REM sleep. The awake EEG is usually abnormal, with common foci in the frontotemporal or centrotemporal regions [8]. In sleep, this becomes nearly continuous, with discharges often demonstrating rapid secondary bilateral synchrony. The normal sleep architecture is disrupted, with decrease in sleep spindles frequently seen [10, 15].

   The frequency of epileptiform discharges in sleep is quantified as the SWI, defined as the proportion of the non-REM sleep record containing them. Methodology for calculating SWI varies, but one practice is to divide the sleep record into 1-second bins and "count" those bins that have at least one epileptiform discharge. Originally it was suggested that the SWI should be at least 85%, but ILAE criteria suggest a figure of 50% [16]. EEG can also be used to help assess treatment efficacy, and there is a strong correlation between improvements in SWI and cognition [17].

4. There have been no randomized controlled trials for treatment in ESES. Cohort studies have reported success with high-dose diazepam, oral and IV steroids, IV immunoglobulin, ketogenic diet, vagus nerve stimulation, conventional antiepileptic agents (valproic acid, ethosuximide, benzodiazepines, levetiracetam, lacosamide, etc.), and surgery, which has included multiple subpial transection, hemispheric surgery, corpus callosotomy, and lobar or multilobar resections [8]. A meta-analysis found that surgery and steroids were superior among these [4]. A recent cohort study demonstrated efficacy of amantadine [18]. Carbonic anhydrase inhibitors have been used successfully, primarily with sulthiame – commercially available in Europe but not in the USA [19, 20] – and acetazolamide [7].

   Treatments to avoid include phenytoin, phenobarbital, carbamazepine, and oxcarbazepine, as these have been reported to lead to worsening of cognitive outcomes and epileptiform discharges. Polypharmacy should be avoided, as it has been reported to worsen symptoms [21].

5. CSWS and LKS are age-related syndromes and resolve spontaneously by puberty [11]. Seizures abate and EEG patterns normalize. Despite this, half or more of patients have long-term neurocognitive disabilities, and a minority attains their previous cognitive baseline. Better outcomes have been reported in cases with unknown etiology, shorter duration of symptoms, and control of seizures [22].

Pearls
- CSWS and LKS are electroclinical syndromes characterized by elevated SWI seen on EEG during sleep (ESES) and developmental regression.
- Predisposing factors for ESES include GRIN2A mutations and thalamic insult.
- Surgery is the most effective treatment option in lesional cases.
- Phenytoin, phenobarbital, carbamazepine, and oxcarbazepine should be avoided in ESES as they have been reported to worsen the EEG and clinical symptoms.
- CSWS and LKS resolve spontaneously by puberty. However, most children are left with residual neurocognitive sequelae.

References

1. Berg AT, et al. Revised terminology and concepts for organization of seizures and epilepsies: report of the ILAE Commission on Classification and Terminology, 2005–2009. Epilepsia. 2010;51(4):676–85.
2. Covanis A. Epileptic encephalopathies (including severe epilepsy syndromes). Epilepsia. 2012;53(Suppl 4):114–26.
3. Kramer U, et al. Epidemiology of epilepsy in childhood: a cohort of 440 consecutive patients. Pediatr Neurol. 1998;18(1):46–50.
4. van den Munckhof B, et al. Treatment of electrical status epilepticus in sleep: a pooled analysis of 575 cases. Epilepsia. 2015;56(11):1738–46.

5. Tovia E, et al. The prevalence of atypical presentations and comorbidities of benign childhood epilepsy with centrotemporal spikes. Epilepsia. 2011;52(8):1483–8.
6. Lee YJ, Hwang SK, Kwon S. The clinical spectrum of benign epilepsy with centro-temporal spikes: a challenge in categorization and predictability. J Epilepsy Res. 2017;7(1):1–6.
7. Fine AL, et al. Acetazolamide for electrical status epilepticus in slow-wave sleep. Epilepsia. 2015;56(9):e134–8.
8. Nickels K, Wirrell E. Electrical status epilepticus in sleep. Semin Pediatr Neurol. 2008;15(2):50–60.
9. Galanopoulou AS, et al. The spectrum of neuropsychiatric abnormalities associated with electrical status epilepticus in sleep. Brain Dev. 2000;22(5):279–95.
10. Bureau M. Continuous spikes and waves during slow sleep, electrical status epilepticus during slow sleep, acquired epileptic aphasia and related conditions. London: John Libbey; 1995.
11. Tassinari CA, et al. The electrical status epilepticus syndrome. Epilepsy Res Suppl. 1992;6:111–5.
12. Sanchez Fernandez I, et al. Continuous spikes and waves during sleep: electroclinical presentation and suggestions for management. Epilepsy Res Treat. 2013;2013:583531.
13. van den Munckhof B, et al. Perinatal thalamic injury: MRI predictors of electrical status epilepticus in sleep and long-term neurodevelopment. Neuroimage Clin. 2020;26:102227.
14. Samanta D, Al Khalili Y. Electrical status epilepticus in sleep (ESES). In: StatPearls. Treasure Island (FL): StatPearls Publishing; 2020.
15. Kobayashi K, et al. Epilepsy with electrical status epilepticus during slow sleep and secondary bilateral synchrony. Epilepsia. 1994;35(5):1097–103.
16. Scheltens-de Boer M. Guidelines for EEG in encephalopathy related to ESES/CSWS in children. Epilepsia. 2009;50(Suppl 7):13–7.
17. van den Munckhof B, et al. Treatment of electrical status epilepticus in sleep: clinical and EEG characteristics and response to 147 treatments in 47 patients. Eur J Paediatr Neurol. 2018;22(1):64–71.
18. Wilson RB, et al. Amantadine: a new treatment for refractory electrical status epilepticus in sleep. Epilepsy Behav. 2018;84:74–8.
19. Wirrell E, Ho AW, Hamiwka L. Sulthiame therapy for continuous spike and wave in slow-wave sleep. Pediatr Neurol. 2006;35(3):204–8.
20. Fejerman N, et al. Sulthiame add-on therapy in children with focal epilepsies associated with encephalopathy related to electrical status epilepticus during slow sleep (ESES). Epilepsia. 2012;53(7):1156–61.
21. Van Lierde A. Therapeutic data. In: Beaumanoir A, Bureau M, Deonna L, Mira L, Tassinari CA, editors. Continuous spikes and waves during slow sleep. London: John Libbey; 1995. p. 225–7.
22. Hempel A, Frost M, Agarwal N. Language and behavioral outcomes of treatment with pulse-dose prednisone for electrical status epilepticus in sleep (ESES). Epilepsy Behav. 2019;94:93–9.

Autonomic Seizures and Panayiotopoulos Syndrome

William O. Tatum and William P. Cheshire

Case Presentation

A 9-year-old boy was evaluated for epilepsy. He had a normal birth, labor, delivery, and development and was well until the previous year, when he experienced a first spell. He was playing outside at a nearby pond. When his mother went to inquire how he was doing, she noted he suddenly developed a weird facial expression and "acted like he was going to be sick." He started repeatedly retching and was profusely sweating for about 10–15 min. He appeared weak and pale and was slow to respond while clutching his abdomen. His mother encouraged him to lie down and rest. She called for his father who arrived and picked up his son. As he lifted him up, he collapsed limply and then vomited. The patient was laid down on the ground, when his eyes rolled up to the left; he became unresponsive, turned his head to the left, and briefly stiffened. After another 10–15 min, he was sleepy and had evidence of urinary incontinence but fully recovered following a 3-hour nap. In the emergency department, a CT brain was normal as were routine laboratory studies and a 12-lead EKG. Subsequently, a brain MRI revealed a left choroid fissure cyst. EEG demonstrated generalized spike-and-slow wave (GSW) discharges. He was diagnosed with absence seizures, and ethosuximide was prescribed, but treatment was declined by the parents since it was only his first episode. A computer-assisted ambulatory EEG captured isolated GSW discharges throughout the recording (Fig. 9.1a).

W. O. Tatum (✉) · W. P. Cheshire
Mayo Clinic, Department of Neurology, Jacksonville, FL, USA
e-mail: tatum.william@mayo.edu; cheshire@mayo.edu

© Springer Nature Switzerland AG 2021
W. O. Tatum et al. (eds.), *Epilepsy Case Studies*,
https://doi.org/10.1007/978-3-030-59078-9_9

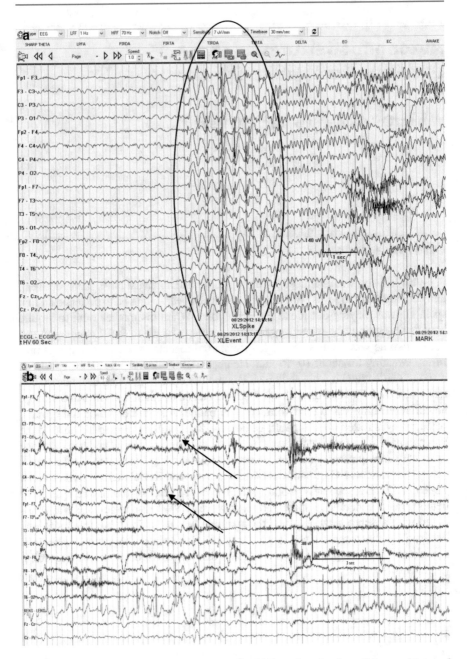

Fig. 9.1 (**a**) EEG demonstrating a 3-Hz generalized bifrontal predominant 2.5 second burst of spike-and-slow waves followed by an arousal without clinical signs (oval) and (**b**) biooccipital spike-and-slow waves (arrows)

Clinical Questions

1. Is this EEG specific for a diagnosis?
2. What is the clinical significance of the seizure?
3. What epilepsy syndrome is suggested?
4. What treatment should be recommended at this point?
5. What is the anticipated prognosis?

Diagnostic Discussion

1. No, an EEG that demonstrates 3-Hz generalized spike-and-slow waves (GSW) is not specific for an epilepsy syndrome. Any of the genetic generalized epilepsies may be associated with GSW on EEG. However, it is the clinical phenomenology that defines the epilepsy syndrome [1]. 3-Hz GSW is most common with absence seizures; however this EEG pattern may be seen with other generalized epilepsies and epilepsy syndromes. Childhood absence epilepsy is most common in this age range and typically presents with multiple daily episodes of brief impaired responsiveness (absences). When absence seizures are associated with myoclonus, epilepsy with myoclonic absences is suggested. When prominent eyelid myoclonia is present with photosensitivity and absences, a diagnosis of Jeavons syndrome should be considered. In the teen years, other generalized seizures (i.e., myoclonus and convulsions) may occur with absence, such as juvenile absence epilepsy and juvenile myoclonic epilepsy [1]. Seizure types can overlap, even evolving from one epilepsy syndrome to another over time [2]. When bursts of GSW are brief, "phantom" absences may be diagnosed when detailed testing such as breath-counting during hyperventilation is performed during EEG. In addition, the finding of GSW may occur in asymptomatic patients when GSW is inherited as a genetic trait independent of an epilepsy phenotype. Also, in a significant minority, GSW may occur in patients with focal epilepsies (such as the genetic focal epilepsies, including benign childhood epilepsy with centrotemporal spikes).
2. The patient's clinical event is characteristic of a prolonged autonomic seizure. Migraine or cyclical vomiting syndrome may be first suspected as the diagnosis, although, when consciousness is impaired and cloinic jerking occurs, the association with seizures becomes more likely. An autonomic seizure is an epileptic seizure characterized by symptoms or signs associated with altered autonomic function. Seizures may appear focal or generalized at the onset with subjective or objective semiology involving signs of dysautonomia. Nausea, vomiting, and other signs of autonomic dysfunction, including changes in pupillary dilation, pallor or flushing, hypersalivation, temperature changes, and incontinence, occur (Table 9.1A). Syncopal episodes may occur and are suggested by limpness, collapse, and pallor. In some children, autonomic seizures with syncope-like episodes precede semiologies more characteristic of seizures with associated hemiclonic jerking or convulsive motor movements [3]. Autonomic seizures

Table 9.1A Clinical signs associated with autonomic seizures	Diaphoresis
	Changes in respiratory rate
	Changes in heart rate
	Changes in blood pressure
	Piloerection
	Flushing
	Pallor
	Cyanosis
	Unpleasant sensation in the abdomen, head, or chest
	Nausea
	Vomiting
	Variable alteration in consciousness
	Pupillary dilation
	Hypotonia
	Posturing

may be quite prolonged, lasting for half an hour or longer and represent autonomic status epilepticus. Typically, autonomic seizures occur during sleep; however, in our patient his initial episode occurred during wakefulness.

3. Panayiotopoulos syndrome (PS) is a recognized childhood epilepsy syndrome with an unusual seizure semiology, which includes autonomic features associated with seizures present in normal children [4]. PS occurs in normal children and is manifested by infrequent autonomic seizures and autonomic status epilepticus [5]. The onset is in childhood, usually before 6 years of age, and presents with symptoms of nausea and vomiting. Autonomic features may be the only symptoms present without the clonic jerking that is more readily associated with epileptic seizures. The nonconvulsive semiology may result in a delay in a diagnosis of epilepsy. Furthermore, EEG may be normal, leading to misdiagnoses. Gastroesophageal reflux, cyclical vomiting syndrome, benign paroxysmal positional vertigo, migraine, and vasovagal syncope should be considered in the differential diagnosis (Table 9.1B) if an episode is unwitnessed. EEG abnormalities demonstrate marked variability with locations that include frontal, centrotemporal, multi-focal, and combinations of focal and generalized epileptiform discharges. When seen, occipital spikes predominate (Fig. 9.1b), are typically high voltage, and can change significantly with repeat EEG recordings. Seizure may show shifting onsets with scalp EEG recording despite similar clinical manifestations.

4. Maintenance antiseizure medications (ASMs) are often not required in PS due to the limited likelihood of recurrence. Most children have fewer than five seizures, though about 5% of cases are recurrent [4]. Many children have only one or two seizures. Treatment may be considered when seizures are prolonged, associated with injury, psychosocially disturbing, or recurrent. While no single ASM appears to show superiority, ethosuximide has activity against absence seizures, though it would not be expected to be beneficial for patients with focal seizures. Video-EEG monitoring may be considered in cases of recurrent events

Table 9.1B Autonomic signs/symptoms in nonepileptic diagnoses

Age	Differential diagnoses	Signs/symptoms
Neonates and infants	Inborn errors of metabolism	Intermittent vomiting, lethargy, apnea
	Breath-holding spells	Emotional triggers, apnea, pallor or cyanosis, apnea, bradycardia
	Sandifer's syndrome	Dystonic posturing, stiffening, apnea, bradycardia, flushing
	Simple gastroesophageal reflux	Hypotonia, apnea, bradycardia, pallor
	Familial dysautonomia	Absence of emotional tears, absence of fungiform papillae of the tongue, episodes of vomiting, sweating, flushing, drooling, increased heart rate and blood pressure
Childhood	Inborn errors of metabolism and breath-holding spells	Symptoms same as above
	Benign paroxysmal positional vertigo	Dizziness, nausea, and pallor that may be precipitated by head movement
	Cyclical vomiting syndrome	Recurrent episodes of vomiting, may occur especially at night
	Sleep disorders/parasomnias	Episodes occur out of sleep, profuse sweating, flushing, tachycardia, anxiety
	Psychiatric/panic attacks	Anxiety, hyperventilation, heart rate and blood pressure elevation, diaphoresis, nausea, vomiting, feeling of dread
	Syncope	Hypotonia, collapse, loss of consciousness, low heart rate and blood pressure, preceding nausea, pallor, diaphoresis
Adolescents/ adults	Syncope, benign paroxysmal positional vertigo, panic attacks, sleep disorders	Symptoms same as above
	Migraine (all ages)	Headache, nausea, vomiting, flushing
	Postural orthostatic tachycardia syndrome	Hypotonia, dizziness, pallor, nausea

or if other seizure types (e.g., "phantom absences") are suggested clinically. Rescue medication with intranasal midazolam or diazepam nasal spray or rectal diazepam gel may be used in the advent of recurrent autonomic status epilepticus. Chronic maintenance ASMs are often not initially prescribed. Lamotrigine was discussed as an option with the patient given its broad spectrum of activity in focal and generalized seizures without producing sedating cognitive adverse effects.

5. The prognosis for PS is excellent, and most remit in several years, although an earlier age of onset may be a negative predictor. The MRI brain was reviewed, and a small choroid fissure cyst was identified. With the clinical presentation and GSW on EEG, it was judged to be asymptomatic and incidental. Children with PS typically demonstrate normal development [4]. PS, like other benign focal epilepsies of childhood, is probably linked to a common, genetically determined, transitory functional derangement of the brain during the maturational process.

A benign childhood seizure susceptibility syndrome has been used to describe a mild and temporary condition that enters remission as the child develops further into adolescence and adulthood [1, 4]. The neuropsychological examination is normal in PS except for visual and visuoperceptual alterations and infrequently minor attention and memory disturbances.

Clinical Pearls
1. Autonomic seizures and autonomic status epilepticus are not uncommon in childhood and may be mistaken for other conditions such as migraine. However, in most cases, the EEG reveals multi-focal, or occipital predominant, high amplitude sharp-and-slow wave complexes.
2. Panayiotopoulos syndrome is a unique childhood epilepsy syndrome with heterogeneous EEG features that carries a favorable prognosis.
3. Many patients with PS do not need treatment with chronic ASM, although rescue medication in the advent of recurrent status epilepticus should be considered.
4. The prognosis for PS is excellent with many episodes occurring as single, nonrepeated events.
5. Despite the prolonged episode and syncopal appearance, seizures may evolve to more obvious focal and convulsive seizures. The overall prognosis for seizures associated with an underlying autonomic instability is good. When ASM are required, most patients respond to treatment and eventually undergo spontaneous remission.

References

1. Panayiotopoulos CP, Chrysostomos P. Typical absence seizures and related epileptic syndromes: assessment of current state and directions for future research. Epilepsia. 2008;49(12):2131–9.
2. Berg AT, Berkovic SF, Brodie MJ, Buchhalter J, Cross HJ, Van Emde BW, et al. Revised terminology and concepts for organization of seizures and epilepsies: report of the ILAE commission on classification and terminology, 2005–2009. Epilepsia. 2010;51:676–85.
3. Koutroumanidis M, Ferrie CD, Valeta T, Sanders S, Michael M, Panayiotopoulos CP. Syncope-like epileptic seizures in Panayiotopoulos syndrome. Neurology. 2012;79(5):463–7.
4. Panayiotopoulos CP, Michael M, Sanders S, Valeta T, Koutroumanidis M. Benign childhood focal epilepsies: assessment of established and newly recognized syndromes. Brain. 2008;131:2264–86.
5. Specchio N, Trivisano M, DiCiommo V, Cappelletti S, Masciarelli G, Volkov J, et al. Panayiotopoulos syndrome: a clinical, EEG, and neuropsychological study of 93 consecutive patients. Epilepsia. 2010;51(10):2098–107.

Genetic Epilepsy with Febrile Seizures Plus

10

William O. Tatum

Case Presentation

A 15-year-old girl was born the second of three children with a normal birth, maternal labor, delivery, and development. Ear infections were recurrent as a child leading to periodic febrile illnesses. At two and one-half years of age, she experienced a convulsion during a fever of 102.7 °F. The seizures were noted to occur with an abrupt onset associated with generalized stiffening of the body and extremities, loss of consciousness, and rhythmic jerking of her arms and legs for about 1–2 min followed by lethargy and recovery without incidence after 10 min. At the hospital she was diagnosed with a febrile seizure (FS). Initially a CT of the brain and lumbar puncture were normal and an EEG was normal. Subsequently, she developed recurrent generalized tonic-clonic seizures whenever she was febrile over the years. This would typically occur when she had ear infections in early childhood though continued until she was 9 years old when an afebrile seizure was noted. There was a past family history of her mother, sister, and maternal grandmother who also had experienced FS as a child. At that time, a CT brain was normal, and she was given a prescription for diazepam rectal gel in case of a prolonged seizure recurrence. She experienced two additional afebrile generalized tonic-clonic seizures, and due to persistent seizures, she was begun on carbamazepine. With carbamazepine a 2nd type of seizure became noted characterized by single body jerk that would lead to brief stiffening with "head nods." A pediatric epileptologist was consulted for evaluation of focal seizures. Brain MRI was normal (see Fig. 10.1a), and EEG (Fig. 10.1b) had a normal background with generalized spike- and polyspike-and-waves. Anti-seizure medication (ASM) was changed from carbamazepine to valproate, and she

W. O. Tatum (✉)
Mayo Clinic, Department of Neurology, Jacksonville, FL, USA
e-mail: tatum.william@mayo.edu

© Springer Nature Switzerland AG 2021
W. O. Tatum et al. (eds.), *Epilepsy Case Studies*,
https://doi.org/10.1007/978-3-030-59078-9_10

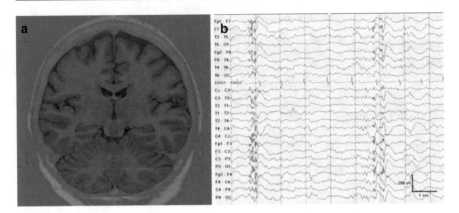

Fig. 10.1 (**a**) Normal brain showing coronal T1-weighted MRI and (**b**) EEG demonstrating a single generalized irregular polyspike-and-wave in second 2 and generalized spike-and-waves in second 7

became seizure-free. At 12 years old, she was changed from valproate to levetiracetam during puberty and retained seizure freedom.

Clinical Questions

1. How often are febrile seizures inherited?
2. What are common epilepsy syndromes that may result?
3. What does the evaluation suggest as the diagnosis in this patient?
4. What is the role of ancillary testing to support the diagnosis?
5. What is the anticipated clinical course and prognosis in this patient?

Diagnostic Discussion

1. Classic febrile seizures (FS) affect 2–4% of children under the age of 6 years and are by far the most common pediatric seizure disorder. Involvement of several family members in our patient suggests an inherited pattern. FS have a strong genetic component with mutations in three main genes (SCN1A, SCN1B, and GABRG2) [1]. However, a single mode of inheritance has not been established for FS. FS occur with approximately a two- to threefold prevalence among the family members of affected children when compared with a similar normal population. If the parents are affected, this increases the risk that FS will occur in their offspring. In addition, the risk is increased when both parents are affected and predicts a greater likelihood of recurrent FS. Asian families in particular are at risk for FS and have demonstrated a population effect. Overall, approximately 1/3 of FS will recur and be more likely when the age of onset is less than 1 year. Most are simple FS without a significance risk for subsequent epilepsy. However,

in 10–20% of children, complex FS and febrile status epilepticus may occur and carry a greater risk of chronic epilepsy especially if there is a prolonged fever, family history, or the presence of a neurological deficit exists.

2. The types of epilepsy that may result include focal and generalized seizures. A minority of patients with FS go on to develop afebrile seizures. Patients with complex FS account for the majority of those who develop subsequent epilepsy. The association with prolonged FS and temporal lobe epilepsy (TLE) due to hippocampal sclerosis that is often drug-resistant is known though a cause and effect relationship remains controversial. Temporal lobe seizures are more likely to remit if a first-degree relative has had a FS. Other generalized seizure types include generalized tonic-clonic with and without absence seizures. Focal epilepsy (TLE) and hemiconvulsion-hemiplegia-epilepsy syndrome with severe febrile status occur with recurrent focal seizures. Generalized epilepsy with a genetic component (i.e., Doose syndrome and myoclonic absence epilepsy) in addition to generalized epilepsy with febrile seizures plus (GEF+) may also be heralded by FS. Genetic epilepsy with febrile seizures plus (GEFS+) occurs in a small proportion of children with FS who either have them extending beyond age 6 and develop epilepsy with afebrile seizures [2]. In this case, a normal mental status makes a malignant epileptic encephalopathy such as Dravet syndrome (severe myoclonic epilepsy of infancy) unlikely to be present. Dravet syndrome is considered part of the GEFS+ spectrum and is the most severe phenotype.

3. The presence of recurrent FS beginning in early childhood that persists beyond the age of 6 years old (the normal cut-off for FS) in addition to the prominent family history and heterogeneous generalized seizures suggests GEF+. GEFS+ is an important childhood genetic epilepsy syndrome to consider due to heterogeneous phenotypes that may occur, including febrile seizures associated with generalized epilepsies comprising variable severity [3]. The family history of FS is the key to suspecting a genetic basis for the clinical diagnosis. The most common phenotypes are FS often associated with afebrile generalized tonic-clonic seizures. In about one third of patients, additional seizure types may occur, such as myoclonic, absences, or tonic/atonic seizures. Focal seizures may also occur in combinations that persist into adolescence or adulthood. The brain MRI and the neurological examination are normal (Fig. 10.1a) though cognitive impairment may be present. The EEG like the phenotype has a wide range of findings, from normal to generalized interictal epileptiform discharges (Fig. 10.1b).

4. Genetic factors are increasing in their importance relative to both diagnosis and treatment of epilepsy. An autosomal dominant mode of inheritance with incomplete penetrance (about 80%) has been demonstrated in GEFS+. However, GEFS+ is a genetically heterogeneous disorder. GEFS+ is genetically heterogeneous and mutations in SCN1B, SCN1A, and GABRG2. Type 1 is associated with SCN1B [4, 5]. Multiple gene mutations with different loci have been identified including several mutations that involve the sodium channel and GABA-A receptor subunit. Sodium channel dysfunction via SCN1A may result in hyperexcitability from inactivation. Sodium gating modulation by SCN2A may lead to interference with the voltage-gated beta subunit encoding. A reduction in the

Table 10.1 Subtypes of GEFS+ with associated genetic heterogeneity

GEFS+ subtype	Gene	Locus
1	SCN1B	19q13, 2q21–33
2	SCN1A	2q24
3	GABARG2	5q34
4	–	2p24
5	GABARD	1p36
6	–	8p23–p21
7	SCN9A	2q24
8	–	6q16.3–q22.31
9	STX1B	16p11
10	HCN1	5p12

Adapted from Ref. [8]

inhibitory effect by a mutation in a subunit of the GABA-A receptor (GABRG2) may interfere with benzodiazepine binding. SCN2A has also been associated with GEFS+. Various subtypes of GEFS+ have been identified based upon the gene mutation involved making diagnosis easier with genetic analysis (Table 10.1). The EEG of GEFS+ may initially be normal as it was in this case. In the EEG, interictal epileptiform discharges may be present. This patient had irregular generalized spike- and polyspike-and-waves with a repetition rate of 2.5 Hz supporting her clinical diagnosis of generalized epilepsy. Focal spikes may also be present in the EEG of patients with GEFS+.

5. Classification systems use terminology and concepts of seizure onset to organize knowledge of the types of epilepsy and predict the clinical course and response to treatment [6]. Patients with GEFS+ express a highly variable phenotype combining FS and generalized seizures often provoked by fever. Absences, myoclonic, or tonic/atonic seizures (drop attacks) may occur with focal seizures and a varying degree of severity. In this case, "pseudo-resistance" to carbamazepine occurred from misclassification of GEFS+ as a focal epilepsy. The treatment course was complicated when seizures were not controlled due to the sodium channel-blocking mechanism associated with carbamazepine's mechanism of action. Genetic generalized epilepsy syndromes such as GEFS+ may not respond to narrow-spectrum ASM used to treat focal seizures and even precipitate new types of seizures (tonic/myoclonic seizures) as in this case. ASM substitution with valproate as a mixed function, broad spectrum, GABAergic ASM may lead to complete control of all seizures. Treatment options include valproate, lamotrigine, topiramate, zonisamide, stiripentol, and clobazam. No ASM may be appropriate in some cases. This stresses the importance of EEG and genetic assessment in the diagnosis and treatment of patients. One third of GEFS+ families tested have a pathogenic variant in a known GEFS+ gene [7]. Because our patient has GEF+ and a mutation of the sodium ion channel, sodium channel-blocking ASM should be avoided.

The prognosis is typically favorable with appropriate treatment and is dependent upon the individual severity of the phenotype. Remission may occur in early adolescence. However, if phenotypes are more characteristic of other epilepsy syndromes then generalized seizures are less likely to remit (i.e., juvenile myoclonic epilepsy, Doose syndrome, or focal epilepsy), and seizures may persist.

Pearls of Wisdom

1. Febrile seizures are the most common seizure disorder seen in early childhood and involve various and complex modes of inheritance with an overall likelihood of developing epilepsy that is <5%.
2. Complex FS are associated with hippocampal sclerosis and focal epilepsies, especially temporal lobe epilepsy. However, generalized seizures may also be associated with FS.
3. GEF+ is a hereditary generalized epilepsy syndrome associated with febrile seizures. It reflects an autosomal dominant mode of inheritance with a clinical course of persistent FS beyond age 6 years evolving into an afebrile heterogeneous group of generalized seizures.
4. Interictal epileptiform abnormalities on EEG may support the clinical diagnosis of a generalized epilepsy though serological testing for SCN1A, SCN1B, and GABRG2 may provide genetic confirmation of a GEFS+clinical diagnosis.
5. Treatment should avoid sodium channel-blocking agents that may aggravate seizures. The prognosis of GEFS+ is usually favorable with seizure control and the potential for spontaneous resolution in adolescence.

References

1. Schubert J, Siekierska A, Langlois M, May P, Huneau C, Becker F, et al. Mutations in STX1B, encoding a presynaptic protein, cause fever-associated epilepsy syndromes. Nat Genet. 2014;46:1327–32.
2. Scheffer I, Berkovic S. Generalized epilepsy with febrile seizures plus. A genetic disorder with heterogeneous clinical phenotypes. Brain. 1997;120(3):479–90.
3. Wallace RH, et al. Febrile seizures and generalized epilepsy associated with a mutation in the Na+-channel β1 subunit gene SCN1B. Nat Genet. 1998;19:366–70.
4. Singh R, Scheffer IE, Crossland K, et al. Generalized epilepsy with febrile seizure plus: a common childhood-onset genetic epilepsy syndrome. Ann Neurol. 1999;45:75–81.
5. Abou-Khalil B, Ge Q, Desai R, et al. Partial and generalized epilepsy with febrile seizures plus and a novel SCN1A mutation. Neurology. 2001;57:2265–72.
6. Berg AT, Berkovic SF, Brodie MJ, et al. Revised terminology and concepts for organization of seizures and epilepsies: report of the ILAE Commission on Classification and Terminology, 2005–2009. Epilepsia. 2010;51(4):676–85.
7. Zhang Y-H, Burgess R, Malone JP, Glubb GC, Helbig KL, Vadlamudi L, et al. Genetic epilepsy with febrile seizures plus: refining the spectrum. Neurology. 2017;89(12):1210–9.
8. https://www.ncbi.nlm.nih.gov/gtr/conditions/C1858672/. Accessed 28 June 2020.

Progressive Myoclonus Epilepsy

11

Katherine Nickels and William O. Tatum

A 15-year-old right-handed girl presented for second opinion of intermittent jerks of her arms upon wakening and while trying to write since age 12 years. At the time of her initial presentation, routine EEG demonstrated activation of generalized atypical spike-and-wave discharges, and she was diagnosed with juvenile myoclonic epilepsy. Valproic acid was initiated with resolution of myoclonic seizures. A single generalized tonic-clonic seizure occurred 2 years later in the setting of subtherapeutic valproic acid level. She experienced no cognitive regression and performed well in school. She notes some worsening of handwriting intermittently. She does not see any myoclonic jerks during that time. However, parents can feel subtle myoclonic jerks if they hold her arms.

Due to complaints of medication side effects from valproic acid, she was transitioned to zonisamide. Unfortunately, myoclonic and generalized tonic-clonic seizures returned. Zonisamide was then transitioned to extended release divalproex with resolution of seizures and without further side effects.

Subsequent EEGs have demonstrated mild to moderate slowing of the background with frequent activation of generalized atypical spike-and-wave discharges and a photoparoxysmal response. MRI brain with epilepsy protocol was normal.

Family history revealed consanguinity; parents were first cousins. Three older sisters had similar presentation as adolescents. Two of her sisters, 10 and 15 years older than the patient, subsequently developed gait difficulties due to frequent

K. Nickels (✉)
Mayo Clinic, Department of Neurology, Rochester, MN, USA
e-mail: Nickels.Katherine@mayo.edu

W. O. Tatum
Mayo Clinic, Department of Neurology, Jacksonville, FL, USA
e-mail: tatum.william@mayo.edu

myoclonus and ataxia and are now wheelchair bound. Both have experienced gradual cognitive decline. The third sister, 3 years older than the patient, has no cognitive or gait difficulties but has continued convulsive seizures.

Clinical Questions

1. Is this history consistent with genetic generalized epilepsy?
2. What etiologies must be excluded?
3. What is the likely etiology?
4. How should she be managed?
5. How will you counsel the family?

Discussion

1. While myoclonic epilepsy presenting in a cognitively normal adolescent is often related to juvenile myoclonic epilepsy, there are multiple concerning findings in this presentation which would suggest this more likely to be related to one of the progressive myoclonus epilepsies. Although she denies cognitive regression, increasing difficulties with handwriting with palpable subtle myoclonus is suggestive of ongoing and worsening myoclonic seizures causing progressive motor impairment. Second, persistent slowing of the background on EEG would suggest encephalopathic features and be inconsistent with juvenile myoclonic epilepsy. Most concerning, however, is the child's family history [1]. All three of her sisters presented similarly and are now more severe, consistent with a progressive epilepsy syndrome.
2. There are multiple progressive myoclonus epilepsy syndromes that present in adolescence. Her unaffected parents have multiple children with similar phenotypes, suggestive of autosomal recessive inheritance. Given that divalproex/valproic acid is commonly used to treat myoclonic seizures, it is essential to exclude mitochondrial disorders as an etiology because valproic acid will worsen the underlying mitochondrial disease and precipitate or worsen hepatic failure [1]. It is also important to remember that mitochondrial proteins encoded by nuclear DNA follow Mendelian genetics and so can also be inherited by autosomal recessive inheritance. Myoclonic epilepsy presenting in adolescence can be due to myoclonic epilepsy with ragged red fibers (MERRF), although these patients typically have multiple neurologic abnormalities not present in our patient [2]. Homozygous or compound heterozygous mutations in polymerase gamma (POLG) often present at a younger age with recurrent prolonged status epilepticus.
3. In addition to mitochondrial disorders, other causes of adolescent-onset progressive myoclonus epilepsy include Lafora disease, juvenile onset neuronal ceroid lipofuscinosis (Batten disease), Unverricht-Lundborg disease, and sialidosis [1]. Lafora disease is often associated with transitory blindness and hallucinations,

multiple generalized seizure types, and progresses to status epilepticus [2]. Juvenile onset neuronal ceroid lipofuscinosis also includes visual symptoms with decreased visual acuity. The dementia with these to syndromes progresses over 8–10 years, faster than what has been demonstrated in our patient's family [2]. Sialidosis Type 1 also presents with slowly progressive visual loss, but without mental deterioration [1, 2]. Our patient has no visual symptoms, and there have been cognitive changes in family members, making these three syndromes unlikely etiologies.

Unverricht-Lundborg disease (EPM1) occurs due to homozygous expansion mutation in the CSTB (cystatin B) gene [3]. It presents in early adolescence with myoclonus and generalized tonic-clonic seizures [1, 2]. The myoclonic jerks are worse upon awakening and can also be action-triggered or stimulus-sensitive, explaining why our patient's myoclonus worsened while trying to write [4]. Ataxia is common when the myoclonus is more intense [4]. The long-term outcome is variable, ranging from independence to a bed-ridden state. Neurocognitive decline can occur over years, but frank dementia would be atypical [1, 3]. The EEG shows generalized slowing (Fig. 11.1), generalized epileptiform discharges (Fig. 11.2), and a photoparoxysmal response (Fig. 11.3), similar to our patient [2, 5].

Indeed, genetic testing confirmed this as the diagnosis for our patient and her sisters.

4. There are no specific treatments for Unverricht-Lundborg disease, and management is symptomatic [1]. Antiseizure medications with efficacy for treating myoclonic seizures are commonly used, including valproic acid, levetiracetam, zonisamide, topiramate, and benzodiazepines [2, 4]. Piracetam at high doses has also been used [2, 4]. Briviteracetam and perampanel are newer potentially

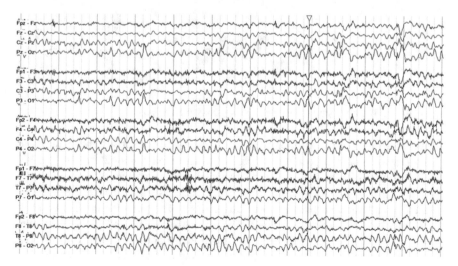

Fig. 11.1 Moderate degree of diffuse slowing of the background on routine EEG (posterior dominant rhythm 5–6 Hz, normal for age 8.5–13 Hz)

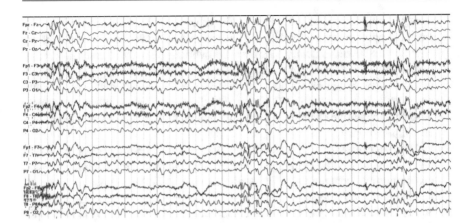

Fig. 11.2 Frequent activation of generalized atypical spike-and-wave discharges during wakefulness on routine EEG

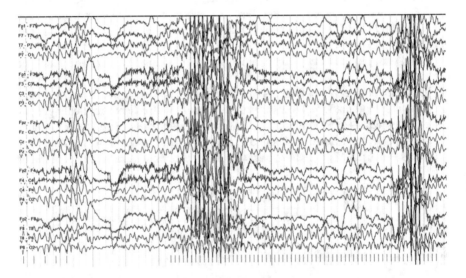

Fig. 11.3 EEG demonstrating generalized photoparoxysmal response

useful options. Patients often require polytherapy [4]. Antiseizure medications known to worsen myoclonus, such as carbamazepine, should be avoided [4]. Other comorbidities should also be managed with supportive care.

5. It is important that this family understands the inheritance pattern, progressive nature, and variable phenotype of this disease. The patient's unaffected older siblings may be carriers, and younger siblings may be affected but not yet symptomatic. From her older siblings, the family has a good understanding that this disease can progress over time. However, this child has been clinically sensitive to valproic acid and has experienced no decline. Due to the variable phenotype, it is not a guarantee that this child will ultimately be as impaired as her sisters. This can provide some hope for our patient.

Pearls of Wisdom

1. The progressive myoclonus epilepsies are a group of structural-metabolic epilepsies manifest as recurrent myoclonic jerks and generalized seizures caused by rare disorders, many of which have a genetic component and debilitating course with a poor outcome.
2. Progressive myoclonus epilepsies are characterized by myoclonic seizures, tonic-clonic seizures, and progressive neurological deterioration, often with cerebellar signs and cognitive deterioration.
3. When diagnosing generalized epilepsy in adolescents, it is important to identify potential features that would suggest a progressive or drug-resistant disease. These include persistent background slowing or generalized slow spike-and-wave on EEG, atypical features during the seizures (such as eyelid myoclonia or myoclonic jerks of the limbs during absence), cognitive decline, progressive motor impairment, cerebellar signs, and myoclonus that is resistant to the appropriate use of antiseizure medication.
4. If a progressive epilepsy syndrome is considered, identification of an underlying mitochondrial disorder is essential in order to avoid treatment with valproic acid. The Cystatin B gene is mutated and may be assayed from serum in patients with Unverricht-Lundborg disease. The presence of the EPM1 may be used to confirm the clinical suspicion.
5. This case stresses the importance of taking a family history which may reveal an inheritance pattern and uncover an autosomal recessive condition such as Unverricht-Lundborg disease. While her initial presentation was consistent with juvenile myoclonic epilepsy, this would be very unlikely with her family history and with neurological deterioration over time.

References

1. De Siqueira LF. Progressive myoclonic epilepsies: review of clinical, molecular and therapeutic aspects. J Neurol. 2020;257(10):1612–9.
2. Shahwan A, Farrell M, Delanty N. Progressive myoclonic epilepsies: a review of genetic and therapeutic aspects. Lancet Neurol. 2005;4(4):239–48.
3. Hypponen J, Aikia M, Joensuu T, Julkunen P, et al. Refining the phenotype of Unverricht-Lundborg disease (EPM1). Neurology. 2015;84:1529–36.
4. Genton P. Unverricht-Lundborg disease (EPM1). Epilepsia. 2010;51(Suppl. 1):37–9.
5. Gargouri-Berrechid A, Nasri A, Kacem I, Sidhom Y, et al. Long-term evolution of EEG in Unverricht-Lundborg disease. Clin Neurophysiol. 2016;46:119–24.

Autoimmune Epilepsies

12

Matthew Hoerth

Case Presentation

A 21-year-old right-handed Caucasian female who 2 months prior to presentation began to have worsening depressive symptoms and later developed nausea and headache. Just prior to presentating for evaluation, her family reported that she had recently been experiencing language difficulties, memory disturbances, as well as auditory hallucinations.

She presented for emergent evaluation because emergency medical personnel were notified after the patient had experienced a nocturnal generalized tonic-clonic seizure. During the first several days after admission, she was noted to be agitated with stereotyped episodes of stiffening and head jerking. She was recognized as potentially having seizures, and antiseizure medication (ASM) was initiated.

Despite this, the patient continued to have frequent seizures during the hospitalization which culminated into non-convulsive status epilepticus that was confirmed by continuous EEG monitoring. The patient was intubated and placed on continuous infusions of several ASMs. For days, multiple different combinations of ASMs were attempted, but she continued to remain in electrographic status epilepticus.

An MRI of the brain, routine laboratory, and urine drug screen were normal. She was healthy other than her present condition and was without any known risk factors for seizures. There was no exposure to drugs or toxins, as well as no sign of systemic or central nervous system infection. She ultimately underwent a lumbar puncture in an effort to determine the etiology for non-convulsive status epilepticus. The results are listed in Fig. 12.1.

M. Hoerth (✉)
Mayo Clinic, Department of Neurology, Phoenix, AZ, USA
e-mail: hoerth.matthew@mayo.edu

© Springer Nature Switzerland AG 2021
W. O. Tatum et al. (eds.), *Epilepsy Case Studies*,
https://doi.org/10.1007/978-3-030-59078-9_12

Fig. 12.1 Cerebrospinal
fluid profile obtained
during NCSE

CSF Fluid Analysis	Result
Appearance	Clear
Color	Colorless
Glucose	66
Protein	31
RBC	18.0 H
Nucleated Cells	16.5 H
Lymph	88% H
Mono	12% L
Oligoclonal Bands	10
IgG index	2.60 H
IgG/Albumin ratio	0.65 H
Synthesis Rate	24.90 H
Blastomyces Antibody	Neg
Cryptococcus Antigen	Neg
Histoplasma Antibody	Neg
VDRL	Neg
Lyme	Neg
West Nile Virus IgG, IgM	Neg
Enterovirus PCR	Neg
HIV Antibody Eval	Neg
Varicella Zoster Virus PCR	Neg
Herpes Simplex-1 PCR	Neg
Herpes Simplex-2 PCR	Neg
CMV PCR	Neg
Parovirus B19 PCR	Neg
Angiotensin Converting Enzyme	Neg
GAD65 Antibody	0.00
ANNA-1	Neg
ANNA-2	Neg
ANNA-3	Neg
Amphiphysin Antibody	Neg
CRMP-5	Neg
Neuronal VGKC Antibody	Neg
Thyroperoxidase Antibody	0.8 (nml <9 .0)
Purkinje Cell Antibody	Neg
Anti-NMDA Receptor Antibody	Positive

Clinical Questions

1. What is the clinical significance of the elevated antibody titer and other CSF results?
2. What neoplasms, if any, are associated with anti-NMDA receptor antibody positivity?

3. Are there any potential alternatives to ASMs for patients in prolonged status epilepticus?
4. Is there any role for immunosuppressant medications in anti-NMDA receptor antibody positivity?
5. What is the prognosis for patients with anti-NMDA receptor antibody encephalitis?

Discussion Points

1. The presence of the anti-N-methyl-D-aspartate (NMDA) receptor antibody solidifies a diagnosis of autoimmune limbic encephalitis. Although multiple different autoantibodies have been implicated in refractory status epilepticus, the anti-NMDA receptor antibody was first reported in 2007 [1]. This cell surface antibody has been postulated to target epitopes on NMDA receptors located in the forebrain and hippocampus. This leads to the development of dyskinesias, autonomic instability, and seizures (often status epilepticus). Prodromal symptoms of headache, low-grade fever, and psychiatric symptoms (anxiety, agitation, hallucinations, paranoia) are often seen and should prompt clinicians to an autoimmune evaluation. The lymphocytic pleocytosis seen in this patient is often found in association with anti-NMDA receptor positivity; however oligoclonal bands are only seen in a minority [1]. Without the positivity of these antibodies, empiric autoimmune treatment could be tried, but aggressive immunosuppression in a critically ill patient would be empiric and risky.
2. Anti-NMDA receptor encephalitis is seen predominantly in females, although not exclusively. Tumors are seen in about half of all patients. Almost all of them have been identified to be reproductive organ tumors (ovarian teratoma and teratoma of the testis), but small-cell lung cancer has also been reported. If a tumor is discovered, resection is the treatment of choice. This can reduce the antibody production and, in turn, the patient's symptoms. Persistence in searching for teratoma is required. It has been reported that not all ovarian teratomas are radiologically evident, and exploratory laparoscopy has been required in some patients [1]. Despite thorough investigation, no tumor was found in this patient.
3. Traditional ASMs are the mainstay for the initial treatment of status epilepticus. When status epilepticus is refractory to multiple ASMs other alternatives should be considered. In this patient, the ketogenic diet was utilized with some degree of success in reducing the dosages of the continuous infusions of ASMs. There are a limited number of case reports describing the use of the ketogenic diet in refractory status epilepticus. In many cases, it has been shown beneficial [2]. Obviously, care should be taken when altering the metabolism in a critically ill patient. In addition to the ketogenic diet, electroconvulsive therapy, and vagus nerve stimulation have been suggested to have beneficial effects in some cases.
4. The potential benefit of immune-modulating therapy is to eliminate the autoantibodies that are operational in producing seizures and status epilepticus.

Initiating treatment involves a costly evaluation and treatment for autoimmune causes. There is yet to be established appropriate guidelines; however suggestions for treatment algorithms have been suggested when considering treatment of autoimmune limbic encephalitis [3–5]. Without an identified tumor, first-line immunotherapy can consist of corticosteroids (usually high dose), intravenous immunoglobulin (IVIg), plasma exchange, or a combination. If these first-line methods are unsuccessful, then rituximab or cyclophosphamide is then considered. It should be noted that relapses can occur in 20–25% of patients, with consideration of repeat immune therapies or longer-term immunosuppression being suggested by some.

5. The prognosis in prolonged refractory status epilepticus is typically poor. It has been suggested in animal models that the anti-NMDA receptor antibodies can cause neuronal dysfunction via inflammation. However, they cause less neuronal damage than other antibodies that may be found to produce autoimmune limbic encephalitis. In the original 100 patients described, 47 were noted to make a full recovery, and 28 people recovered with mild stable neurological deficits [1]. This was despite a median length of hospitalization of 2.5 months. Early tumor identification and removal were found to be predictive of a better outcome [3]. Although when screening for tumors, a comprehensive screen is suggested. However, specific antibodies suggest a higher likelihood for certain tumor types [4]. A list of antibodies associated with tumors is noted in Table 12.1. It should be noted that cases without an identified antibody does not exclude the possibility of an autoimmune etiology. It has been suggested that

Table 12.1 Tumors associated with certain antibodies

Antibody	Tumor
ANNA-1	Small-cell lung
Ma1	Breast, colon, testicular
Ma2	Testicular
Amphiphysin	Small-cell lung, breast
GAD65	Thymoma, renal cell, breast, colon
LGI1, Caspr2	Small-cell lung, thymoma, breast, prostate
NMDA receptor	Ovarian teratoma, testicular germinoma, neuroblastoma
AMPA receptor	Thymoma, lung, breast
GABA-B receptor	Small-cell lung, neuroendocrine
mGluR5 receptor	Hodgkin lymphoma
gAChR	Adenocarcinoma, thymoma, small-cell lung

ANNA-1 antineuronal nuclear antibody type 1, *GAD65* glutamic acid decarboxylase 65, *LGI1* leucine-rich glioma inactivated protein I, *Caspr2* contactin-associated protein-like 2, *NMDA,* N-methyl-D-aspartate, *AMPA* α-amino-3-hydroxy-5-methyl-4-isoxazolepropionic acid, *GABA-B* γ-aminobutyric acid-B, *mGluR5* metabotropic glutamate receptor 5, *gAChR* neuronal ganglionic nicotinic acetylcholine receptor

with a clinical suspicion of autoimmune encephalitis, empiric therapy with immune suppressive medications can be trailed in those who no other etiology is identified [5].

Pearls

1. The ability to identify specific antibodies in autoimmune limbic encephalitis is helpful in the evaluation of refractory status epilepticus. This opens opportunities for immune therapies in the treatment of status epilepticus.
2. When status epilepticus is refractory or super-refractory, then consideration of other treatment modalities, other than ASM should be considered. The ketogenic diet and other non-medication approaches may show some beneficial effect.
3. Aside from ASMs, immune-modulating therapies should be considered if a case of autoimmune limbic encephalitis is identified. In many cases, success in patient outcome is a result of having a high clinical suspicion and the willingness to consider other therapies besides standard ASM.
4. Immune therapies that should be considered for autoimmune-mediated encephalitis/epilepsy could include IVIg, plasmapheresis, or high-dose intravenous steroids.
5. For cases of antibody identified autoimmune encephalitis, an evaluation to search for an underlying tumor should be undertaken. Even in cases that an antibody is not identified, with a high enough suspicion, tumor evaluation could be considered.

References

1. Guasp M, Dalmau J. Encephalitis associated with antibodies against the NMDA receptor. Encefalitis por anticuerpos contra el receptor de NMDA. Med Clin (Barc). 2018;151(2):71–9. https://doi.org/10.1016/j.medcli.2017.10.015.
2. Nam SH, Lee BL, Lee CG, Yu HJ, Joo EY, Lee J, Lee M. The role of ketogenic diet in the treatment of refractory status epilepticus. Epilepsia. 2011;52(11):e181–4.
3. Wang H. Efficacies of treatments for anti-NMDA receptor encephalitis. Front Biosci (Landmark Ed). 2016;21:651–63. Published 2016 Jan 1. https://doi.org/10.2741/4412.
4. Toledano M, Pittock SJ. Autoimmune epilepsy. Semin Neurol. 2015;35(3):245–58. https://doi.org/10.1055/s-0035-1552625.
5. Dubey D, Singh J, Britton JW, et al. Predictive models in the diagnosis and treatment of autoimmune epilepsy. Epilepsia. 2017;58(7):1181–9. https://doi.org/10.1111/epi.13797.

Electroclinical Localization and Treatment

13

William O. Tatum

A 21-year-old right-handed female had drug-resistant epilepsy. She had failed several anti-seizure medications (ASM) as single agents due to poor tolerability and had been maintained on oxcarbazepine for years. She was otherwise born via an uncomplicated delivery and was without any known risk factors for epilepsy. Seizure onset began at 9 years of age manifest as "petit mal" seizures. These occurred weekly and were worse after she started her menstrual period at menarche occurring with monthly frequency around the time of menses. She was initially begun on ethosuximide after an EEG demonstrated "petit mal seizure discharges" though had incomplete improvement in her episodic staring spells. Subsequently "grand mal" seizures developed within the year following puberty, and she was changed to valproate. She continued with intermittent "grand mal" and rare "petit mal" seizures recurring monthly despite failing six trials of ASM she was maintained on lacosamide 600 mg/day. TPM and LEV lead to side effects of "memory problems" and severe anxiety. She was disabled by frequent seizures and was unable to attend college. She was seen for another opinion. Seizures began without a warning; she would turn her head slightly to the right, have impaired consciousness and ability to respond, and then evolve to a generalized tonic-clonic seizure (GTC). Her neurological examination was normal. A high-resolution 3-T brain MRI with an epilepsy protocol was normal. EEG demonstrated single complexes and brief bursts of 3-Hz generalized spike-and-wave discharges (Fig. 13.1).

After initial discussion, she was admitted to the epilepsy monitoring unit for classification of seizures. Intermittent left lateralization was present for three typical seizures with ictal EEG demonstrating bilateral irregular spike-and-wave at onset and clear left lateralization after 30 s in one of the thred seizures. Head version to

W. O. Tatum (✉)
Mayo Clinic, Department of Neurology, Jacksonville, FL, USA
e-mail: tatum.william@mayo.edu

© Springer Nature Switzerland AG 2021
W. O. Tatum et al. (eds.), *Epilepsy Case Studies*,
https://doi.org/10.1007/978-3-030-59078-9_13

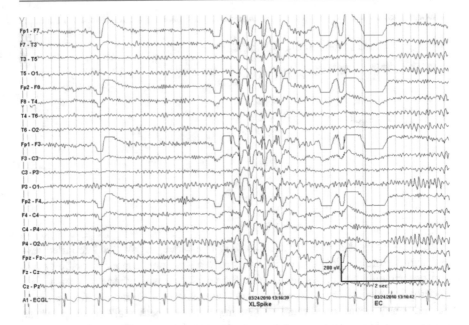

Fig. 13.1 Interictal EEG demonstrating a 1-s burst of irregular generalized anterior predominant bilateral 3-Hz generalized spike-and-wave discharge. EEG: longitudinal bipolar montage, sensitivity 7 uv, filters 1–70 Hz

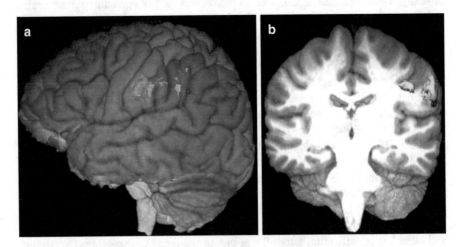

Fig. 13.2 FDG-PET co-registered to MRI (**a**) sagittal image and (**b**) coronal image. Note the left central-parietal region of hypometabolism. (Images courtesy of Dr. Ed Faught)

the right occurred prior to recording two focal to bilateral tonic-clonic seizures. Focal epilepsy was diagnosed and an epilepsy surgery evaluation requested by the patient. A subsequent FDG PET scan demonstrated left parietal hypometabolism (Fig. 13.2). Magnetoencephalography revealed a left superior-posterior temporal

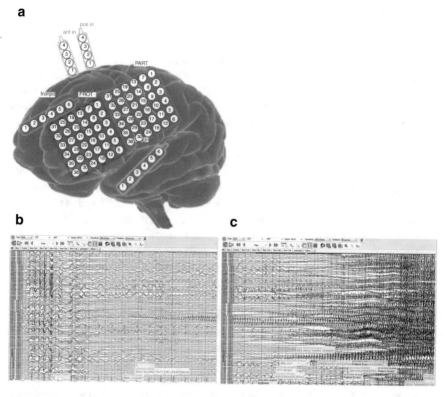

Fig. 13.3 Invasive EEG array (**a**) depicted by intracranial electrodes and (**b**) seizure onset and (**c**) seizure propagated pattern. Despite the 3-Hz generalized spike-and-wave interictal epileptiform abnormalities, a focal onset was present on invasive EEG recording

dipole cluster. She subsequently underwent left craniotomy with broad placement of subdural grids and strip electrodes over the left hemisphere. Seizure onset was focal in seizure #3 (Fig. 13.3), and electrocortical brain stimulation for functional mapping was performed. Her site of seizure onset was identified at the electrode site of onset and surrounding area within the primary sensory-motor strip. She was implanted with the responsive neurostimulator but it was without benefit.

Clinical Questions

1. Does the electroclinical localization in this patient suggest "petit mal" seizures?
2. How do the ancillary tests help classify the staring spells in this patient?
3. What type (classification) of epilepsy does this patient have?
4. What if the best approach to treatment?
5. Can patients have both focal and generalized seizures?

Diagnostic Discussion

1. This patient does not have true "petit mal" (aka absence seizures) [1]. Episodes of staring may be differentiated by a sudden stare for 10–15 s in absence, while focal seizures with impaired consciousness (focal impaired awareness seizures) typically last 30–40 s and may manifest with a warning (focal aware seizure or aura) at seizure onset. Distinctions may blur the dichotomy between focal and generalized seizure semiology [2]. Lateralizing signs and localizing signs carry diagnostic implications for focal epilepsy though may also occur in patients with generalized epilepsies. True absence seizures begin and end abruptly, while focal impaired awareness seizures usually exhibit postictal disorientation and lethargy. Our patient had focal seizures suspected clinically that was supported by PET scan and confirmed by video-EEG monitoring. Many patients refer to staring episodes as "petit mal," yet this misapplication of terminology reflects only the non-convulsive nature of the events often used by patients and not precise classification by epilepsy clinicians.

2. The interictal EEG demonstrated 3-Hz generalized spike-and-waves (GSW) which normally suggests a genetic generalized epilepsy though subtle asymmetries are common. Generalized interictal epileptiform discharges (IEDs) may occur in patients such as ours due to secondary bilateral synchrony in the EEG. Another possibility is that generalized spike-and-waves in the interictal EEG occurred as a concomitant inherited trait without the phenotype involving clinical seizures. However, GSW as an incidental finding is present in a small minority of patients and therefore is a highly specific marker for epilepsy. A generalized EEG pattern may be seen in patients with extratemporal epilepsies due to rapid propagation of epileptiform activity through the corpus callosum to diffusely affect both hemispheres. There may be a "lead in" to generalized discharges that appear, and the generalized spikes (or polyspikes) usually have a repetition rate of <3 Hz when secondary bilateral synchronous discharges occurs from a focal seizure. In this case, focal and lateralized epileptiform activity was present on invasive EEG supporting classification of the epilepsy syndrome as focal epilepsy in this case.

3. This patient has focal epilepsy manifest as brief focal impaired awareness seizures and predominantly focal to bilateral tonic-clonic seizures. Semiological classification systems have been designed to identify seizure onset, symptoms due to propagated patterns, and seizure offset [3]. Focal seizures that evolve to convulsions may be rapid and therefore difficult to classify and localize with standard EEG in patients with focal epilepsy. In addition, lateralized semiology and EEG features may occur in patients with generalized seizures associated with genetic generalized epilepsy (i.e., JME) in up to 50% of people. Terminology and concepts for re-organization of the epilepsies were recently performed to identify seizures that are focal, generalized seizures, and unknown relative to seizure onset [1]. Overlap between generalized and focal seizures may rarely occur. The "petit mal" (absence) reported by the patient, especially

with a 3-Hz GSW pattern on EEG in a patient with additional convulsions suggests one of the genetic generalized epilepsies. However, our patient had semiology, PET, and secondary bilateral synchrony on the EEG later proven to have a focal onset on invasive EEG.

4. Treatment is predicated upon proper seizure and epilepsy classification. Narrow-spectrum ASM such as carbamazepine and phenytoin may aggravate seizure control or worsen some generalized seizure types (absence and myoclonic seizures) [4]. Similarly, some ASM for generalized seizures (ethosuximide) may be ineffective for the treatment of focal seizures. EEG is fundamental to seizure classification when semiology is unclear such as those with staring episodes and convulsions. Even EEG may be challenging when a lack of defining interictal epileptiform discharges or secondary bilateral synchronous epileptiform discharges is present. Brain MRI may reveal a focal lesion that supports the localization for seizure onset and guide ASM selection. Most ASM are available for treatment of focal seizures. Following the failure of two appropriate ASM for the appropriate seizure type (in this case broad spectrum ASM was not effective), used for an adequate time period portends drug-resistance with substitution or addition of alternative agents that carries a low yield of success. When ASM fails, epilepsy surgery should be considered. In this case because of seizure onset overlapping functional (aka eloquent) cortex, neuromodulation was attempted albeit without benefit.

5. The International League Against Epilepsy (ILAE) Classification of the Epilepsies has been updated to reflect our gain in understanding of the epilepsies and their mechanisms following major scientific advances that have taken place recently [5]. Classification of seizures was revised to categories of focal, generalized, and unknown onset with further subdivisions based on their motor versus nonmotor characteristics. Epilepsy syndromes consist of specific constellations of similar semiologies, EEG abnormalities, etiologies, and comorbidities. The epilepsies were also reclassified as focal, generalized, combined generalized and focal, or unknown in type. However, patients may also have both generalized and focal seizure types. This is common in patients with mixed seizure disorders (i.e., Lennox-Gastaut syndrome and Dravet syndrome). They may also have interictal EEG findings that are focal, generalized or multi-focal accompanying either or both seizure types. Unknown seizure onset is used to identify people with epilepsy, but it is not possible to denote the precise classification of the epilepsy syndrome. This results when there is insufficient information or discordant information. Typically, this occurs when the semiology, MRI brain, EEG, and ancillary information is normal or uninformative. In our patient the GSW on scalp EEG was in striking contrast to the focal onset identified on invasive EEG. This illustrates the point that significant variation may exist from what is present on scalp EEG and what actually exists when invasive EEG (electrocorticography) is performed. Current classification systems are a framework and are not designed to reflect overlap or a spectrum of the epilepsies as seen in this patient.

Pearls of Wisdom

1. In adults who report "petit mal" and "grand mal" seizures beginning after adolescence, it is important to consider lay terminology. When used, these terms may potentially reflect a focal epilepsy with focal seizures with/ without impaired awareness and focal to bilateral tonic-clonic seizures instead of generalized seizure types.

2. EEG is the most useful test when the brain MRI is normal or non-specific. When clear focal or generalized interictal epileptiform discharges are present, this supports the electroclinical diagnosis of epilepsy and supports a generalized or focal mechanism for the recurrent seizures. However, an EEG with secondary bilateral synchrony in patients with extratemporal focal epilepsy may be difficult to differentiate from epileptiform discharges associated with the generalized epilepsies.

3. Broad-spectrum anti-seizure medication is useful for treatment of patients when the classification of the seizures and epilepsy type is unknown. These agents are effective for both focal and generalized seizures and do not aggravate a specific seizure type.

4. Drug resistance is a definable entity and a pre-requisite to disabled patients who may be amenable to undergo an epilepsy surgery evaluation. Even when a patient is motivated and the surgical target is identifiable, the lesion may reside in eloquent cortex that precludes surgery due to the risk of incurring a neurological deficit despite potentially achieving seizure freedom.

5. Electroclinical localization to classify seizures reflects an epilepsy diagnosis and etiology and directs therapy for the patient's specific disease. Generalized IEDs may occur from an extemporal source in patients with focal epilepsies and may reflect focal or widespread epileptogenicity.

References

1. Berg AT, Berkovic SF, Brodie MJ, Buchhalter J, Cross JH, van Emde BW, Engel J, French J, Glauser TA, Mathern GW, Moshe SL, Nordli D, Plouin P, Scheffer IE. Revised terminology and concepts for organization of seizures and epilepsies: report of the ILAE Commission on Classification and Terminology, 2005–2009. Epilepsia. 2010;51:676–85.

2. Fisher RS, Cross JH, French JA, et al. Operational classification of seizure types by the International League against epilepsy: position paper of the ILAE Commission for Classification and Terminology. Epilepsia. 2017;58:522–30.

3. Luders HO, Acharya J, Caumgartner C, et al. Semiological seizure classification. Epilepsia. 1998;39(9):1006–13.

4. Brodie MJ, Dichter MA. Antiepileptic drugs. N Engl J Med. 1996;334:168–75.

5. Scheffer IE, Berkovic S, Capovilla G, et al. ILAE classification of the epilepsies: position paper of the ILAE Commission for Classification and Terminology. Epilepsia. 2017;58(4):512–21.

Brain Tumor-Related Epilepsy

14

Anteneh M. Feyissa

Case Presentation

A previously healthy 36-year-old right-handed man presented with a 4-week history of dizziness upon waking in the morning. On the morning of his presentation, he also had intermittent brief twitching involving his right arm and hand. An avid guitar player, he noticed difficulty playing simple songs with his guitar for 1 week.

Head CT was unremarkable but a brain MRI disclosed an infiltrative non-enhancing lesion in the left posterior-superior frontal sulcus (Fig. 14.1a, b). An EEG was unrevealing, but he was placed on oral levetiracetam, given the concern for focal aware motor seizures. Functional MRI showed strong left hemispheric dominance for language and revealed right-hand motor cortex was located posterior and lateral to the left frontal tumor (Fig. 14.1c). During neuropsychological testing, the patient was able to play various songs with his guitar without difficulty.

A week later, the patient underwent left-sided supratentorial awake craniotomy for tumor resection and motor mapping. Intraoperative direct cortical electrical stimulation (DCES) assisted with electrocorticography (ECoG) using a customized 22-contact circular grid identified the right-hand motor cortex abutting the left frontal tumor. DCES also induced brief focal motor seizures involving the right hand (Fig. 14.1d). During DCES and throughout the tumor resection, the patient was tasked to play different songs with his guitar. Given the findings of DCES, he underwent subtotal resection of the left superior frontal tumor, sparing the right-hand motor cortex. Pathology revealed diffuse astrocytoma with tumor cells exhibiting diffuse and strong isocitrate dehydrogenase-1 (IDH1) positivity (Fig. 14.1e).

A. M. Feyissa (✉)
Mayo Clinic, Department of Neurology, Jacksonville, FL, USA
e-mail: Feyissa.Anteneh@mayo.edu

© Springer Nature Switzerland AG 2021
W. O. Tatum et al. (eds.), *Epilepsy Case Studies*,
https://doi.org/10.1007/978-3-030-59078-9_14

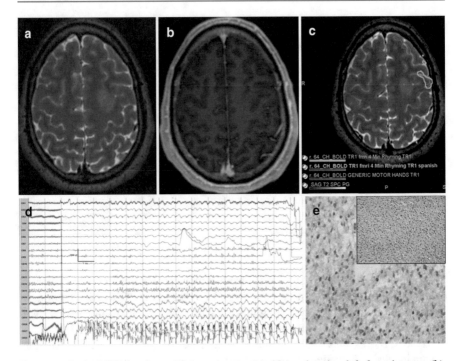

Fig. 14.1 Brain MRI showing a T2 hyperintense (**a**). Non-enhancing left frontal tumor (**b**). Functional MRI showing the hand motor area posteriorolateral to the left frontal tumor (**c**). Intraoperative ECoG recording using a 22-contact circular grid captured stimulation-induced focal seizure in contacts overlying the posterior margins of the left frontal tumor (**d**). Photomicrographs showing diffuse astrocytoma (HE, ×20) [black box] with tumor cells exhibiting diffuse and strong IDH1-R132H positivity (immunohistochemistry, ×20) (**e**)

Clinical Questions

1. How common is brain tumor-related epilepsy (BTRE)?
2. What is the mechanism of epileptogenesis in BTRE?
3. What are the risk factors for BTRE?
4. What is the role of intraoperative electrocorticography during brain tumor surgeries?
5. What is the long-term clinical outcome of BTRE?

Discussion

1. Epileptic seizures often develop in patients with primary (and metastatic) brain tumors (40–70%), and approximately 30% are drug-resistant [1]. Brain tumor-related epilepsy (BTRE) is characterized by symptomatic seizures manifesting as focal aware or focal impaired awareness and focal to bilateral tonic-clonic

seizures. Increased seizure burden and drug-resistant seizures affect quality of life, causes cognitive deterioration, and imparts significant morbidity in this patient population [1].

2. The exact mechanism of BTRE remains poorly understood but appears to be multifactorial. Disturbances at the cellular level, including alterations in synaptic and neuronal function, connectivity, and excitotoxicity, are proposed mechanisms that have recently gained traction [2]. Among these, glutamate-induced excitotoxicity and disruption of intracellular communication have garnered the most attention for patients with primary brain tumors (i.e., glioma) [3].

3. The incidence of seizures is lower in high-grade brain tumors such as glioblastoma multiforme and primary CNS lymphoma and higher in low-grade tumors [2–4]. The probability of developing epilepsy ranges from 10% in primary lymphomas to nearly 100% in patients with dysembryoplastic neuroepithelial tumors (DNETs). Seizures also occur more commonly in patients with tumors located in cortical regions as opposed to subcortical areas, highest in tumors located in the frontal peri-rolandic and temporo-insular regions [4]. However, recent studies suggest that epileptogenesis may be more associated with tumor molecular genetic markers than tumor grade or location. For example, tumors with an IDH1 mutation are more likely to cause seizures than IDH1 wild-type tumors [1–3].

4. Intraoperative electrocorticography (iECoG) is widely utilized for electrical mapping of the epileptogenic zone and eloquent cortex during or before brain tumor surgeries [5]. Intraoperative cortical mapping requires a high level of patient cooperation; hence, it is generally performed on awake patients under local anesthesia (awake craniotomy). The primary role of iECoG during DCES is to confirm the absence of after-discharges since their absence is necessary to validate the results of the functional cortical mapping. iECoG may also help identify and delineate the cortex with epileptic activity, although this remains controversial. However, iECoG may help recognize electrographic or subtle clinical seizures that may not otherwise be recognized [5].

5. Management of BTRE requires a multidisciplinary approach involving the use of anti-seizure medications (ASMs), surgical resection aided by iECoG, and adjuvant chemoradiation. The introduction of an ASM should be made after a first clinical seizure due to the lesional etiology and high likelihood of recurrence [1]. Prophylactic or perioperative ASMs are not generally recommended regardless of tumor type. The choice of ASM is typically based on several individual patient characteristics, including age, sex, weight, seizure type, and comorbidities. There is a general agreement to avoid enzyme-inducing ASMs (e.g., phenytoin, carbamazepine, and phenobarbital) despite their good anticonvulsant efficacy, as they can alter the pharmacokinetics of anti-neoplastic agents [1]. Valproate and levetiracetam are generally favored given their potential to influence seizures and primary brain tumor biology [1]. Brain tumor surgery aims not only to improve survival through reduction of tumor burden but also by achieving seizure freedom. Gross-total tumor resection, including the peritumoral epileptogenic foci, provides the highest chance of seizure freedom and reduced ASM requirement.

Clinical Pearls

1. BTRE is characterized by recurrent symptomatic seizures due to the presence of a brain tumor. Increased seizure burden and drug-resistant seizures in patients with BTRE affect the quality of life, causes cognitive deterioration, and significant morbidity.
2. The exact mechanism of BTRE remains poorly understood but appears to be multifactorial.
3. The incidence of seizure is higher in patients with slow-growing tumors than rapidly growing tumors and tumors located in the frontal peri-rolandic and temporo-insular regions. Recent studies suggest epileptogenesis is more associated with tumor molecular genetic markers than tumor grade or location.
4. The primary role of iECoG during brain tumor surgery is to confirm the absence of after-discharges during DCES. iECoG may also identify the epileptogenic zone and guide the surgical strategy in some patients to improve postoperative seizure control.
5. Management of BTRE involves the use of ASMs, surgery aided by iECoG, and adjuvant chemoradiation. Gross-total resection aims not only to improve survival through reduction of tumor burden but also by achieving seizure freedom.

References

1. Goldstein ED, Feyissa AM. Brain tumor related-epilepsy. Neurol Neurochir Pol. 2018;52(4):436–47.
2. Tatum WO 4th, Quinones-Hinojosa A. Onco-epilepsy: more than tumor and seizures. Mayo Clin Proc. 2018;93(9):1181–4.
3. Huberfeld G, Vecht CJ. Seizures and gliomas – towards a single therapeutic approach. Nat Rev. 2016;12:204–16.
4. Englot DJ, Berger MS, Barbaro NM, Chang EF. Factors associated with seizure freedom in the surgical resection of glioneuronal tumors. Epilepsia. 2012;53(1):51–7.
5. Yao P, Zheng S, Wang F, Kang DZ, Lin YX. Surgery guided with intraoperative electrocorticography in patients with low-grade glioma and refractory seizures. J Neurosurg. 2018;128:840–5.

Head Trauma and Seizures

Gregory D. Cascino

Case Presentation

A 32-year-old man who is a self-employed welder had a severe traumatic brain injury following a motor vehicle accident. The patient was unresponsive at the time of initial presentation in a local emergency department and required intubation for airway protection. A CT head was performed shortly after admission and revealed multiple intracerebral hematomas, maximal in the left frontal lobe (Fig. 15.1). The neurological examination at the time of admission showed the patient to be unresponsive with preservation of pupillary and brainstem reflexes. There were no definite focal neurological signs. Within 24 h after admission, the patient had a 3–5 min tonic-clonic seizure. Initially, he had a focal motor seizure involving the right upper extremity that evolved into a bilaterally convulsive tonic-clonic seizure. He received intravenous lorazepam and intravenous levetiracetam as an acute antiseizure treatment. He was then placed on maintenance levetiracetam and remained seizure-free during the hospital stay. The traumatic brain injury did not require any neurosurgical intervention. Physical therapy and rehabilitation were conducted in hospital over 4–6 weeks. At the time of dismissal from hospital to home, the patient was awake and alert and had no focal neurological findings on examination. He did complain of "short-term memory loss" and "irritability." The patient was discharged on levetiracetam 1500 mg twice daily and was cautioned "for now" not to operate a motor vehicle or return to work. A follow-up appointment to be seen in the neurology clinic was scheduled to occur in 1–3 months.

EEG studies in hospital were performed. The initial EEG 24 h following the seizure showed diffuse intermixed delta slowing and multifocal sharp wave discharges, maximal left frontal. An EEG performed 3 weeks later revealed mild and intermittent diffuse theta slowing without epileptiform discharges. CT head prior to

G. D. Cascino (✉)
Mayo Clinic, Department of Neurology, Rochester, MN, USA
e-mail: gcascino@mayo.edu

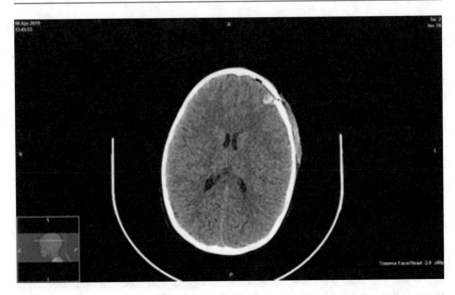

Fig. 15.1 Head CT showing traumatic brain injury associated with a left frontal skull fracture and small cortical intraparenchymal hemorrhage

dismissal showed the expected reduction in the size of the intracranial hemorrhages consistent with prior head trauma.

The patient returned to the neurology clinic 2 months after dismissal. He remained seizure-free but noted cognitive impairment and adverse mood changes. There had been no other new neurological problems. The patient has two questions when seen: How long do I have to take the levetiracetam? When can I drive and go back to work?

Clinical Questions

1. Does this patient have PTE?
2. Is there an indication for long-term antiseizure medication (ASM)?
3. What is the likelihood of seizure recurrence with withdrawal of ASM?
4. Should the patient's ASM be changed because of potential side-effects of "irritability"?
5. Should this patient be permitted to drive and work?

Diagnostic Discussion

1. This patient had an acute symptomatic or post-traumatic seizure that occurred 24 h following a traumatic brain injury. This would not indicate he has PTE or a seizure disorder [1–3]. The single seizure may relate to the severity of his head injury. The acute medical treatment with ASM was appropriate. The presence of

a post-traumatic seizure is a risk factor for the development of PTE [3]. The prolonged seizure may be life-threatening and warranted effective therapeutic intervention.

2. It is difficult to know with medical certainty the long-term outcome following an acute symptomatic seizure related to a traumatic brain injury. The severity of the post-traumatic seizure and the risk of a second seizure may be sufficiently high to warranted initial medical therapy [2]. The factors predictive of seizure recurrence in this patient may include the CT head-identified changes with intracerebral hemorrhages, the focal onset seizure, the abnormal EEG study with epileptiform discharges, and the prolonged seizure duration. Not uncommonly, patients are "observed" on ASM for a "period of time" prior to considering medication withdrawal. There is little evidence to support the extended long-term use of ASM after an early post-traumatic seizure as medical therapy may not preclude the occurrence of PTE [2].

3. The risk of further seizure activity at present is unclear. It has been approximately 3–4 months since his head injury and single seizure episode. PTE may develop weeks to months to years after the head trauma [3, 4]. The majority of patients will have the onset of PTE within 1–2 years [4]. It would be reasonable to obtain a levetiracetam trough level to see if the patient is compliant with his ASM. A standard EEG with standard activating procedures should be performed if there is a consideration withdrawing ASM to assess recurrence risk and the presence or absence of epileptiform discharges.

4. The two main complaints at present include memory deficits and "irritability." The etiology of the mood disorder could be multifactorial including the head trauma, use of levetiracetam, as well as the psychosocial problems that could result from an inability to drive and work. It may be appropriate to consider neuropsychological studies remote from the head injury to see if the patient has a neurocognitive disorder. The complaint of "memory loss" is not specific and can be a presenting symptom of depression or mood disorder. If the patient has evidence for a neurocognitive impairment following a head injury, an MRI head study should also be performed. This would assist in imaging the medial temporal lobe regions. A mood disorder consult with psychiatry should be considered if the symptoms are significant. Interviews with family members may be helpful. A multidisciplinary "brain rehabilitation" program may be appropriate to evaluate this patient who had a severe traumatic brain injury and has neurocognitive complaints [5]. Importantly, irritability can be a treatment-emergent adverse effect of levetiracetam. If an ASD is considered necessary, then a change in ASM should be considered if the judgement after the above evaluation is that he is experiencing levetiracetam-induced mood changes. An alternative ASM such as lamotrigine or oxcarbazepine could be considered if ASM is to be continued.

5. The patient will need to comply with the driving laws specific for his individual state. Driving laws are sufficiently variable from one state to the next so that no one answer is uniform to encompass all of them. The patient's cognitive issues should also be considered when evaluating the ability to operate a motor vehicle. There are no occupational laws regarding the patient's employment as a welder. The neurological examination may abnormalities that assist in determining the safety of his occupation.

Clinical Pearls

1. Post-traumatic seizures may occur following head trauma. These may be "early," within a few hours of the injury, and often represent focal to bilateral tonic-clonic seizures.
2. ASMs are appropriate in the management of post-traumatic seizures. Unfortunately, medical therapy using currently available ASM does not preclude the onset of PTE.
3. The important risk factors in that predict development of PTE include the severity of the traumatic brain injury and the presence of post-traumatic seizures.
4. PTE may develop remote from the acute head trauma and require evaluation and management with ASM.
5. Multidisciplinary care of patients with severe head trauma is often required because of the significant neurocognitive and psychosocial issues that may be present.

References

1. Ritter AC, Wagner AK, Fabio A, et al. Incidence and risk factors of posttraumatic seizures following traumatic brain injury: a traumatic brain injury model systems study. Epilepsia. 2016;57:1968.
2. Temkin NR. Risk factors for posttraumatic seizures in adults. Epilepsia. 2003;44(Suppl 10):18.
3. Chang BS, Lowenstein DH, Quality Standards Subcommittee of the American Academy of Neurology. Practice parameter: antiepileptic drug prophylaxis in severe traumatic brain injury: report of the quality standards subcommittee of the American Academy of Neurology. Neurology. 2003;60:10.
4. Annegers JF, Hauser WA, Coan SP, Rocca WA. A population-based study of seizures after traumatic brain injuries. N Engl J Med. 1998;338:20.
5. Wilson CD, Burks JD, Rodgers RB, Evans RM, Bakare AA, Safavi-Abbasi S. Early and late posttraumatic epilepsy in the setting of traumatic brain injury: a meta-analysis and review of antiepileptic management. World Neurosurg. 2018;110:e901–6.

First Seizure and Epilepsy

16

William O. Tatum

Case Presentation

A 32-year-old man presented for evaluation after his first unprovoked seizure. The seizure was described as "grand mal" by his wife and occurred while they were sleeping at night approximately 5:30 a.m. His wife awoke when she felt jerking movement in the bed. She estimated the seizure duration was about 5 min though admitted that she was afraid and that her estimate was unreliable. She immediately called 911. When she turned on the light following the seizure, she found that the patient was struggling to breath though gradually recovered awareness of his environment. There was blood on his pillow and evidence that he had bitten the left side of his tongue. He did not have a history of seizures or predisposing neurological conditions or comorbidity that would have increased his likelihood of experiencing a seizure. The only possible risk factor to experience a seizure was a mild concussion that he sustained when he was playing sports in high school. In addition, there was a cousin with seizures though they also had a "drug problem." The patient was taking no medication at the time of the seizure. He was married with two children, worked for a business manufacturing office equipment, drank alcohol socially on the weekend, had no recent foreign travel or exposures, denied illicit drug use, and drove down the street to work every day. Upon evaluation in the emergency department, he was post-ictal with a left posterior-lateral tongue laceration. His general and neurological examination were within normal limits without focal findings. A CT of the head and a subsequent brain MRI were normal. He was admitted overnight with "new-onset seizures." An EEG was performed later that day (Fig. 16.1). Other than complaining of a mild headache, myalgias, and a "sore tongue" he recovered by the following morning and was discharged home.

W. O. Tatum (✉)
Mayo Clinic, Department of Neurology, Jacksonville, FL, USA
e-mail: tatum.william@mayo.edu

© Springer Nature Switzerland AG 2021
W. O. Tatum et al. (eds.), *Epilepsy Case Studies*,
https://doi.org/10.1007/978-3-030-59078-9_16

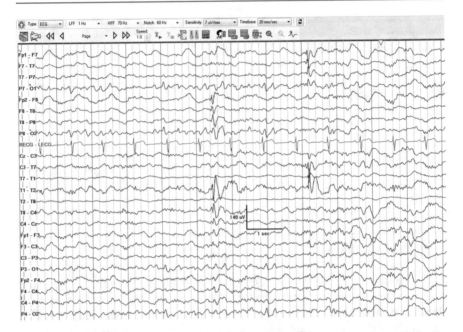

Fig. 16.1 EEG demonstrating independent bitemporal epileptiform discharges. Parameters of recording include sensitivity of 7 μV/mm; display speed 30 mm/s; and filter settings of 1–70 Hz

Clinical Questions

1. What are his chances that seizures will recur? Does he have epilepsy after a single seizure?
2. What clinical risk factors increase the chance of recurrence?
3. What is the best treatment approach?
4. What should the patient be told about driving a motorized vehicle?
5. What is the overall prognosis?

Discussion

1. A first seizure provoked by an acute brain insult is unlikely to recur (3–10%). However, adults with an unprovoked first seizure should be informed that their seizure recurrence risk is 21–45% and greatest early within the first 2 years [1]. Approximately two-thirds of patients will experience a third seizure after two spontaneous unprovoked seizures have occurred. Because of the nocturnal occurrence and an epileptiform EEG, this patient has a >60% likelihood of experiencing a seizure recurrence and therefore a working diagnosis of epilepsy (according to the current definition of epilepsy).
2. Clinical risk factors that may increase the likelihood of recurrent seizures include a prior brain insult or evidence of neurological injury (Level A), an EEG with

epileptiform abnormalities (Level A), a significant brain-imaging abnormality (Level B), and a nocturnal seizure (Level B) as in our patient [1]. Overall, an EEG and MRI are crucial to obtain to assess whether patients possess an epileptiform discharge on EEG or a structural lesion on neuroimaging given the high likelihood of seizure recurrence that may be inferred from these non-invasive tests. An EEG with epileptiform abnormalities is associated with a relative rate increase for seizure recurrence at 1–5 years of 2.16 (95% CI 1.07–4.38) as compared with patients without such EEG abnormalities [2].

3. The use of antiseizure medication (ASM) to prevent seizure recurrence after a single unprovoked seizure needs to be individualized. ASM has been shown in clinical studies to reduce the risk of seizure recurrence during short term follow-up. One study determined that immediate ASM treatment was preferable to deferred treatment in adult first-seizure patients over a wide and clinically relevant range of variables [3]. Furthermore, the analysis suggested that the 10-year seizure recurrence rate with ASM (38.0%) was substantially lower than the 60% threshold used in the current definition of epilepsy [3]. Without high-risk features, the potential benefit of ASM therapy needs to be contrasted with the clinical confidence of experiencing a seizures and the potential adverse effects of medication. Important issues in patients who are treated with ASM include considering the duration of therapy and the need for drug-level monitoring. Patient compliance and their acceptance of medical therapy should also be considered when making a treatment decision.

4. Following a seizure, patients should be informed not to drive or operate a motorized vehicle. Documentation should be included in the chart to reflect this conversation. However, the duration of restriction by law is determined by each state. The "seizure-free" duration period may range from 3 months to 1 year. Most states require 6 months of seizure freedom though following a first seizure, this may be shortened to 3 months if an EEG is normal in some states. Self-reporting is required by patients in some states though others still require mandatory reporting by the clinician. Medical forms may need to be completed prior to the individual being permitted to operate a motorized vehicle. Clinicians should discuss driving and other safety issues with the patient and review individual state driving laws.

5. The clinical course is variable in patients who present with a single unprovoked seizure. Deciding whether to treat patients who have experienced a first seizure can be challenging. This is true especially when the clinical history is unclear, and no provoking factors or abnormalities on ancillary tests such as MRI and EEG are found. Because the reported seizure recurrence rates in patients with a first unprovoked seizure is <50% in the first 2 years, many patients will not have another seizure, and the practical result in those with a "negative workup" is delaying treatment with ASM [4, 5]. Conditions where treatment may be warranted in adults include a prolonged focal seizure or status epilepticus, the presence of an immediate family history, a neurological deficit, an abnormal MRI or EEG, and a personal history of remote seizures. From an individual patient perspective, those with high-risk jobs or an individual inability to accept a second seizure may warrant considering initial treatment. The occurrence of a second

seizure usually warrants ASM and careful monitoring of the patient for ongoing seizures and side-effects. Most patients with focal epilepsy have a favorable outcome with ASM with two-thirds who are rendered seizure-free. It is even better for patients who have genetic generalized epilepsy with seizure freedom approaching 80–85% with appropriate ASM. The overall prognosis is related to the underlying epilepsy syndrome, and etiology, with patients who have focal epilepsy due to a structural lesion and those with epileptic encephalopathies often requiring long-term or even life-long therapy.

Clinical Pearls

1. Single unprovoked seizures do not always indicate the onset of epilepsy. Overall, after a first seizure, patients have a 21–45% likelihood of seizure recurrence. This reflects a <50% likelihood of experiencing a seizure recurrence within the first 2 years. The likelihood is lowest when crucial studies such as MRI and EEG are normal or unrevealing for clear abnormalities. When a nocturnal seizure and/or an epileptiform EEG is present in a person with a first seizure, as in our patient, the likelihood of recurrence is >60% and provides a working diagnosis of epilepsy.

2. Level A evidence exists for clinical risk factors that may increase the likelihood of recurrent seizures after a first seizure. Patients with a prior brain insult or evidence of neurological injury and an epileptiform EEG abnormality (our patient) are at high risk of recurrence. Level B evidence is present when a significant brain-imaging abnormality and a nocturnal seizure has occurred (our patient). Most individuals will have recurrent seizures during the first year following an unprovoked seizure, with the highest risk being in the initial 3 months.

3. The use of ASM to prevent seizure recurrence after a single unprovoked seizure should be individualized and involve the patient in the decision-making process. Patients who are at high risk due to risk factors (our patient) or at significant environmental risk from employment or recreation should be considered for initial treatment with ASM. The evidence does not permit determination for the length of treatment duration or indicate a specific ASM.

4. In general, the longer a patient remains seizure-free after a single unprovoked seizure, the less likely there will be seizure recurrence. However, individuals who experience a first seizure should be educated to modify their behavior in an effort to avoid proconvulsant activities such as sleep-deprivation, skipping ASM, and use of illicit drugs and alcohol, as these provocative factors may increase the likelihood of seizure aggravation. Similarly, some prescription medication should be avoided or used with caution.

5. The clinical course is variable from the time a patient experiences a first seizure. When the clinical history is unclear for a seizure diagnosis and no provoking factors or abnormalities are found on ancillary tests such as MRI and EEG, most patients will have a favorable outcome with respect to recurrence risk. When ASM is required, it will render two-thirds of high-risk patients seizure-free. The response rate to ASM is even better for patients with genetic generalized epilepsy and approaches 80–85%. The overall prognosis is related to the underlying epilepsy syndrome. Patients with focal epilepsy due to a structural lesion, and some patients with generalized epilepsies (i.e., juvenile myoclonic epilepsy, juvenile absence epilepsy, generalized tonic-clonic seizures-alone) and those with epileptic encephalopathies often requires long-term or even lifelong therapy.

References

1. Krumholz A, Wiebe S, Gronseth GS, Gloss DS, Sanchez AM, Kabir AA, et al. Evidence-based guideline: management of an unprovoked first seizure in adults. Report of the guideline development subcommittee of the American Academy of Neurology and the American Epilepsy Society. Neurology. 2015;84(16):1705–13.
2. Hauser WA, Rich SS, Annegers JF, Anderson VE. Seizure recurrence after a 1st unprovoked seizure: an extended follow-up. Neurology. 1990;40:1163–70.
3. Bao EL, Chao L-Y, Ni P, Moura LM, Cole AJ, Cash SS, et al. Antiepileptic drug treatment after an unprovoked first seizure: a decision analysis. Neurology. 2018;91(15):e1429–39.
4. Jacobs CS, Lee JW. Immediate vs delayed treatment of first unprovoked seizure: to treat, or not to treat? Neurology. 2018;91(15):684–5.
5. Bergey GK. Management of a first seizure. Continuum (Minneap Minn). 2016;22:38–50.

Starting Antiseizure Medication

17

Amy Z. Crepeau

Case Presentation

A 19-year-old right-handed college student was seen in clinic after being seen in the emergency department for a first-time seizure. The seizure occurred while he was working out in the gym. He states he had no warning before the seizure and the onset was described as a sensation of falling backwards. He reportedly had generalized convulsions lasting approximately 60 s, and he did not begin responding again until he was being transported to the emergency department. He has no recall of any of the events until he was seen in the emergency department. In the emergency department, a complete blood count and comprehensive metabolic profile, was performed and was normal. A urine drug screen was negative. A head CT and 12 lead EKG were both normal. He was discharged from the emergency department with a prescription for levetiracetam 500 mg twice daily.

Further history was obtained during the clinic appointment. He has no epilepsy risk factors. He denies any history of febrile seizures, CNS infections, significant head trauma, or family members with epilepsy. There was no identifiable preceding illness or injury associated with the seizure. He has no significant past medical history and was on no medications. He did not start levetiracetam after being discharged from the emergency department.

On further questioning, he reported a 3-year history of recurrent unusual events. He stated that these would consist of a sudden blood taste in his mouth and a feeling as though he was "in his own little world." He had been told that he would stare off during these events but was unclear as to whether or not he would lose awareness. He estimated that these events had been occurring 2 or 3 times per week for the past 3 years.

A. Z. Crepeau (✉)
Mayo Clinic, Department of Neurology, Phoenix, AZ, USA
e-mail: Crepeau.amy@mayo.edu

© Springer Nature Switzerland AG 2021
W. O. Tatum et al. (eds.), *Epilepsy Case Studies*,
https://doi.org/10.1007/978-3-030-59078-9_17

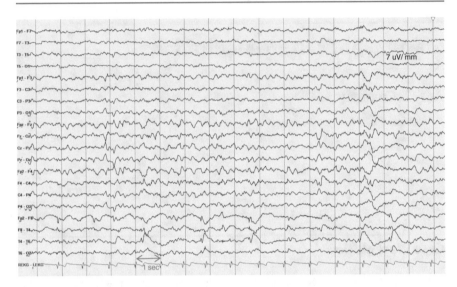

Fig. 17.1 Standard outpatient EEG. Right temporal spike-and-wave discharges and focal delta slowing seen during sleep

A standard outpatient EEG was completed, which showed right temporal spikes and sharp waves (Fig. 17.1). An brain MRI was normal.

Clinical Questions

1. What additional test should be considered to determine risk of seizure recurrence?
2. Which aspects of the clinical history suggest this patient is at risk for further seizures?
3. What is the risk of seizure recurrence if an antiseizure drug is started?
4. How should a first ASM be chosen?
5. What is the risk of starting ASM after a first-time seizure?

Discussion

1. When assessing the risk of seizure recurrence, and ultimately a decision whether not to start ASM antiseizure drug (ASD), the first question to ask is whether or not this was a provoked seizure. In this case example, the emergency department evaluation and the clinical history obtained in the clinic were able to determine that this was an unprovoked seizure. The relevant details included screening for any significant electrolyte abnormalities or illicit substances in the emergency department with basic lab work. The head CT excluded an acute structural cause, such as an intracranial hemorrhage or mass lesion. The clinical history did not suggest any preceding infection or illness or medication use that

would have potentially provoked the seizure. There is a significant difference in risk of seizure recurrence after a first-time seizure depending upon whether it was provoked or unprovoked. Population studies demonstrate approximately 20% risk of seizure recurrence at 10 years if it was a provoked seizure versus an approximately 65% risk of seizure recurrence at 10 years in the unprovoked setting [1]. When seizures are determined to be unprovoked, additional testing can assist with determining the risk of further recurrence. The American Academy of Neurology Practice Management Guideline recommends an outpatient standard EEG after a first-time seizure. If this initial EEG shows epileptiform activity, the associated risk of seizure recurrence within the first year is increased, estimated between 30% and 70%. An MRI of the brain is recommended as the gold standard for imaging in the evaluation of a first-time seizure, as it can better visualize mesial temporal structures and cortical abnormalities [2]. A potentially epileptogenic structural lesion, which is concordant with the described seizure semiology, would increase the risk of seizure recurrence and likely favor initiating an ASM.

2. The clinical history obtained is also important in assessing the risk of further seizure recurrence. There has been some association with the timing of a first-time seizure and recurrence risk. A seizure arising out of sleep has been associated with elevated risk of recurrence [2]. Another common scenario is that while a patient presents with a first-time recognized seizure, there has been a history of unrecognized seizures in the past. In this specific case, the patient presented after having a witnessed generalized tonic-clonic seizure, but he also described additional recurrent, stereotyped events, that were highly suspicious for focal seizures with and without impaired awareness. The number of unprovoked seizures the patient experienced in the past is associated with the risk of future recurrence [3]. After two or three unprovoked seizures, ASM should be initiated.

3. In a patient with a single unprovoked seizure, the next question is how initiating ASM would change the risk of recurrence. A prospective study was performed in the United Kingdom investigating immediate versus deferred treatment for first-time seizure patients. This study determined that immediate treatment did significantly reduce the risk of seizure recurrence during the first 2 years, but did not impact long-term seizure control past 5 years. The 2-year seizure recurrence risk was 32% in those with immediate treatment versus 39% in those with deferred treatment. The number needed to treat was 14 [4]. These data were also able to stratify risk factors for seizure recurrence. More than one seizure prior to presentation, abnormal EEG, and an underlying neurologic disorder deficit were all associated with increased risk of seizure recurrence (Table 17.1). The high-risk

Table 17.1 Risk factors associated with seizure recurrence	Unprovoked seizure History of prior seizures Concordant intracranial structural lesion Epileptiform discharges on routine EEG Prior neurologic insult or injury Seizure arising from sleep

group did have a significant increased probability of seizures at 1, 3, and 5 years if treatment was delayed [5].

4. Once a decision is made to initiate treatment with ASM, a specific medication needs to be selected. The goal of treatment is for the patient to have no further seizures and no significant side effects from the medication. The first consideration is seizure classification: focal or generalized onset. If there is not definite evidence of the seizure being focal onset, a broad-spectrum ASM should be chosen. A generalized tonic-clonic seizure without an aura which can be recalled by the patient raises the likelihood of generalized onset. In this case, reasonable ASMs to consider ASD would be levetiracetam, lamotrigine, zonisamide, topiramate, or valproate. However, if the patient has a clinical history or laboratory findings consistent with focal onset seizures then narrow-spectrum ASMs such as oxcarbazepine, carbamazepine, or lacosamide would be appropriate. Next, medical comorbidities, such as of mood disorder, liver or kidney disease, or cardiac arrhythmias should be considered, as some ASMs can impact these underlying conditions. Finally, urgency of reaching a therapeutic dose should be considered, as some ASMs can be titrated rapidly, but others, such as lamotrigine, require a prolonged titration schedule. If after initiation of the ASM the patient either has continued seizures or significant side effects, the initial ASM that was selected should be reassessed [6].

5. The goal for seizure management with ASM is for the patient to have no significant side effects, however, there are risks associated with starting medication. In patients who were immediately started on an ASM after the first-time seizure, there was a higher rate of adverse side effects compared to those patients with deferred treatment. Adverse effects included depression, anxiety, dizziness, fatigue, headache, and cognitive complaints [4]. Each ASM also carries its own potential side effect profile. These potential side effects need to be weighed against the risk and implications of further seizures and patients should be monitored once therapy is initiated.

Clinical Pearls
- The initial evaluation and clinical history are necessary to determine if a seizure was provoked or unprovoked.
- Careful history needs to be obtained to determine if the presentation is truly a first-time seizure or the first clinically recognized seizure.
- In patients with elevated risk of seizure recurrence, ASM should be considered after a first-time seizure.
- When choosing an ASM, if it cannot be determined whether a seizure is focal or generalized in onset, a broad-spectrum ASD should be selected.
- The goal of treatment is for the patient to have no further seizures and no significant side effects from treatment.

References

1. Hesdorffer DC, Benn EK, Cascino GD, Hauser WA. Is a first acute symptomatic seizure epilepsy? Mortality and risk for recurrent seizure. Epilepsia. 2009;50(5):1102–8.
2. Krumholz A, Wiebe S, Gronseth GS, Gloss DS, Sanchez AM, Kabir AA, et al. Evidence-based guideline: management of an unprovoked first seizure in adults: report of the guideline development subcommittee of the American Academy of Neurology and the American Epilepsy Society. Epilepsy Curr. 2015;15(3):144–52.
3. Hauser WA, Rich SS, Lee JR, Annegers JF, Anderson VE. Risk of recurrent seizures after two unprovoked seizures. N Engl J Med. [Research Support, U.S. Gov't, P.H.S.]. 1998;338(7):429–34.
4. Marson A, Jacoby A, Johnson A, Kim L, Gamble C, Chadwick D. Immediate versus deferred antiepileptic drug treatment for early epilepsy and single seizures: a randomised controlled trial. Lancet. [Clinical Trial Comparative Study Multicenter Study Randomized Controlled Trial Research Support, Non-U.S. Gov't]. 2005;365(9476):2007–13.
5. Kim LG, Johnson TL, Marson AG, Chadwick DW. Prediction of risk of seizure recurrence after a single seizure and early epilepsy: further results from the MESS trial. Lancet Neurol. [Clinical Trial Comparative Study Multicenter Study Randomized Controlled Trial Research Support, Non-U.S. Gov't]. 2006;5(4):317–22.
6. Crepeau AZ, Sirven JI. Management of adult onset seizures. Mayo Clin Proc. [Review]. 2017;92(2):306–18.

Stopping Antiseizure Medication

18

Amy Z. Crepeau

Case Presentation

A 38-year-old woman presents to Epilepsy Clinic for a new visit. She has a history of two seizures in her lifetime: at ages 20 and 22. Both seizures were described as generalized tonic-clonic seizures that occurred in the morning. Each one occurred after staying up late to study for final exams while she was in college. She has been on levetiracetam since the second seizure. She reported seeing a neurologist in her early 20s but since that time has been maintained on levetiracetam monotherapy administered through her primary care physician. She has been unable to obtain the records from her initial evaluation but recalls having an MRI and routine EEG and does not recall being told of any abnormalities.

She has no other significant past medical history and is on no other medications. She has no history of febrile seizures, CNS infections, significant head trauma, or family members with seizures. Other than the two described generalized tonic-clonic seizures, she denies any other type of events suggestive of focal, absence, myoclonic, or generalized tonic-clonic seizures.

She asked for consultation to discuss the need to continue an antiseizure medication (ASM). If possible, she would like to discontinue levetiracetam and is wondering if this could be done with a relative degree of safety.

Questions

1. What clinical features are suggestive of seizure relapse after ASM withdrawal?
2. When should ASM be withdrawn in childhood epilepsy?
3. Can patients with genetic generalized epilepsies be successfully withdrawn?

A. Z. Crepeau (✉)
Mayo Clinic, Department of Neurology, Phoenix, AZ, USA
e-mail: Crepeau.amy@mayo.edu

© Springer Nature Switzerland AG 2021
W. O. Tatum et al. (eds.), *Epilepsy Case Studies*,
https://doi.org/10.1007/978-3-030-59078-9_18

4. What is the risk of seizure recurrence after ASM withdrawal following epilepsy surgery?
5. How risky is ASM withdrawal after an acute symptomatic seizure?

Discussion

1. The International League Against Epilepsy defines "resolved epilepsy" as an age dependent epilepsy that has remitted, or a patient who has been seizure-free for 10 years and successfully off ASM for 5 years [1]. Per the definition, it is the successful withdrawal of ASM that allows epilepsy to be considered resolved, which makes it challenging to determine at what point a trial should be initiated. Some important clinical details should be obtained prior to initiating a trial of ASM withdrawal. The patient should be carefully questioned to determine that they have in fact been seizure-free for several years. This includes insuring that they have not had focal aware seizures, absence seizures, or unwitnessed seizures. Details regarding the circumstances around the initial seizures, including potential provoking factors, should also be considered. It is important to review any imaging. If the patient has an underlying structural lesion, such as a prior cerebral infarction, mesial temporal sclerosis, or focal cortical dysplasia, which is concordant with her seizure semiology, there should be greater caution in withdrawing ASM, despite a prolonged period of seizure freedom due to the higher risk of relapse. Prior to a trial of tapering ASM to discontinuation, a standard EEG should be obtained. Interictal epileptiform discharges suggest an elevated risk for seizure recurrence.

2. There is not a definite consensus on how long the patient should remain seizure-free before considering a trial of ASM withdrawal. A single center study followed 336 patients who were seizure-free for 4 years, underwent a planned withdrawal of ASM, and had 3 years of follow-up. Nearly 65% of patients experienced seizure relapse, with no significant differences between those patients who relapsed while being tapered off of ASM and those who relapsed after the taper was complete. The features that were significantly associated with relapse were seizures persisting more than 10 years, seizure onset before age 20, and people with focal epilepsy [2]. In a study of childhood epilepsy, 18% of patients relapsed after a trial of ASM withdrawal. The features that were associated with seizure freedom were a seizure-free interval of at least 3 years and genetic epilepsy. Juvenile myoclonic epilepsy or absence epilepsy like patients with epilepsy due to a structural-metabolic cause were associated with the highest risk of relapse [3]. In a meta-analysis of five randomized clinical trials involving children, a seizure freedom lasting more than 2 years was a favorable sign. Intellectual disability, frequent seizures, and a history of status epilepticus were associated with higher risk of seizure relapse after ASM withdrawal. Seizure onset before age 2 or after age 10 also carried a higher risk [4].

3. In general, common genetic generalized epilepsies, other than specific childhood syndromes such as childhood absence epilepsy, are thought to entail a lifelong

predisposition to seizures. Many of these patients will have long spans of time between seizures, making it difficult to determine what the necessary seizure-free interval would be to consider ASM withdrawal. A German study followed patients with longstanding genetic generalized epilepsy who attempted ASM discontinuation. Among 84 patients who attempted discontinuation, 46% had seizure recurrence, with a short period of seizure remission. Among those patients who were seizure-free for greater than 5 years prior to a trial of ASM withdrawal, only one-third had seizure recurrence, compared to two-thirds having seizure recurrence if they had had fewer than 5 years of seizure freedom [5].

4. After successful epilepsy surgery, many patients are eager to come off of ASM. It can be challenging to decide when a taper should be initiated. The TimeToStop trial, examining ASM ASD withdrawal after pediatric epilepsy surgery, determined that early withdrawal did not affect long-term outcome, but instead unmasks an incomplete surgical success compared to if the child had been maintained on an ASM [6]. Among children who underwent resection of a focal cortical dysplasia, incomplete resectino and ongoing epileptiform discharges on the postoperative EEGs were predictors of seizure recurrence after ASM withdrawal [7] a meta-analysis of ASM withdrawal in both medically and surgically treated patients determined that in the surgically treated group, nearly 50% of seizure relapses occurred within the first year after ASM withdrawal. No consistent predictors of seizure relapse were able to be identified in this analysis [8].

5. Patients who had an acute symptomatic seizure, such as at the time of an acute cerebral infarction or intracranial hemorrhage, in the immediate post-neurosurgical period, or in the setting of meningitis, are often discharged from the hospital on an ASM. In the outpatient setting, the challenge is to determine at what time the ASM can be withdrawn, assuming the patient has remained seizure-free. There is no standard for the period of time patients should be maintained on an ASM in this setting. It is important to first ensure that the underlying provoking cause has resolved. For example, if the seizure occurred in the setting of an intracranial hemorrhage, serial monitoring to ensure resolution of the acute blood products would be appropriate. A standard EEG can help as an adjunct to withdrawal when it has excluded epileptiform discharges. If the patient presented with status epilepticus, greater caution should be used prior to attempting ASM withdrawal. If a seizure occurs during or after withdrawal, this may represent an underlying predisposition for seizures and need for long-term ASM.

Clinical Pearls
1. ASM withdrawal can be considered after 2–5 years of seizure freedom, though specific clinical features need to be carefully considered with patient input.
2. Factors that would raise concern for seizure relapse after ASM withdrawal include seizures occurring over several years, an underlying structural lesion, and ongoing epileptiform discharges on the EEG.

3. After epilepsy surgery, incomplete resection and continued epileptiform discharges on EEG are negative prognosticators of successful ASM withdrawal.
4. Many genetic generalized epilepsies except childhood absence epilepsy imply the need for long-term treatment with ASM, especially if generalized spike- and polyspike- and- wave discharges are present.
5. After an acute symptomatic seizure, it is reasonable to consider ASM withdrawal following resolution of the underlying provoking cause and the results of an EEG demonstrate lack of ongoing epileptiform discharges.

References

1. Fisher RS, Acevedo C, Arzimanoglou A, Bogacz A, Cross JH, Elger CE, et al. ILAE official report: a practical clinical definition of epilepsy. Epilepsia. [Case Reports Review]. 2014;55(4):475–82.
2. Park S, Lee DH, Kim SW, Roh YH. Prognostic analysis of patients with epilepsy according to time of relapse after withdrawal of antiepileptic drugs following four seizure-free years. Epilepsia. 2017;58(1):60–7.
3. Karalok ZS, Guven A, Ozturk Z, Gurkas E. Risk factors for recurrence after drug withdrawal in childhood epilepsy. Brain and Development. 2020;42(1):35–40.
4. Strozzi I, Nolan SJ, Sperling MR, Wingerchuk DM, Sirven J. Early versus late antiepileptic drug withdrawal for people with epilepsy in remission. Cochrane Database Syst Rev. [Meta-Analysis Review Systematic Review]. 2015;11(2):CD001902.
5. Vorderwulbecke BJ, Kirschbaum A, Merkle H, Senf P, Holtkamp M. Discontinuing antiepileptic drugs in long-standing idiopathic generalised epilepsy. J Neurol. [Observational Study]. 2019;266(10):2554–9.
6. Boshuisen K, Arzimanoglou A, Cross JH, Uiterwaal CS, Polster T, van Nieuwenhuizen O, et al. Timing of antiepileptic drug withdrawal and long-term seizure outcome after paediatric epilepsy surgery (TimeToStop): a retrospective observational study. Lancet Neurol. [Multicenter Study Research Support, Non-U.S. Gov't]. 2012;11(9):784–91.
7. Choi SA, Kim SY, Kim WJ, Shim YK, Kim H, Hwang H, et al. Antiepileptic drug withdrawal after surgery in children with focal cortical dysplasia: seizure recurrence and its predictors. J Clin Neurol. 2019;15(1):84–9.
8. Lamberink HJ, Otte WM, Geleijns K, Braun KP. Antiepileptic drug withdrawal in medically and surgically treated patients: a meta-analysis of seizure recurrence and systematic review of its predictors. Epileptic Disord. [Meta-Analysis Review Systematic Review]. 2015;17(3):211–28.

Classification of Epilepsy

19

William O. Tatum

Case Presentation

A 19-year-old, right-handed, white female had uncontrolled seizures despite unsuccessful trials of antiseizure medications (ASMs). She failed two ASMs due to unacceptable side effects and was maintained on carbamazepine for years. No early risk factors for epilepsy were present, and she otherwise developed normally as an "A" student in high school. "Petit mal seizures" began at 9 years of age and were described as an abrupt stare with and impaired awareness. During this time, her mom would touch her though she would not respond. The patient's mother reported that an early EEG was reported to be abnormal with "spikes everywhere." She was initially placed on ethosuximide which reduced her seizure frequency from 2–3 times per week to 2–3 times per month, worsening around her menstrual period. When she experienced a "grand mal" seizure a year later during puberty, a repeat standard EEG was normal. She was changed to levetiracetam. However, it was rapidly discontinued due to side effects. Lacosamide worsened her "petit mal" seizures and a follow-up sleep-deprived EEG was also normal (though only drowsiness was obtained). She continued with intermittent "petit mal" seizures on a weekly basis while "grand mal" seizures were controlled. She had a total of three convulsions and these occurred at 9 years old, at 12 during menarche, and one when she failed to take her ASM during her freshman year of high school. Trials of ASMs included levetiracetam, lacosamide, and oxcarbazepine. All ASM were ineffective or poorly tolerated. Lacosamide resulted in headache and depression though it was effective for controlling her seizures. Levetiracetam resulted in severe anxiety and suicidal behavior and was rapidly discontinued. She was then seen for another opinion regarding pregnancy and driving. At that time, she was taking PHT 400 mg PO q HS

W. O. Tatum (✉)
Mayo Clinic, Department of Neurology, Jacksonville, FL, USA
e-mail: tatum.william@mayo.edu

© Springer Nature Switzerland AG 2021
W. O. Tatum et al. (eds.), *Epilepsy Case Studies*,
https://doi.org/10.1007/978-3-030-59078-9_19

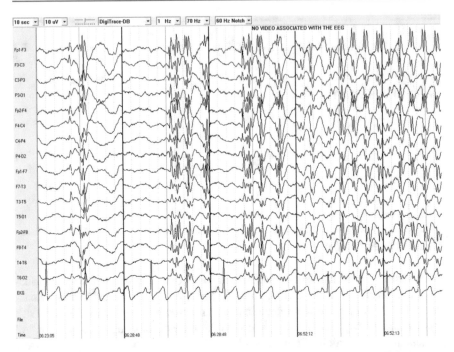

Fig. 19.1 Interictal computer-assisted ambulatory EEG demonstrating generalized bifrontal predominant polyspike-and-wave complexes and 3-Hz generalized spike-and-wave bursts during sleep

which had provided her the best control though around her menstrual period she complained of feeling "twitchy" and continued to experience "petit mal" seizures. Her neurological examination was normal. A high-resolution brain MRI with an epilepsy protocol was normal. A computer-assisted ambulatory EEG is demonstrated in the Fig. 19.1.

Clinical Questions

1. Does this patient have focal or generalized seizures?
2. How do the ancillary tests help classify staring spells?
3. What syndromic classification is present in this patient?
4. What antiseizure medication is most appropriate for the epilepsy syndrome?
5. What is the best course of management when drugs fail?

Diagnostic Discussion

1. This patient does have true "petit mal" (a.k.a. absence seizures). One clinical clue to the diagnosis of seizures is that the patient was unresponsive to tactile stimulation during the event. Other conditions such as daydreaming and inattention or

preoccupation may simulate absence though with these events, patients are alerted and responsive to touch. Episodes of staring due to absence seizures may be distinguished by a sudden stare for approximately 10–20 s associated with impaired awareness or responsiveness, while focal impaired awareness seizures and impaired consciousness typically last 30–40 s that may begin with a warning (or aura) [1]. Absence seizures begin and end abruptly while focal seizures often exhibit post-ictal disorientation and lethargy. Automatisms commonly occur in focal seizures but also occur, albeit less frequently, in patients with absence seizures. Our patient is manifesting absence seizures and is supported by a generalized epileptiform abnormality on EEG. Many patients refer to staring episodes as "petit mal" because they are meant to reflect the non-convulsive nature of the events. In this case the EEG supports the use of the terminology "petit mal."

2. The EEG shows generalized bifrontal predominant polyspike- and generalized spike-and-waves during sleep. Generalized epileptiform discharges in patients with generalized epilepsies may become activated during sleep. If sleep is not captured during EEG recording, then no epileptiform discharges may provide an inconclusive evaluation. In this case, the computer-assisted ambulatory EEG was able to capture generalized polyspike-and-waves and generalized spike-and-waves during sleep to classify the patient with poorly classified epilepsy and repeatedly normal EEGs. The window to capture epileptiform abnormalities on standard EEG is brief, and the yield of a single EEG is low (overall about one-third are abnormal). Among the activation procedures, sleep is the most effective method. Ambulatory EEG with overnight recording is superior to sleep-deprived EEG may provide a higher yield in capturing epileptiform discharges as well as ictal events [2]. Infrequently, a generalized EEG pattern may occur in patients with focal epilepsies such as occurs when seizures arise from the mesial frontal lobe. There may be a "lead in" to generalized discharges that can appear, and the generalized spikes (or polyspikes) in this case usually have a repetition rate of <3 Hz when it occurs. In our case, the bilateral symmetrical polyspikes and spikes without lateralization and the 3 Hz interspike interval suggest a genetic generalized epilepsy. Prolongation of the EEG recording to include overnight assessment of sleep using ambulatory EEG monitoring can help to identify characteristic features associated with epilepsies [3].

3. This patient has one of the genetic generalized epilepsies manifest as recurrent absence and generalized tonic-clonic seizures. In addition, myoclonic seizures were noted around the time of her menstrual period. Catamenial exacerbation of seizures may occur in patients with generalized epilepsies, and menarche is a common time of seizure onset. With the combination of seizure types, the best syndromic classification for our patient is juvenile absence epilepsy. Generalized seizures such as absence and myoclonic seizures may increase immediately prior to a convulsion though in contrast to patients with focal epilepsies, an "aura" and post-ictal state do not occur (Table 19.1). However, occasionally a prodrome may occur as a nonepileptic preceding sense that a seizure is likely to occur. Prodromes are symptoms that encompass a broad range of preictal symptoms that may be experienced by the patient for a duration lasting minutes or up to several days persisting until seizure onset occurs. The International League Against Epilepsy has updated the classification of the epilepsies recently to assist

Table 19.1 Differences between absence seizures (generalized epilepsies) and focal impaired awareness seizures (focal epilepsies) presenting as staring spells with impaired consciousness

Features	Absence seizures	Focal impaired awareness seizures
Onset	Sudden onset and offset (4–10 y with CAE; 9–13 y with JAE)	Onset and offset may be gradual (any time of life)
Aura	No	Yes
Stare	Yes	Yes
Impaired awareness	Yes	Yes
Automatisms	Infrequently and simply	Frequently and simple or complex
Seizure duration	3–20 s	30–60 s
Post-ictal confusion	No	Yes
Frequency	Daily (CAE) to weekly (JAE)	Weekly to monthly
Pathology	None (thalamocortical dysfunction)	Focal pathology (i.e., hippocampal sclerosis, cortical dysplasia, tumors, vascular malformations, normal, etc.)
MRI	Normal	Often abnormal
EEG	Rarely normal, >3 Hz polyspike-and-waves and spike-and-waves	Focal spikes with/without after-going slow-waves (often unilateral or bilateral temporal)
Provocative factors	Hyperventilation, intermittent photic stimulation	Sleep-deprivation may have unique triggers reflexively
Gene alterations	Calcium (CACNA1A), potassium (KCNMB3), and GABA (GABRB3)	DEPDC5, LGI1, PCDH19, SCN1A, and GRIN2A
Treatment	ASM (VPA, LTG, ETH) and neuromodulation when resistant	ASM (LTG, OXC, LEV) and epilepsy surgery (resection, ablation, neuromodulation)
Prognosis	Good response to ASM treatment (about 2/3rds to 85%), CAE resolves by 18 y; JAE is life-long	1/3 of patients are drug-resistant, may become self-limited following successful medical/surgical treatment

CAE childhood absence epilepsy, *JAE* juvenile absence epilepsy, *s* seconds, *Hz* hertz, *ASM* antiseizure medication, *VPA* valproate, *LTG* lamotrigine, *ETH* ethosuximide, *OXC* oxcarbazepine, *LEV* levetiracetam, *y* years

with treatment [4]. The classification system is designed to provide flexibility with use of descriptive terms (i.e., motor vs nonmotor) and even free text descriptions are encouraged to more thoroughly classify seizures and the epilepsies.

4. Treatment is dependent upon proper seizure and epilepsy classification. Narrow-spectrum ASMs such as carbamazepine and phenytoin may aggravate seizure control or worsen some generalized seizure types (i.e., absence and myoclonic seizures). Similarly, some ASMs for used for the successful treatment of generalized seizures, such as ethosuximide, may be ineffective or even aggravate seizures in patient treated for focal seizures. EEG is fundamental to seizure diagnosis as well as classification. Semiology may be unrevealing. Staring episodes and convulsions may not allow proper identification of a focal or generalized epilepsy. EEG may be unhelpful when a lack of defining interictal discharges are present. Occasionally brain MRI may reveal a focal lesion that supports a focal epilepsy syndrome and additionally guide selection of ASM useful for treating focal seizures. Most ASMs have been approved by the U.S. Food and Drug Administration for clinical use in the treatment of focal seizures [5].

Valproate, lamotrigine, topiramate, levetiracetam, zonisamide, lacosamide, and perampanel have demonstrated efficacy in patients with generalized seizures of focal and non-focal origin. Ethosuximide is probably the most effective absence treatment though it does not effectively treat convulsions. Genetic variation plays a role in the proper treatment of generalized epilepsy syndromes with a differential drug response exhibted based upon seizure type (i.e., absence vs myoclonus vs generalized tonic-clonic seizures) [6]. The barbiturates and benzodiazepines may also demonstrate a broad spectrum of usage in patients with focal and generalized seizure types though sedation often limits usage.

5. The best course of action for this patient with genetic generalized epilepsy is to achieve success with the initial approach to treatment using an effective well-tolerated ASM monotherapy. Unlike most absence epilepsies that have a high rate of remission, juvenile absence epilepsy carries a low likelihood of remission and implies the need for life-long treatment similar to Jeavons syndrome (eyelid myoclonia with absence), generalized tonic-clonic seizures-alone, and juvenile myoclonic epilepsy. Following the failure to reach seizure control with two appropriate antiseizure drugs (present in 20–25% of patients), patients who have taken ASMs at optimal doses for an adequate period of treatment time, making further changes in ASM by substituting or adding another agent carries a lower yield of success. Pursuing trials of broad-spectrum ASM and polytherapy with a synergistic combination (i.e., valproate and lamotrigine) or additive combinations effective for absence seizures (ethosuximide and lamotrigine) may be necessary. Our patient was treated with lamotrigine and valproate and remained seizure-free. Other options include the ketogenic diet (see separate chapter) and neuromodulation (see separate chapter) such as vagus nerve stimulation.

Clinical Pearls

1. Petit mal is a common colloquialism used by patients to reflect non-convulsive staring spells and does not reliably reflect absence seizures as many patients use this term to reflect staring associated with focal seizures. Common terms patients use to describe seizures are grand mal and petit mal though they are often used loosely to refer to witnessed semiologies.

2. EEG is the most useful test when the brain MRI and clnical history is normal or nonspecific. When clear generalized interictal epileptiform discharges are present, this supports the diagnosis of generalized epilepsies as the mechanism for recurrent seizures. Genetic etiologies usually have an interspike interval with a frequency of 3 Hz or greater.

3. Absence seizures beginning in early adolescence are often accompanied by generalized tonic-clonic seizures (and infrequent myoclonus) in juvenile absence epilepsy syndrome. Unlike other types of genetic generalized epilepsies, juvenile absence epilepsy merits long-term consideration of treatment.

4. Broad-spectrum, antiseizure medications are useful treatments when the classification of the seizures and epilepsy type is generalized or unknown. These agents are effective for both focal and generalized seizures and do not aggravate a specific seizure type.

5. Drug-resistance is a definable entity when two or more ASMs appropriate for the patient's seizure type are given in an adequate dose for an appropriate time period. Genetic influences play a role in differential drug response and is dependent upon seizure type. Unlike focal epilepsy that is potentially amenable to epilepsy surgery, patients with genetic generalized epilepsies are not candidates for excisional epilepsy surgery though may be responsive to various forms of neuromodulation.

References

1. Berg AT, Berkovic SF, Brodie MJ, Buchhalter J, Cross JH, van Emde BW, Engel J, French J, Glauser TA, Mathern GW, Moshe SL, Nordli D, Plouin P, Scheffer IE. Revised terminology and concepts for organization of seizures and epilepsies: report of the ILAE Commission on Classification and Terminology, 2005–2009. Epilepsia. 2010;51:676–85.
2. Baldin E, Hauser WA, Buchhalter JR, Hesdorffer DC, Ottman R. Utility of EEG activation procedures in epilepsy: a population-based study. J Clin Neurophysiol. 2017;34(6):512–9.
3. Seneviratne U, Mohamed A, Cook M, D'Souza W. The utility of ambulatory electroencephalography in routine clinical practice: a critical review. Epilepsy Res. 2013;105(1–2):1–12.
4. Scheffer IE, Berkovic S, Capovilla G, Connolly MB, French J, Guilhoto L, et al. ILAE classification of the epilepsies: position paper of the ILAE Commission for Classification and Terminology. Epilepsia. 2017;58(4):512–21.
5. Abou-Khalil BW. Update on antiepileptic drugs 2019. Neurology. 2019;25(2):508–36.
6. Glauser TA, Holland K, O'Brien VP, Keddache M, Martin LJ, Clark PO, et al. Pharmacogenetics of antiepileptic drug efficacy in childhood absence epilepsy. Ann Neurol. 2017;81:444–53.

Seizures in the Intensive Care Unit

20

Jason Siegel and W. David Freeman

Case Presentation

A 66-year-old right-handed female, with past medical history of orthotopic liver transplant (OLT), was admitted for seizures. She had received the OLT 3 months prior to presentation and was recently admitted 1 week prior to presentation for headache, confusion, blurry vision, hypertension, and a supratherapeutic tacrolimus level. She was diagnosed with posterior reversible encephalopathy syndrome (PRES). Magnetic resonance imaging (MRI) of her brain at that time was negative, though her blood pressure and tacrolimus levels had been corrected.

Five days after discharge, she was found unconscious by her significant other and taken to an outside hospital where she developed left upper extremity rhythmic movements. Brain MRI revealed patchy T2 hyperintensities in both hemispheres, involving both white and grey matter, concerning for PRES. Cerebrospinal fluid analysis was negative, tacrolimus was discontinued, and she was transferred to our facility. On arrival, she continued to have left upper extremity rhythmic movements and right gaze deviation. An electroencephalogram (EEG) was diagnostic for non-convulsive status epilepticus (NCSE) (Fig. 20.1), a brain MRI was consistent with PRES (Fig. 20.2), and treatment was initiated (Fig. 20.3). CSF analyses on hospital days 9, 61, and 67 all had normal cell counts, protein, and glucose. Comprehensive infectious and autoimmune panels were also negative.

J. Siegel (✉) · W. D. Freeman
Mayo Clinic Florida, Departments of Critical Care Medicine, Neurology, and Neurosurgery, Jacksonville, FL, USA
e-mail: Siegel.jason@mayo.edu; Freeman.william1@mayo.edu

© Springer Nature Switzerland AG 2021
W. O. Tatum et al. (eds.), *Epilepsy Case Studies*,
https://doi.org/10.1007/978-3-030-59078-9_20

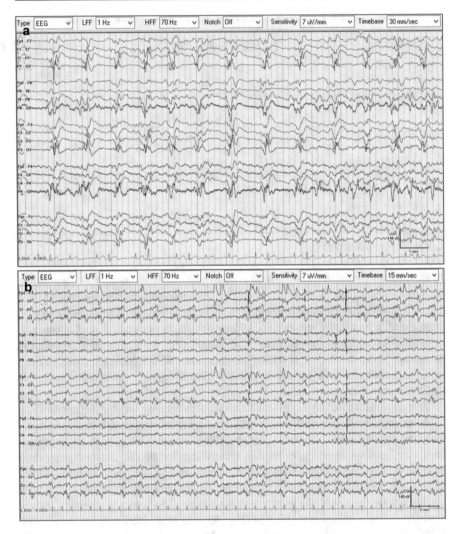

Fig. 20.1 Samples of EEG findings during hospitalization. (**a**) Presence of 1 Hz, generalized periodic discharges with left posterior quadrant predominance. They were associated with left upper limb jerking with and without head deviation. (**b**) Presence of lateralized periodic epileptiform discharges with fast activity at 1–1.5 Hz. There is maximum electronegativity in the left occipital head region

She had a long, protracted hospitalization including super-refractory status epilepticus, prolonged intubation with tracheostomy and gastrojejunostomy tube placement, labile blood pressure fluctuations (between hypertensive emergency and shock), pneumonia, sepsis, and cardiac dysrhythmia. Ultimately, with no overall improvement and a poor prognosis, she was admitted to hospice care on hospital day 113. Note the difference between the bolded star representing clinical seizures and the open star denoting electrographic seizures.

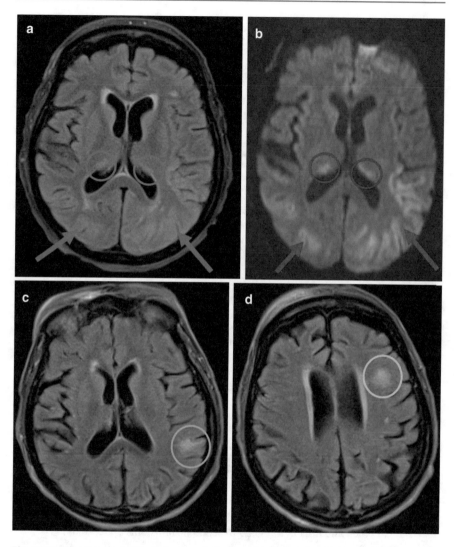

Fig. 20.2 Sample brain MRIs during hospitalization. (**a**) T2-weighted fluid-attenuated inversion recovery (FLAIR), day 2, with T2 hyperintensity and edema in bilateral occipital and parietal lobes (blue arrows), as well as bilateral posterior thalami (blue circles). (**b**) Diffuse-weighted imaging (DWI), day 2, with correlative areas of restricted diffusion of the same areas with cortical ribbon-ing (red arrows) and thalami (red circles). (**c, d**) T2-weighted FLAIR, day 57, with emergence of new cortical and subcortical hyperintensities of the left parietal lobe (green circle) and left frontal lobe (orange circle)

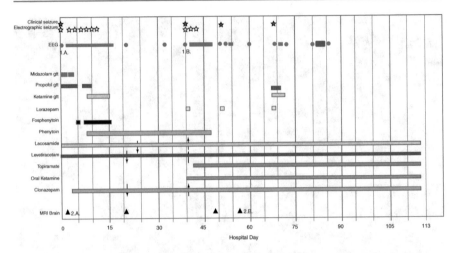

Fig. 20.3 Course of neurological events during hospitalization. Days with seizures are demarcated with the stars. The clinical seizures appear in red and electrographic seizures in yellow. Days with 20-min EEGs (circles) or prolonged EEGs (bars) are depicted in blue. Note that EEGs from day 1 and 40 correlated with Fig. 20.1a, b, respectively. Antiseizure medication is depicted by solid bars. Down-pointing arrows refer to a de-escalation in dose due to encephalopathy. Up-pointing arrows refer to reescalation of these drugs due to seizures. Days with brain MRI are demarcated in triangles. MRIs on days 2 and 57 were abnormal and correlate with Fig. 20.2a/b, c/d, respectively. Of note is that the two interval MRIs were unremarkable for acute pathology. gtt=continuous infusion

Clinical Questions

1. What is the frequency of seizures and status epilepticus in critical care?
2. How is nonconvulsive status epilepticus diagnosed?
3. What features constitute the ictal-interictal continuum?
4. What is the strategy for treatment in super-refractory status epilepticus in the intensive care unit?
5. What is PRES, and how is it related to seizures and status epilepticus?

Diagnostic Discussion

1. Clinical and subclinical seizures are common problems in all intensive care units (ICU). In the neurocritical care unit, seizures are commonly associated with traumatic brain injury, stroke, intracerebral hemorrhage, and subarachnoid hemorrhage. In medical and surgical ICUs, they are commonly associated with sepsis, electrolyte abnormalities, renal failure/uremia, and liver failure/hyperammonemia. It is estimated that seizure incidence ranges from 8% to 34%, but when considering ICU patients with altered mental status, about 20% will have seizures on continuous EEG (cEEG) monitoring [1–3]. The rate of seizure

detection depends on the duration of the cEEG. Only 4% of seizures are detected at the onset during standard EEG, which increases to 42% within 20 min and 92% within 24 h. There is a slight increase in incidence to 97% seizure detected within 48 h.

There are four primary reasons to escalate EEG monitoring from a 20-min standard EEG to a continuous EEG (cEEG) [3]:

(a) Detection of EEG seizures – In patients deemed high risk based on history, risk factors, or findings on the standard EEG (including seizures or epileptiform discharges).

(b) Characterization of unexplained encephalopathy – cEEG can elucidate the cause of encephalopathy (metabolic cause or subclinical seizures), can trend the degree of encephalopathy over time, and can help in prognostication.

(c) Detection of cerebral ischemia – Analysis of cEEG and quantitative EEG (trending), especially regarding the alpha/delta ratio (the ratio of normal alpha activity to slower delta ratio) in patients with aneurysmal subarachnoid hemorrhage and are at risk for vasospasm and delayed cerebral ischemia.

(d) Classify abnormal hyperactive movements and differentiate them from seizures. ICU patients often have myoclonus, fasciculations, asymmetrical weakness, and abnormal eye movements which are driven by a variety of metabolic derangements, including severe electrolyte abnormalities, hyperammonemia, uremia, hypoxia, hypercarbia, and hypoglycemia. In these cases, ruling out seizures can prevent patients from receiving unnecessary antiseizure medications.

2. By definition, nonconvulsive status epileptics (NCSE) has no to minimal clinical signs. Nystagmus, eye deviation, and subtle hand or face twitching could be clinical signs of seizures or completely unrelated to seizure activity and furthermore can be easily missed my bedside clinicians and nurses. The only way to diagnose NCSE is by EEG; unfortunately, our appreciation of the ictal-interictal continuum is still evolving. In 2013, a working diagnosis of NCSE was created and EEG criteria consist of [4]:

(a) Patients without known epileptic encephalopathy
   i. Epileptiform discharges >2.5 Hz
   ii. Epileptiform discharges ≤2.5 Hz or rhythmic delta or theta activity (>0.5 Hz) *and* one of the following:
      1. EEG and clinical improvement after intravenous antiseizure medication
      2. Subtle clinical ictal phenomena correlating with an ictal EEG
      3. Typical spatiotemporal evolution

(b) Patients with known epileptic encephalopathy
   i. Increase in prominence of frequency of the features mentioned above, when compared to baseline with observable change in clinical state
   ii. Improvement of clinical and EEG features with intravenous antiseizure medication

3. cEEG can reveal other abnormalities that do not strictly fit the definition of NCSE yet could portend ongoing cerebral malfunction and the propensity of

seizure development. The meaning of these often rhythmic or periodic interictal discharges is still under investigation, but recent efforts have attempted to standardize terminology [5]. All patterns require two main terms.

(a) Main Term 1: Generalized, lateralized, bilateral independent, and multifocal
(b) Main Term 2: Periodic discharge, rhythmic delta activity, and spike-and-wave or sharp waves

Terminology specifies these further by prevalence, duration, frequency, sharpness, amplitude, polarity, stimulus-induced, evolving or fluctuating, or plus (+) other additional features (superimposed fast, rhythmic, or sharp activity). In general, the sharper, faster, and more complex the pattern, the higher correlation with the patient developing seizures [6]. Like NCSE, a trial of fast-acting antiseizure medication can help determine if long-term treatment is warranted. If a benzodiazepine challenge clinically improves the patient and the EEG, they should be treated with longer-acting and maintenance medications. Commonly, benzodiazepines will abate any potentially ictal patterns on EEG, but the patient does not clinically improve, possibly because of benzodiazepine sedation. In this case, the clinical picture should be followed very closely, and further sedation should be avoided.

4. Super-refractory status epilepticus (SRSE) is defined as SE not controlled by third-line agents. About 10–15% of patients with SE will progress into SRSE [7]. The standard progression of SE treatment is tiered from a choice of one first-, second-, or third-line medication:

(a) First-line – lorazepam, diazepam, and midazolam
(b) Second-line – fosphenytoin, lacosamide, levetiracetam, phenobarbital, phenytoin, topiramate, and valproic acid
(c) Third-line continuous anesthetic infusion – midazolam, propofol, pentobarbital, thiopental, ketamine, and isoflurane

SRSE, though, emerges or continues despite anesthesia. At this point, there are several unproven strategies including surgery (lesionectomy, vagus nerve stimulator, deep brain stimulator), immunosuppression (methylprednisolone, intravenous immune globulin, plasmapheresis, allopregnanolone), noninvasive stimulation (electroconvulsive therapy, repetitive transcranial magnetic stimulation), or metabolic strategy (ketogenic diet, magnesium, pyridoxine). Of these, the ketogenic diet has likely shown the most promise [8, 9].

5. PRES is a condition of endothelial and blood-brain barrier damage leading to vasogenic edema. It has been reported that about 77% of patients with PRES will have seizures [9, 10]. Hypertensive emergency accounts for about 35% of cases, with pharmacologic immunosuppression involved in 58% of patients. Solid organ transplant patients are at increased risk because of the usage of calcineurin inhibitors, though the overall incidence is low. On EEG, generalized slowing is the most common feature (97.3%), followed by interictal discharges (11–28.9%). Only 0–5% of patients have seizures more than 1 month beyond hospitalization for PRES.

Pearls
- Critically ill patients are at high risk for seizures, especially nonconvulsive seizures with no, minimal, or easily missed clinical signs.
- Four indications for cEEG monitoring in the ICU are the detection of seizures, the characterization of encephalopathy, the detection of cerebral ischemia, and the diagnosis of abnormal hyperactive movements.
- 24 h of cEEG has a yield of >90% in diagnosing seizures, and therefore not much additional information is gained extending it to record 48 h.
- The meaning of the ictal-interictal continuum relative to outcome is still being discovered. Like NCSE, a trial of short-acting benzodiazepine ("benzodiazepine challenge") can help elucidate the impact of an abnormal EEG containing interictal discharges.
- Super-refractory NCSE is rare but has high morbidity. Appropriate treatments are still under investigation.

References

1. Privitera M, Hoffman M, Moore J, Jester D. EEG detection of nontonic-clonic status epilepticus in patients with altered consciousness. Epilepsy Res. 1994;18(2):155–66. Retrieved 21 May 2020, from https://ncbi.nlm.nih.gov/pubmed/7957038.
2. Claassen J, Mayer SA, Kowalski RG, Emerson RG, Hirsch LJ. Detection of electrographic seizures with continuous EEG monitoring in critically ill patients. Neurology. 2004;62(10):1743–8. Retrieved 21 May 2020, from https://ncbi.nlm.nih.gov/pubmed/15159471.
3. Newey CR, Kinzy TF, Punia V, Hantus S. Continuous electroencephalography in the critically ill: clinical and continuous electroencephalography markers for targeted monitoring. J Clin Neurophysiol. 2018;35(4):325–31.
4. Beniczky S, Hirsch LJ, Kaplan PW, Pressler R, Bauer G, Auerlien H, Brogger JC, Trinka E. Unified EEG terminology and criteria for nonconvulsive status epilepticus. Epilepsia. 2013;54(Suppl. 6):28–9.
5. Hirsch LJ, LaRoche SM, Gaspard N, Gerard E, Svoronos A, Herman S, Mani R, Arif H, Jette N, Minazad Y, Kerrigan J, Vestpa P, Hantus S, Claassen J, Young GB, So E, Kaplan PW, Nuwer MR, Fountain NB, Drislane FW. American Clinical Neurophysiology Society's standardized critical care EEG terminology: 2012 version. J Clin Neurophysiol. 2013;30:1–27.
6. Rubinos C, Reynolds AS, Claassen J. The Ictal-Interictal continuum: to treat of not to treat (and how)? Nuerocrit Care. 2018;29:3–8.
7. Kantanen AM, Reinikainen M, Parviainen I, Ruokonen E, Ala-Peijari M, Backlund T, Koskenkari J, Laitio R, Kalvaiainen R. Incidence and mortality of super-refractory status epilepticus in adults. Epilepsy Behav. 2015;49:1313–4.
8. Cervenka MC, Hocker S, Koenig M, Bar B, Henry-Barron B, Kossoff EH, Hargman A, Probasco JC, Benavides D, Venkatesan A, Hagen EC, Dittrich D, Stern T, Radzik B, Depew M, Caserta FM, Nyquist P, Kaplan PW, Geocadin RG. Phase I/II multicenter ketogenic diet study for adult superrefractory status epilepticus. Neurology. 2017;88(10):938–43.
9. Shah Z, Moran BP, McKinney AM, Henry TR. Seizure outcomes of posterior reversible encephalopathy syndrome and correlations with electroencephalographic changes. Epilepsy Behav. 2015;48:70–4.
10. Kastrup O, Gerwig M, Frings M, Diener HC. Posterior reversible encephalopathy syndrome (PRES): electroencephalographic findings and seizure patterns. J Neurol. 2012;259:1383–9.

Epilepsy in Older Adults

21

Joseph I. Sirven

Case Presentation

A 75-year-old man with hypertension, hyperlipidemia, and recent transient ischemic attack (TIA) presented to the neurology clinic with the chief complaint of worsening memory. The patient's family was concerned because despite a slow decline in his memory over the past 6 months, he recently has been found "staring quietly out the window." These new periods were associated with momentary lapses in attention lasting between 1 and 2 min at a time and occurring sporadically anytime of the day. There was no convulsive activity that was noted during these episodes of staring, and the patient was amnestic for the events. These newer spells affecting his memory began approximately 4 weeks after the patient had been discharged from the hospital for a TIA. There were no new medications that were begun other than low-dose aspirin. His current medications included hydrochlorothiazide and atorvastatin. There was no family history of any similar type of spells. Prior to the patient's admission to the hospital for a possible stroke which presented with changes in speech, there had been no other similar problems in the past. The patient denied smoking but occasionally enjoyed one mixed drink every week. The patient is a retired attorney who loves to do crossword puzzles and read books. His wife in particular is quite concerned that his short-term memory has significantly worsened since the onset of these events.

His neurological examination was otherwise normal. Magnetic resonance imaging of the brain was unrevealing. His EEG is displayed in Fig. 21.1.

The patient's wife has two specific questions: What are these episodes? And does my husband have Alzheimer's disease?

J. I. Sirven (✉)
Mayo Clinic, Department of Neurology, Jacksonville, FL, USA
e-mail: Sirven.Joseph@mayo.edu

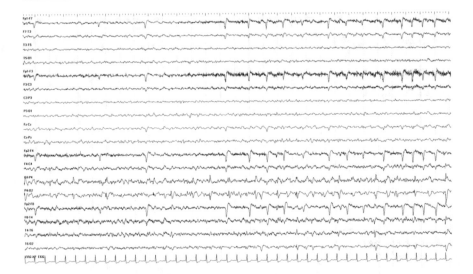

Fig. 21.1 EEG of the patient having a staring event during the EEG. There are frequent sharp waves at the F7 electrode that evolves into an electro clinical. The EEG clinched the diagnosis (partial seizure = focal seizure; simple partial = focal aware, GTC and partial seizure = focal to bilateral tonic-clonic and focal seizure)

Clinical Questions

1. How common are seizures in older adults?
2. Can seizures in older adults present with cognitive difficulties, and how do seizures vary between older and younger adults?
3. What should occur during an evaluation of seizures in older adults?
4. Are there any differences in the treatment of seizures in older adult as compared to younger adults?
5. Is there a correct choice of antiseizure drug in the older adult?

Diagnostic Discussion

1. Age in of itself is a risk factor for developing a first seizure and recurrent seizures or epilepsy. For people over age 60 years, the risk of a first seizure (1.27 in 1000) is almost twice as high as the risk in adults under age 60 years (0.52–0.59 in 1000). Seizure recurrence rates are also higher in adults over age 60 years (79% at 1 year and 83% at 3 years) compared with those under age 60 years (38–40%) [1].
2. Acute symptomatic seizures are more common in older adults, and focal impaired awareness seizures are the most common seizure type, followed by generalized tonic-clonic seizures (Fig. 21.2). Seizure presentation is also different in adults over age 60 in some very important ways. Auras are reported less often by older

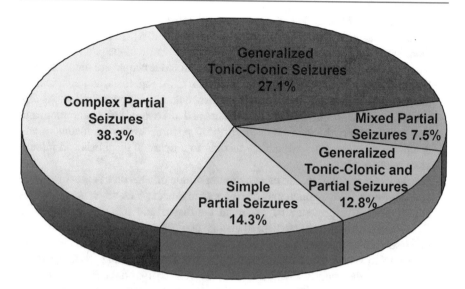

Fig. 21.2 Frequency of seizure types in older adults

individuals, and when they are, they tend to be nonspecific. When auras are appreciated, older people describe a nonspecific feeling of dizziness before a seizure event and have a greater tendency to have amnesia around the event. This may occur in patients with or without comorbid mild cognitive impairment, Alzheimer's disease, or dementia that is common in the elderly population. Auras may be reported less frequently because they are not able to be remembered or because of the seizure type or location of seizure onset. Typical auras present in younger adults with temporal lobe epilepsy, often described as a déjà vu, experiential, abdominal sensation, and fear or panic, are often not reported by older adults [2].

Older adults often have more extratemporal lobe epilepsies in the frontal and parietal lobes and less often arise from temporal lobe foci. Individuals with focal impaired awareness seizures tend to present with altered responsiveness, episodes of subtle staring, and confusion. The subtle presentation makes signs and symptoms associated with epileptic seizures difficult to tease out from other conditions. This is a hallmark of epilepsy and seizures that occur in older individuals. For example, older individuals who are hospitalized for urinary tract infections, pneumonia, or other medical conditions independent of preexisting seizures often have altered cognition, staring, or confusion. These patients with focal seizures might be literally staring us in the face, but because they have other conditions that present in a similar way, their seizures may go unrecognized [2].

The postictal state, the time that it takes for a person to recover after a seizure, is prolonged in approximately 14% of older individuals with epilepsy and may last as long as 24 h. Todd's paralysis, a postictal state that appears as localized paralysis and lasts for 15–24 h, occurs more frequently [2, 3]. Seizures can be more injurious in older individuals with epilepsy because of the relative frailty of older people. For example, falls from seizures in older people are more likely to lead to fracture because of the higher incidence of osteoporosis, and this, in turn, leads to higher levels of functional dependence and institutionalization. As discussed, amnesia around the time of a seizure and afterward is more common, and less recall means there is less reporting of seizures to family members and healthcare professionals, ultimately leading to a delay in diagnosis and incomplete treatment [4].

3. For the older population, the most common mimic of a seizure is syncope when consciousness is lost though may also appear to reflect a TIA when focal features are evident. The presence of post-ictal confusion and lethargy or cognitive changes is a fundamental element of history-taking for older individuals to separate a seizure from syncope or a TIA. Therefore, the evaluation of the older adult suspected of seizures is to obtain a carefully detailed history and physical examination. Enlisting family members and observers is important in providing an accurate history since the patient is often amnestic for recurrent events. It is important to inquire about recent changes in medications as well as investigate other systemic illnesses like infections and other common conditions that can cause seizures in older adults. The diagnostic evaluation with brain MRI, EEG, and laboratory testing is similar to that of younger aged patients with seizures to assess for systemic illnesses. In some cases, tilt table testing and event monitoring may be helpful to assist cardiac evaluation for abnormalities responsible for syncope [5, 6].

4. The considerations in the treatment of an older adult with seizures have to do with the many comorbidities that occur, including Alzheimer's disease and dementias, TIA and stroke, brain tumor, and other age-specific conditions seen in the elderly. Oftentimes, the situation is complicated by complex polypharmacy adding to altered memory and changes in mental status. For this reason, when starting ASM, many of which have cognitive side effects, it is critical to keep in mind the interactions and adverse effects that can occur. Older adults are more susceptible to cognitive side effects from medication. Tolerability is often dictated by a narrower therapeutic window due to normal metabolic changes that occur with aging (e.g., slower hepatic metabolism, decreased protein binding, and delayed renal clearance). Older adults are also prone to noncompliance with treatment because of memory dysfunction and other cognitive deficits and/or multiple sensory deficits (seeing, hearing, sensorimotor issues that may be present (e.g., difficulty reading the drug bottle label or trouble remembering to take medication as scheduled)). Drug bioavailability may also be influenced by other medications with similar metabolic clearance or protein binding. Specifically, anticoagulants (e.g., warfarin) and some of antihypertensives and statins can also have interactions with ASM. Complicating matters further, the serum levels that

we often check in younger adults may not be applicable to older adults because these come from studies of younger populations excluding older adults during regulatory trials.

5. Although studies have been done comparing certain ASM to assess which drug is best suited to older adults, results have shown that literally any ASM is appropriate for an older adults if one remembers the adage of "Start low and go slow" relative to initiation and titration.

A study of effective doses of ASM in older adults showed that many achieve freedom from seizure at doses lower than typically found to be effective in younger people. Older adults are also less likely to have epilepsy resistant to medical treatment. A tip in tripping elderly patients is to start the ASM dose low—half to two-thirds of initial dose recommended in younger adults—and go slow with longer periods of time in between dosage increases. This often allows for a lower total effective dose and is also far less likely to cause intolerable side effects. Use as few doses of ASM per day as possible, because the less often a drug is taken, the less often it can be forgotten. Remember that drug levels considered standard in younger individuals may not apply to older adults, and stay vigilant for clinical signs of clinical toxicity and least encountered side effects. Evaluate and reevaluate the medication regimen, and continue only those drugs for which a clear need can be established. This is done to potentially lessen the greater tendency toward polypharmacy. This is common in older adults and may be further complicated during and by treatment with ASM. Consider tapering and discontinuing ASM after a stroke or other acute symptomatic precipitating event to minimize the consequences of polypharmacy, and limit the cost of added medication in an older individual.

Clinical Pearls

1. Seizures are very common in older adults and may present with complaints of memory loss and recurrent subtle or vague spells.
2. Evaluation of the older adult with seizures is facilitated by speaking with family members to obtain an accurate history given the patients is often amnestic for seizures after they occur.
3. Diagnostic testing is similar to that of a younger adult and is etiology specific. Due to its greater frequency, additional studies such as tilt table testing may be required in order to differentiate between syncope and seizures.
4. "Start low and go slow" when selecting an ASM in older adults as oftentimes doses used for younger adults are excessive for aging patients.
5. Be aware of the numerous drug interactions that can occur between ASM and other medications used for comorbid conditions that are commonly seen in older adults.

References

1. Sapkota S, Kobau R, Pastula DM, et al. Close to 1 million US adults aged 55 years or older have active epilepsy-National Health Interview Survey, 2010, 2013, and 2015. Epilepsy Behav. 2018;87:233–4.
2. Cloyd J, Hauser W, Towne A, et al. Epidemiological and medical aspects of epilepsy in the elderly. Epilepsy Res. 2006;68(Suppl 1):S39–48.
3. Arif H, Buchsbaum R, Pierro J, et al. Comparative effectiveness of 10 antiepileptic drugs in older adults with epilepsy. Arch Neurol. 2010;67(4):408–15.
4. England MJ, Liverman CT, Schultz AM, Strawbridge LM, editors. Epilepsy across the spectrum: promoting health and understanding. Washington, DC: Institute of Medicine of the National Academies of Medicine; 2012.
5. LaRoche S, Taylor D, Walter P. Tilt table testing with video EEG monitoring in the evaluation of patients with unexplained loss of consciousness. Clin EEG Neurosci. 2011;42(3):202–5.
6. Lawn N, Kelly A, Dunne J, et al. First seizure in the older patient: clinical features and prognosis. Epilepsy Res. 2013;107(1–2):109–14.

Seizures and Renal/Liver Failure

22

David B. Burkholder

Case Presentation

A 42-year-old man with end-stage renal disease (ESRD) on intermittent hemodialysis presents with seizures. He's had 8 in the past 18 months. These are all described as generalized tonic-clonic seizures. All have occurred at the end of dialysis, or not long after. His mother felt it may be due to low blood sugar, so they gave him snacks before and during dialysis without benefit. Adjustments to dialysis, including more gradual dialysis, failed to impact seizures. He was placed on levetiracetam but continued to have seizures in the same pattern. He was previously on the kidney transplant list but was removed until his seizures could be controlled. MRI of the brain was normal. EEG showed bifrontal sharp waves.

Examination showed very-low-amplitude multi-directional twitches of the fingers, consistent with polyminimyoclonus, and was otherwise normal.

Clinical Questions

1. What can cause seizures in renal and hepatic disease?
2. What drug properties dictate pharmacokinetics?
3. How are pharmacokinetics affected in renal and hepatic disease?
4. What are the pharmacokinetic properties of antiseizure drugs?
5. How does ASD dosing change depending on renal and hepatic disease?

D. B. Burkholder (✉)
Mayo Clinic, Department of Neurology, Rochester, MN, USA
e-mail: burkholder.david@mayo.edu

© Springer Nature Switzerland AG 2021
W. O. Tatum et al. (eds.), *Epilepsy Case Studies*,
https://doi.org/10.1007/978-3-030-59078-9_22

Discussion

1. Epilepsy aside, seizures may occur in either liver or renal disease, with a common cause being an accumulation of toxins. Seizures occur in about one-third of patients with uremic encephalopathy due to kidney disease [1]. In ESRD, hemodialysis can also cause seizures related to rapid shifts in concentrations of urea. This is more likely to be problematic in new dialysis patients or patients who are resuming dialysis after missed sessions, or rapid dialysis. Dialysis dementia is a progressive dialysis-related complication caused by aluminum use as a phosphate binder, but this is now rarely seen due to use of non-aluminum phosphate binders. Seizures are uncommon in hepatic disease but can occur related to cerebral edema or effects on neurotransmission from hyperammonemia [2]. While there appeared to be association with dialysis in our patient, changes to his dialysis did not change his seizures, so treatment would be advisable.

2. While many factors impact drug concentrations, for clinical purposes, focus can be maintained on clearance (CL), volume of distribution (V_d), and elimination half-life ($t_{1/2}$). Table 22.1 provides definitions for these terms [3]. CL of a drug may be through hepatic, renal, and other mechanisms. CL is often a combination of all of these pathways. Steady-state concentration is particularly correlated with CL rate. V_d relies on multiple factors including body composition, drug properties, and protein binding – which may be related to drug properties or affected by pathophysiologic processes. Drugs that are widely diffused throughout tissues and therefore have a high V_d are more lipophilic, less ionized, and less protein bound and so are more able to diffuse out of plasma. Only drug present in plasma is available to be eliminated.

    Elimination $t_{1/2}$ is directly affected by both CL and V_d, outlined by the equation:

$$t_{1/2} = 0.693 \times V_d/CL$$

   The relationship between factors is intuitive. CL has an inverse relationship with $t_{1/2}$ such that as CL increases (i.e., drug is cleared more quickly), $t_{1/2}$ decreases. Conversely, V_d has a direct relationship with $t_{1/2}$, so as V_d declines (i.e., drug is readily available in plasma to be eliminated), so does $t_{1/2}$.

3. *Kidney Disease*

    Kidney disease is a common entity with numerous potential causes, a wide range of severity, and a variable time profile in that it can be acute and reversible or chronic and progressive. With such a complex disease, understanding its impact on ASDs is critical to providing appropriate management and anticipating the need for changes.

Table 22.1 Definition of pharmacokinetic terms

Clearance (CL)	Amount of plasma volume entirely cleared of drug by unit time
Volume of distribution (V_d)	The theoretical volume required to produce the same drug concentration found in plasma after an oral or parenteral dose
Elimination half-life ($t_{1/2}$)	Amount of time required for half of a concentration of drug to be cleared from the body

Drug CL is impacted by kidney disease in different ways depending on the mechanism by which the drug is cleared. The simplest cause-effect association occurs in drugs that are primarily eliminated renally. In acute and chronic kidney disease, glomerular filtration is reduced, and renal drug transport may be impaired, leading to slower CL and accumulation of drug or active metabolites. However, ASDs that are primarily metabolized through hepatic enzymatic activity may also be affected. Uremic toxicity can result in enzymatic inhibition even in patients with healthy livers, which in turn can also act to reduce CL and increase drug concentrations. Enzymatic activity in this scenario may be repaired by uremia correction through renal replacement therapy, but that may itself affect ASD dosing requirements [3].

V_d also has kidney-dependent changes. Some of this has to do with the above mechanisms but also is dependent upon body composition. Fluid retention may increase the V_d of a drug so that plasma concentrations are relatively reduced, thereby requiring higher dosing to achieve desired plasma levels. Protein function may be impaired, leading to an increase in free drug in plasma and in general an associated increase in V_d [3].

Liver Disease

Hepatic CL via enzymatic metabolism is the way that most drugs in general are removed from circulation. The liver is also important to the production of proteins and filtering of non-drug toxins. Predictably, liver disease results in many changes that can affect ASD dosing.

A decrease in hepatic CL occurs through multiple mechanisms. Hepatopathies result in decreased enzymatic activity in both cytochrome P450 (CYP) and UDT-glucuronosyltransferase (UGT) pathways related to decreased perfusion through multiple mechanisms. It is possible that UGT pathways are less affected, but not entirely spared, compared to CYP-mediated metabolism. CYP dysfunction also appears to depend on the severity of hepatic dysfunction and the specific CYP isoform. In chronic hepatic disease, porto-systemic shunting results in a bypass of hepatic circulation back into systemic circulation without being exposed to liver filtration, thereby reducing both first-pass and subsequent metabolisms. These porto-systemic shunts may be disease-related (e.g. esophageal varices or splenorenal shunting) or iatrogenic to reduce portal hypertension (transjugular intrahepatic porto-systemic shunt, or TIPS) [4].

V_d is affected by both protein and fluid-related changes. An injured liver has a reduced capacity to produce albumin and other proteins in terms of both amount and efficiency, leading to less available and lower-quality circulating proteins and therefore more unbound drug. Chronic liver disease can also result in ascites due to portal hypertension. Increased availability of unbound drug and accumulation of extravascular fluid can both result in an increase in V_d [4].

In some cases, patients with cirrhosis or liver failure can develop hepatorenal syndrome, where renal failure is ultimately caused by preceding hepatic disease [4]. This creates more complicated considerations for ASM dosing due to the effects that renal function has on drug elimination outlined earlier in this chapter.

4. The pharmacokinetic properties of ASMs vary significantly between drugs. Table 22.2 outlines the different properties of common and newer ASMs as provided by the Food and Drug Administration-approved package insert.
5. In patients with kidney or hepatic disease, special attention should be paid to the known pharmacokinetic properties of ASDs being considered or continued in conjunction with the severity of their disease. Most dosing recommendations are based on disease severity. For kidney disease, severity is stratified by creatinine clearance. In liver disease, the Child-Pugh score is most commonly used to stratify severity (Table 22.3).

Dosing recommendations, when applicable, uniformly call for a reduced dose based on the anticipation of decreased CL and changes in V_d related to the properties of the ASM used and organ system affected [5]. Dosing recommendations depend on clinical conditions; however, providers should be aware that most ASMs do not have studied dosing strategies for end-organ disease [4]. Therefore, the most important rule is to be attentive when treating patients with epilepsy and either kidney or liver dysfunction. Table 22.4 indicates which ASDs are recommended to have dosing adjustments in kidney or hepatic disease, or post-dialysis supplemental dosing.

In the case of ESRD on intermittent hemodialysis, the V_d and protein binding properties of the ASD used must be carefully considered in order to anticipate

Table 22.2 Common and newer antiseizure medication pharmacokinetics

	Primary elimination	% unchanged in urine	% protein bound	V_d	$t_{1/2}$ (hours)
Brivaracetam	Hydrolysis, CYP2C19	<10	<20	0.5 L/kg	9
Carbamazepine (ER)	CYP3A4	3	70–80	0.8–2 L/kg	12–17
Cenobamate	UGT	6	60	40–50 L	50–60
Clobazam	CYP3A4 (active metabolite CYP2C19)	2	80–90	100 L	36–42
Divalproex sodium	Multiple	<3	73–92	11 L	9–16
Eslicarbazepine	UGT, renal	66	<40	61 L	13–20
Ethosuximide	CYP3A4	10–20	–	0.6–0.7 L/kg	17–56
Lacosamide	CYP2C19	40	<15	0.6 L/kg	13
Lamotrigine	UGT	10	55	0.9–1.3 L/kg	25–33
Levetiracetam	Renal	66	<10	0.7 L/kg	6–8
Oxcarbazepine (metabolite)	UGT	27	40	49 L	9
Perampanel	CYP3A4	–	95–96	–	105
Phenobarbital	CYP2C9/2C19	25	45–50	0.5–1 L/kg	70–140
Phenytoin	CYP2C9	<5	90–95	0.5–1 L/kg	14–22
Topiramate	Renal	70	15–41	0.6–0.8 L/kg	21
Zonisamide	CYP3A4	35	40	1.45 L/kg	63

Table 22.3 Child-Pugh score for liver disease severity

	Points		
	+1	+2	+3
Total bilirubin (mg/dL)	<2	2–3	>3
Albumin (g/dL)	>3.5	2.8–3.5	<2.8
INR	<1.7	1.7–2.3	>2.3
Ascites	Absent	Mild	Moderate-severe
Encephalopathy	None	Grade 1–2	Grade 3–4

Class A = <7 points – mild
Class B = 7–9 points – moderate
Class C = >9 points – severe

Table 22.4 Need for dosing change or supplementation for common and newer antiseizure medications

	Is dose adjustment recommended?		
	Kidney disease	Post-dialysis supplementation	Hepatic disease
Brivaracetam			✓
Carbamazepine			✓ (probably)
Cenobamate			✓
Clobazam			✓ (probably)
Divalproex sodium			NR
Eslicarbazepine	✓	+/−	NR in severe disease
Ethosuximide	+/−	+/−	+/−
Lacosamide	✓	✓	✓
Lamotrigine			✓ in moderate-severe disease
Levetiracetam	✓	✓	
Oxcarbazepine	✓ if CrCl <30 mL/min		
Perampanel	NR if CrCL <30 mL/min	NR	✓
Phenobarbital			✓ (probably)
Phenytoin			✓ (probably)
Topiramate	✓		+/−
Zonisamide	+/−; NR if GFR <50 mL/min		+/−

✓ dose change or supplementation recommended, +/− use with caution, NR use not recommended, CrCl creatinine clearance, GFR glomerular filtration rate

when drug is dialyzed and therefore may require post-dialysis supplemental dosing. Similarly, patient-related factors may dictate that a non-dialyzed ASD be used, requiring prescriber awareness of these factors. Some ASDs may or may not require supplemental dosing after dialysis [1]. If unsure as to the need for supplementation, a drug level (including free and total, when applicable) may be drawn after dialysis and at the same time on a non-dialysis day and compared. If the post-dialysis level is significantly lower than the non-dialysis level, and falls below the threshold level desired by the prescribing provider, then supplemental dosing may be useful.

Older non-dialyzed drugs, like phenytoin and valproate, have largely been replaced by newer ASMs that have more favorable drug-drug interaction profiles, including levetiracetam. However, the timing of seizures with our patient is important to consider in his treatment. His seizures were strictly at the end of or shortly after dialysis, so dialyzed drugs like levetiracetam would be less likely to be effective at preventing his seizures as the drug would be at its nadir exactly at the time that the patient's seizure risk would be highest. He was started on phenytoin and, with close monitoring, had his dose adjusted until his free drug level was within the reference range (1–2 mcg/mL) with a corresponding total level of 8 mcg/mL (usual reference range 10–20 mcg/mL). He remained seizure-free thereafter.

Pearls of Wisdom
- Pharmacokinetic properties are altered by kidney and liver disease, resulting in impaired CL and V_d changes that usually increase $t_{1/2}$ and drug concentrations.
- ASM dose adjustments may be required depending on the drug used and the diseased organ system. When problems are anticipated, an ASM can be selected that allows for use without adjustment in certain circumstances.
- In cases where the V_d is increased due to fluid retention, like ascites or edema, a higher than usual loading dose of an ASM may be needed acutely to achieve adequate levels. In that case, levels should be closely monitored to ensure appropriate dosing.
- The Child-Pugh score is most often used to assess severity of liver disease as it pertains to ASM dosing adjustments.
- Supplemental dosing after dialysis is needed for some ASMs, particularly levetiracetam and lacosamide.

References

1. Titoff V, Moury HN, Titoff IB, Kelly KM. Seizures, antiepileptic drugs, and CKD. Am J Kidney Dis. 2018;73(1):90–101.
2. Ferenci P. Hepatic encephalopathy. Gastroenterol Rep (Oxf). 2017;5(2):138–47.
3. Lea-Henry TN, Carland JE, Stocker SL, Sevastos J, Roberts DM. Clinical pharmacokinetics in kidney disease: fundamental principles. Clin J Am Soc Nephrol. 2018;13:1085–95.
4. Verbeeck RK. Pharmacokinetics and dosage adjustment in patients with hepatic dysfunction. Eur J Clin Pharmacol. 2008;64:1147–61.
5. Asconapé JJ. Use of antiepileptic drugs in hepatic and renal disease. Handb Clin Neurol. 2014;119:417–32.

Antiseizure Drugs and Seizure Aggravation

23

Matthew Hoerth

Case Presentation

A 21-year-old female presents with a history of seizures beginning at about the age of 5. Her seizures had variable control over the years. Currently, the seizures have been occurring about twice a month and have been associated with her menstrual cycle. Additionally, they seem to also be exacerbated by lack of sleep and alcohol use. She had occasions where she experienced an aura that she could not describe well, but states that with her seizures she "blanks out." The patient states that she has convulsions that typically occur at night or in the early morning hours. Other seizures she describes are events where "everything goes black." She has not had an EEG or brain MRI in the last 5 years.

Since her seizure diagnosis, she has been on multiple antiseizure medications. She believes that she was on phenytoin earlier in life. At one point in time, she remembers valproic acid was added to her regimen and she ended up in the hospital with status epilepticus. More recently, she has been taking carbamazepine for the past 7 years. Seizure control fluctuated over her lifetime, but she has never been seizure-free. The patient's seizures had worsened ever since she began her menstrual cycles beginning at the age of 12. The patient brings some previous laboratory studies. Her carbamazepine level 6 months ago was reported as 5.6 mcg/mL (normal 4.0–12.0 mcg/mL). She states that at the time of this previous lab test, she was taking 400 mg of the extended release formulation twice a day. The patient explains that after this level, her previous neurologist increased the dose to 600 mg twice a day in an attempt to get her blood levels close to the high therapeutic range, since she was still having both "auras" multiple times per week and generalized tonic-clonic seizures every other month.

M. Hoerth (✉)
Mayo Clinic, Department of Neurology, Phoenix, AZ, USA
e-mail: hoerth.matthew@mayo.edu

© Springer Nature Switzerland AG 2021
W. O. Tatum et al. (eds.), *Epilepsy Case Studies*,
https://doi.org/10.1007/978-3-030-59078-9_23

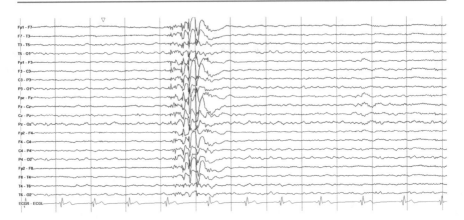

Fig. 23.1 Example of EEG findings demonstrating a brief burst of generalized spike-and-wave discharges

Currently, the patient states that the "auras" have actually been worse in the last 6 months. She attributes the worsening seizures to increased stress of moving, but then explains that she is quite happy with her new job that she obtained after graduation. The move and transition went very smoothly. Her laboratory studies were rechecked on the day of presentation, with a carbamazepine level of 7.3 mcg/ml. She reports that she has been compliant with her ASM, and, since graduating college, she has established a regular sleep schedule. In this patient's case, a repeat MRI was normal with a routine EEG demonstrating generalized spike-and-wave discharges during light sleep (Fig. 23.1).

Questions

1. From the patient's clinical history, what type of epilepsy does this patient have?
2. Why did the patient have the episode of status epilepticus after valproate was added to her regimen?
3. Why did the carbamazepine level only increase a mild degree when the dose was increased significantly?
4. What is the reason that the patient's seizures continue and potentially even worsen despite increasing doses of ASM?
5. What is the best treatment choice for the patient at this point?

Discussion Points

1. The first step to approaching a new patient for the evaluation of seizures is to determine if the patient is having epileptic seizures. Ruling out seizure mimics is the first priority. When epilepsy is diagnosed, the next step is to determine the seizure type or types [1, 2]. The patient in this case has a diagnosis of genetic

generalized epilepsy and sporadic tonic-clonic seizures and absence seizures. This may not have been completely apparent from the patient's initial case presentation; however, certain features may have brought this suspicion. These features include the nocturnal nature of the events and the early onset in life. The patient described "auras" and "blank outs" though despite their relationship to focal seizures, in our patient they likely represent absence seizures. Patient terminology should not always be taken at face value. Even though the patient had been taken care of by a previous neurologist, the diagnosis should be re-evaluated. Previous records should be obtained or, if appropriate, repeat testing would be justified. The EEG with generalized spike-and-waves supports a clinical diagnosis of a genetic generalized epilepsy with the age of onset suggesting the epilepsy syndrome of childhood absence epilepsy persisting into adulthood with recurrent absence and generalized tonic-clonic seizures.

2. The fact that the patient did poorly when valproate was added to existing phenytoin can be explained by drug-drug interactions. With phenytoin and other seizure medications including valproate, drug-drug interactions can be complex as both antiseizure medications are highly protein bound. It is not predictable whether the drug level of phenytoin would increase, decrease, or stay the same [3]. Drug monitoring in this case would be helpful to determine the extent of the interaction, rather than simply stating that valproate worsened the patient's seizures as shifts in free fractions may have increased free phenytoin levels to aggravate seizures.

3. The choice of carbamazepine for this patient should also be avoided (see Table 23.1). Carbamazepine is an enzyme-inducing ASM metabolized by the hepatic P450 system and may also aggravate generalized seizures [1–4]. Further carbamazepine undergoes autoinduction and by 6 weeks has the effect of reducing its own serum concentration. This explains why the patient's carbamazepine level was lower than intended despite a significant dosage increase. Monitoring of the serum concentration of antiseizure medication (especially first-generation drugs) can be helpful [3].

Table 23.1 Effectiveness of antiseizure drugs relative to specific seizure types

Efficacy	Focal	Generalized tonic-clonic	Absence	Myoclonic
Carbamazepine	X		May worsen	May worsen
Phenytoin	X		May worsen	May worsen
Levetiracetam	X	X	X	X
Valproate	X	X	X	X
Lamotrigine	X	X	X	May worsen in some patients
Topiramate	X	X	X	X
Ethosuximide			X	
Most all other antiseizure medications	X			

4. Ultimately, carbamazepine is not a good long-term choice of ASM for this patient with other non-enzyme inducing ASMs available. When seizure classification is unclear, a ASM that is effective for all or nearly all seizure types (broad spectrum) should be chosen [5]. Since there is a suspicion for a genetic generalized epilepsy, avoidance of certain ASMs such as carbamazepine and phenytoin that could aggravate seizure control in patients with genetic generalized epilepsies including absence and myoclonic seizures should be attempted. This was evidenced with this patient in that her seizure control worsened with the increased dose.
5. A medication such as lamotrigine would be a better consideration for this patient [5]. Although several other choices exist, lamotrigine is an effective broad-spectrum ASM, showing efficacy for our patient's seizure types. Additionally, there is a relatively low side effect profile as well as a relatively lower risk of teratogenicity. As always, counseling regarding birth control should be completed.

Pearls
1. When seizures are not under control, especially after multiple ASM, reconsider the diagnosis and confirm with video-EEG monitoring if necessary.
2. The interaction between phenytoin and other ASMs can be complex due to zero-order pharmacokinetic, and the potential for a drug-drug interaction that is high. When valproate is combined with phenytoin, it may decrease, increase, or not change the levels of total (bound) and free (unbound) fractions of the phenytoin concentration.
3. Carbamazepine is a strong hepatic enzyme-inducing ASM and may reduce the serum drug concentrations of other medications and also induce its own metabolism.
4. Most ASMs (please note exceptions exist) are effective for focal seizures. When a patient has generalized seizures related to genetic generalized epilepsies, ASMs such as carbamazepine and phenytoin may aggravate seizure control and worsen absence and myoclonic seizures.
5. It is ideal to know the specific epilepsy diagnosis, or at least the seizure types, in order to prescribe the appropriate ASM. When the seizure types are unknown, consider a broad-spectrum (works for most/all seizure types) ASM.

References

1. Abou-Khalil BW. Antiepileptic drugs. Continuum (Minneap Minn). 2016;22(1 Epilepsy):132–56. https://doi.org/10.1212/CON.0000000000000289.
2. Abou-Khalil BW. Update on antiepileptic drugs 2019. Continuum (Minneap Minn). 2019;25(2):508–36. https://doi.org/10.1212/CON.0000000000000715.

3. Patsalos PN, Spencer EP, Berry DJ. Therapeutic drug monitoring of antiepileptic drugs in epilepsy: a 2018 update. Ther Drug Monit. 2018;40(5):526–48. https://doi.org/10.1097/FTD.0000000000000546.
4. French JA, Gidal BE. Antiepileptic drug interactions. Epilepsia. 2000;41(Suppl 8):S30–6. https://doi.org/10.1111/j.1528-1157.2000.tb02944.x.
5. Kanner AM, Ashman E, Gloss D, et al. Practice guideline update summary: efficacy and tolerability of the new antiepileptic drugs I: treatment of new-onset epilepsy: report of the guideline development, dissemination, and implementation Subcommittee of the American Academy of Neurology and the American Epilepsy Society. Neurology. 2018;91(2):74–81. https://doi.org/10.1212/WNL.0000000000005755.

Driving and Epilepsy

24

Joseph F. Drazkowski

Case Presentation

The patient is a 24-year-old male who presents to the emergency room (ER) for a history of recurrent "spells" while working the overnight shift at a local casino as card dealer. As observed by co-workers, the spell consisted of the patient staring off into space for about 30 s and being unresponsive to questions with no abnormal movements. Upon arrival in the ER, the patient was noted to be awake but was having difficulty answering questions. The patient's vital signs were normal as was a computer tomography (CT) of the brain. Routine lab tests including CBC, CMP, Mg, EKG, and urine drug screen were all normal. Thirty minutes after admission, the patient was back to baseline physically and cognitively. The patient was given the diagnosis of transient altered awareness and instructed to see a neurologist as soon as possible. No discussion about driving restrictions due to altered awareness occurred in the ER. The patient's motor vehicle license was issued in a state that requires the healthcare provider to report to the driving authorities for altered awareness and seizures. Driving restrictions in the patient's state requires a seizure-free interval of 6 months before returning to drive.

Two weeks later, the patient was evaluated by the neurologist. Upon further questioning, the neurologist noted that the patient was actually having similar attacks for the last 6 months occurring about once a week. The patient did report a 5–10 s aura of déjà vu before 80% of his attacks. The neurologist suggested a magnetic resonance image (MRI) with high-resolution cuts through the temporal lobes which later showed imaging characteristics of mesial temporal sclerosis in the right hemisphere. The patient was given a prescription for medication to treat the seizures. During the evaluation and office visit, the neurologist diligently discussed the

J. F. Drazkowski (✉)
Mayo Clinic, Department of Neurology, Phoenix, AZ, USA
e-mail: Drazkowski.Joseph@mayo.edu

co-morbidities and the social consequences of epilepsy. In the conversation, there was appropriate discussion of anti-seizure medication side effects, safety, sudden unexpected death in epilepsy, mood disorders, and finally driving motor vehicles. During the conversation the neurologist informed the patient that the patient was restricted from driving for 6 months as long as he remained seizure-free. The patient was then informed that according to state law the clinician is required to report the patient to the Department of Motor Vehicles and he should immediately stop driving. The patient was visibly disappointed and upset about the inability to legally drive and especially about the fact that the motor vehicle department would be informed. The inability to drive back and forth to work was especially troubling to the patient, being worried about possible loss of employment and independence. The office visit was going well until the discussion about driving, after which the patient stormed out of the office. A 6-month follow-up visit was scheduled.

After leaving the office, the patient continued to be upset, especially about the driving restrictions placed on him by state law. The patient tried the medication for seizures and was doing well without noting any seizures except for a rare aura. After about 3 months, the patient noted possible side effects in addition to the auras. He was reluctant to call the neurologist to discuss his situation as he was concerned about the possible extension of the driving restrictions. He never did call for advice and lowered the dose of the medication unilaterally and felt better. The patient noted no definite seizures 2 months later and made the decision on his own to begin driving to work as he was having difficulty getting rides from friends. Taxis and ride share services in his area were expensive and public transportation was lacking, especially for night shift workers. Four months later, while at work on the night shift, the patient while on break was found on the floor unconscious and EMS was called. The patient slowly began to awaken and remained confused for several minutes and on the way to the ER he returned to baseline. In the ER, he was evaluated and noted to be normal without injury. The patient informed the provider that he felt he was dehydrated after working in the yard for several hours in the heat earlier in the afternoon. Being at baseline the patient was released and told to follow-up with his primary care physician as soon as possible. No discussion of driving restriction occurred at this visit. On discharge from the hospital, the patient took a taxi ride back to his workplace, his shift was now over, and he proceeded to gather his things to go home. He got in his car, and on the way home, he was involved in a single vehicle car crash and hit a bridge abutment. The patient was rescued and was admitted to the ICU for the next month due to numerous serious injuries.

Clinical Questions

1. What is the risk for motor vehicle crashes due to seizure/epilepsy?
2. What is the obligation for the clinician to report the person with epilepsy to driving authorities?
3. How important is the ability to operate a motor vehicle to the person with epilepsy (PWE)?

4. How good is the medical community at informing patients about driving restriction?
5. How does the driving risk for people with epilepsy (PWE) compare to other medical conditions, and what are the characteristics of car crashes due to seizures?

Discussion

1. The risk of a vehicle crash for the PWE of having a crash due to a seizure is historically low. The actual crash rates for the PWE remain elusive as published reports are retrospective. The actual number of PWE driving illegally is largely unknown but probably represents a significant minority. Other factors that complicate the issue are that PWE may drive against medical advice as in this case [3]. The ability to be independent and sometimes keep a job depends on the ability to drive. The number of crashes due to seizure directly is likely low as most all counties, and all the states in the USA have specific restrictions for the person with recent seizures from driving. Most patients will follow the law, and thus the overall numbers of seizure-related crashes remain low. For example, in a retrospective study looking at crashes related to medical conditions, the number of crashes in Arizona related to seizure was 0.04%.
2. The legal obligation to report the PWE to driving authorities is variable from state to state [3]. Some states, as in this case, require providers to report the PWE to driving authorities (Table 24.1). The reporting requirement has been shown to impair the communication between the physician and patient. In this case, the fear of being reported to authorities is a powerful motivator for patients to not to report all seizures or concerns to treating physician. In the ER the attending physician and the neurologist were not informed largely motivated by a fear of being reported to the authorities. In this case, the ER physician was not fully informed by the patient of the very important history of seizures.
3. The privilege to legally drive a motor vehicle is a major determinant of quality of life for many PWE. In some locations the desire to drive is not as strong as in other areas. For example, many major metropolitan areas may have well-developed public transportation systems that are accessible and affordable. Rural locations with less well-developed public transportation options may have more motivation to

Table 24.1 States that require physicians to report PWE to their State Medical Transportation Board	Delaware
	California
	Nevada
	New Jersey
	Oregon
	Pennsylvania
	See https://www.epilepsy.com/driving-laws (Accessed 5 Jan 2020) for up-to-date driving regulations [4]

obtain a license to drive. The seizure-free interval (SFI) is still the gold standard used by the states to be allowed to drive and ranges from as little as 3–12 months with several states having variable SFI. It should also be emphasized that the PWE must also pass all the typical required reading and physical requirements to pass standardized written and on road testing. The SFI defines the minimum time required not to drive and should be followed per local regulations. It should be remembered that sometimes other factors should be considered in the decision of driving or not. A patient history of non-compliance, lack of trust, medication toxicities, or even other co-morbidities should be taken into account when making a decision.

4. A clinician (typically a neurologist) who treats PWE is often well versed in having discussions about driving. In this case, during the two ER visits, the patient was not counselled about driving on either occasion. Although we typically strive to do treat the patient to the best of our ability, counselling the person presenting with altered mental status about driving after an event with altered mental status sometimes is not accomplished in practice. Advocating for our patients sometimes means giving advice not to drive for the safety of the patient and other drivers on public roads. In general, the neurologist is better than other providers at giving driving advice in the ER after an episode of altered awareness, but there is room for improvement for all providers. The discussion should be documented when it does occur.

5. The risk of PWE crashing while driving has been studied and compares to the general population and to people with other medical conditions. Restrictions placed on PWE ability to drive should be based on what is known about the actual risks. The risks for the PWE have been shown to be similar to drivers with medical conditions including diabetes, cardiovascular disease, and even mental health disorders. Old age (>80Y/O) and young males both have significantly higher relative risks of causing crashes than the PWE, and society permits these people to drive despite the higher crash risk.

Clinical Pearls
1. Physicians familiar with PWE and driving issues often face disappointment from the patient when told they are not legally able to drive due to seizures. This decision can have implications for independence, going to school, and sometimes working. The discussion necessarily requires time, understanding of the requirements, and enough time during the visit to explain and discuss the situation thoroughly. When there is trust between clinicians and the PWE, there is a better chance meaningful communication and thorough understanding of what needs to happen with a better chance of it occurring. The sometimes one visit is not enough to make such an important decision, especially with complex cases. Reminding the PWE of the potential consequences of driving illegally often persuades the PWE.

2. There are patterns and characteristics of car crashes due to seizures. The crashes due to seizures are more often single vehicle crashes, striking objects such as the abutment as in our case. The crashes caused by the PWE as a result of seizure are associated with injury more often than not, often serious injury [5, 6]. Often the patient does not express concern about their own safety caused by crashes due to seizures. Appealing to their sense of responsibility if they were to injure another person often helps lead to the correct decision about driving or not driving. Alternatives to driving can also be discussed, such as public transportation, and even ride sharing services may soften the blow, when no driving is suggested/required. We should also recall that we as practitioners for the most part do not make the ultimate decision about who drives and who does not. In most cases, the ultimate decision falls to local driving authorities.

3. Epilepsy is often a dynamic disease, and therefore the driving discussion is as well. Practitioners who treat epilepsy know this all too well. Sometimes stable epilepsy patients have break through seizures. The driving laws vary from state to state. If the recurrence is explainable such as a non-recurring illness or being prescribed a proconvulsant medication, the situation may be handled differently than non-compliance or unprovoked seizure recurrence. Check and know your local regulations.

4. Many states have official forms (medical assessment forms) that need to be filled out when patients are applying or re-applying for reinstatement of driving privileges. The forms often require signatures from applicant (PWE) and the physician. The forms are legal documents and should be treated accordingly. Many caregivers find such things time consuming and frustrating. This part of the job is important for the patient applying to retain or begin driving for improved quality of life; your patients will appreciate the effort. Many states have required follow-up forms to be filled out through annual or other specified visits.

5. The ability to drive a motor vehicle for the PWE is a privilege and not a right. Thus, the patient and the practitioner both must understand and participate in the process about driving legally. The decision is one of the most important ones to be made and affects quality of life, going to school, and impacting family plans and employment in many cases. Mutual trust and individualizing delivery of this information is a must [7].

References

1. Drazkowski J, Fisher R, et al. Seizure related motor vehicle crashes in Arizona before and after reducing the driving restriction from 12 to 3 months. Mayo Clin Proc. 2003;78:819–25.
2. Neiman E, Drazkowski J, et al. Frequency of physician counseling and attitudes towards driving motor vehicles in people with epilepsy: comparing a mandatory –reporting with a voluntary reporting state. Epilepsy Behav. 2010;19(1):52–4.

3. Shareef Y, McKinnon J, et al. Counseling for driving restrictions in epilepsy and other causes of temporary impairment of consciousness: how are we doing? Epilepsy Behav. 2009;14:550–2.
4. Epilepsy.com States Driving Laws; Accessed 13 Apr 2020.
5. Sheth S, Krauss G, et al. Mortality and epilepsy: driving fatalities vs. other causes of death in patients with epilepsy. Neurology. 2004;63:1002–7.
6. Neal A, et al. Characteristics of motor vehicle crashes associated with seizures. Neurology. 2018;91(12):e1102.
7. Tatum WO, Worley A, Selenica M-L. Disobedience and driving in epilepsy. Epilepsy Behav. 2012;23(1):30–5.

Frontal Lobe Epilepsy

25

Lily C. Wong-Kisiel and Gregory A. Worrell

Abbreviations

EEG	Electroencephalography
FDG	Fluorodeoxyglucose
MRI	Magnetic resonance imaging
MEG	Magnetoencephalography
PET	Positron emission tomography
SEEG	Stereoelectroencephalography
SPECT	Single-photon emission computed tomography
SPM	Statistical parametric mapping

Case Presentation

A 16-year-old right-handed teenager with seizure onset at age 11 years had habitual seizures from sleep where he would suddenly arouse and sit up, kicking his legs in bicycling movement around 30 s, and poorly responsive afterward up to a minute. Initial EEG showed nonspecific slowing in the bifrontal region, maximal over the right frontocentral head region. Prolonged video EEG showed bifrontal spike and sharp waves with a hypermotor seizure from sleep with indeterminate EEG onset. MRI brain 3 T showed an asymmetry of the lateral ventricles, increased ventricle size in the right, and nonspecific T2 signals in the subcortical white matter in the left frontal lobe. His epilepsy remained refractory to oxcarbazepine, lacosamide, and zonisamide. There is no family history of epilepsy.

L. C. Wong-Kisiel (✉) · G. A. Worrell
Mayo Clinic, Department of Neurology, Rochester, MN, USA
e-mail: wongkisiel.lily@mayo.edu; worrell.gregory@mayo.edu

© Springer Nature Switzerland AG 2021
W. O. Tatum et al. (eds.), *Epilepsy Case Studies*,
https://doi.org/10.1007/978-3-030-59078-9_25

Epilepsy surgery evaluation at age 16 years included prolonged video EEG which showed no interictal discharges. Electroclinical seizures were characterized by arousal from sleep and hyperkinetic movements including bilateral bicycling leg movements, grunting and vocalization, restlessness, and unresponsiveness. The ictal EEG onset was either non-localized or arose from the right frontotemporal head region (Fig. 25.1). Interictal magnetoencephalography (MEG) dipoles associated with epileptiform discharges were detected bilaterally in the frontal, posterior temporal, and posterior insular head regions. Repeat MRI brain 7 T MRI showed no definitive epileptogenic focus. Statistical parametric mapping with single photon emission computed tomography (SPECT) with ictal SPECT injected at 23 s during a habitual seizure lasting 59 s indicated an area of hyperperfusion near the right insular region. PET-MRI was non-localizing. Multidisciplinary epilepsy surgery conference consensus recommended phase 2 monitoring with stereoEEG electrodes (SEEG) targeting the bilateral frontal network including the most posterior interictal MEG dipoles in the bilateral insula and temporal lobes.

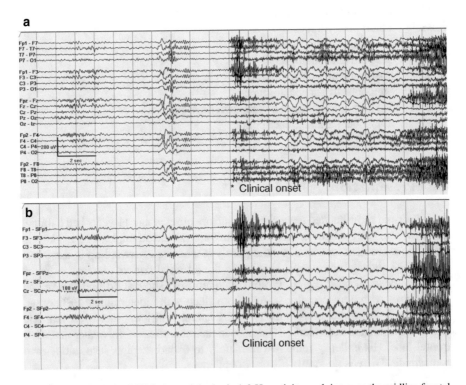

Fig. 25.1 (a) Scalp ictal EEG showed rhythmic 1-2 Hz activity evolving over the midline frontal and midline central head regions during an event, indicative of a seizure (LFF 5 Hz, HFF 50 Hz, Notch 60 Hz). (b) The "coned down" view with arrows demonstrating the evolution during the event

Clinical Questions

1. What are the features of frontal lobe epilepsy?
2. Why are the EEGs normal in frontal lobe epilepsy?
3. What is sleep-related hypermotor epilepsy?
4. What are the differential diagnoses of sleep-related hypermotor epilepsy?
5. What are the diagnostic evaluations and management for drug-resistant frontal lobe epilepsy?

Diagnostic Discussion

1. Frontal lobe seizures are typically frequent, brief, often occurring in clusters, predominantly nocturnal, and often without significant loss of awareness during the seizure and brief postictal symptoms [1]. Clinical characteristics depend on the brain regions generating the seizures. Seizures from the primary motor cortex present with contralateral clonic movements or dystonic posturing. Supplementary motor area involvement manifests as synchronous, asymmetric tonic seizures that may include the fencer's posture (forced head turn to the side of extended arm contralateral to the side of seizure onset and ipsilateral arm elevation and elbow flexion). If awareness is impaired, recovery is quick without prolonged postictal confusion. Seizures involving the mesial frontal lobe may exhibit bizarre automatism and pronounced hypermotor activity such as running around in circles, rock back and forth, leg bicycling, jumping out of bed, and spitting. Vocalization including yelling, swearing, and screaming may occur in up to 30% of patients. The bizarre and emotional semiology is what suggests a psychiatric origin to the behavior (aka pseudoseizure), yet this seizure is epileptic (pseudo-pseudoseizure). Rotational body movement can occur so that the patient appears to turn in a circle (version). Depending on the propagation, orbitofrontal seizures can present as hypermotor seizures or appear similar to mesial temporal lobe seizures demonstrating oral and manual automatism with altered awareness. Frontal polar seizures may also present with hypermotor seizures [2].
2. Frontal lobe seizures (especially focal seizures without impaired consciousness) may elude detection by the scalp EEG in up to 30% of patients who do not demonstrate interictal epileptiform discharges on repeat recordings. The reason is that many patients with frontal lobe seizures may have a generator that is cortically based in the frontal lobe where low-voltage fast frequencies are generated (and only seen at the cortical surface) or the generator is deep in the midline structures that is not amenable to routine scalp EEG recording. Antiepileptic drug discontinuation may be necessary to elicit more frequent and more intense seizures to reveal ictal EEG findings on scalp monitoring. Even a normal ictal EEG does not exclude the possibility of frontal lobe epilepsy. Frontal lobe epilepsy can be challenging to diagnose, even with simultaneous EEG and video analysis because the EEG is often obscured by muscle artifact or at the scalp may

appear normal. When juxtaposed frame by frame, frontal lobe seizures for an individual patient follow the same stereotyped sequence and motor repertoire.

3. Sleep-related hypermotor epilepsy (SHE) is a distinct electroclinical syndrome and replaces the historic terminology "nocturnal frontal lobe epilepsy." Seizures are brief <2 min, and usually clusters, and occur primarily in non-REM sleep [3]. Seizures occur during sleep and therefore more likely nocturnal but can occur in daytime or nighttime sleep. Hyperkinetic motor behaviors are the predominant features, but asymmetric or symmetric tonic and dystonic movements have been observed. Preserved awareness is not uncommon. Interictal EEG abnormalities may be absent. SHE may originate from the frontal lobe and about a third of patients with seizure onset from extrafrontal areas: insulo-opercular, temporal, and parietal lobes. Early nonmotor manifestations can be helpful in localizing extrafrontal seizure onset zone. Etiology is unknown for majority of patients. Structural etiology may be due to focal cortical dysplasia, malformation of cortical development, or anatomic abnormalities from acquired injuries. Genetic causes can contribute to both familial and sporadic SHE such as pathogenic mutations in genes encoding the subunits of the nicotinic acetylcholine receptor *CHRNA4, CHRNB2,* and *CHRNA2.* Individuals with pathogenic mutations in *KCNT1* a sodium-activated potassium channel, *DEPDC5* a repressor of the mammalian target of rapamycin (mTOR) pathway, have also been identified.

4. Paroxysmal events can be epileptic or nonepileptic. Nonepileptic childhood onset paroxysmal events due to physiologic causes may include jitteriness, movement disorder, self-stimulation, syncope, transient metabolic disorders, gastroesophageal reflux (Sandifer syndrome), or sleep disorders. Terminology for paroxysmal nonepileptic events due to psychological cause has changed from the term "pseudoseizures" due to negative connotation. Psychogenic nonepileptic attacks (PNEA) is now a frequently used term reflected in the current literature to avoid the implication of being false that the prefix "pseudo" implies [4]. Epileptic seizures may be mistaken as nonepileptic if the semiology includes psychiatric symptoms. Mesial temporal lobe seizures may be associated with psychic symptoms such as anxiety, panic attacks, déjà vu, jamais vu, and auditory or visual hallucination. Frontal lobe seizures may be brief and occur without postictal confusion. They may manifest as bizarre behaviors with prominent vocalization and complex bimanual-bipedal motor automatisms. Epilepsy and psychiatric illness frequently co-exist which make the diagnosis more challenging.

5. Clinical features of PNEA and nonepileptic events vary and lack consistency in the episodic behavior within an individual patient. Prolonged events, a waxing and waning or "on-off" course, non-stereotypical writhing motor movements or flailing, thrashing, side-to-side head movements, asynchronous body movements, forward pelvic thrusting, and eye closure with resistance to passive eye opening are concerning symptoms for PNEA. PNEA do not arise from sleep and may be intensified by a bystander. Epileptic seizures are stereotypic. Eye closure can rarely occur with epileptic seizures, but it is typically not seen during the entirety of the seizure. Tongue bites are located posterior-laterally in patients with epileptic seizures. Frontal lobe seizures can present with complex and bizarre motor movements, but

these seizures are brief 5–20 s and tend to cluster in sleep. Prominent axial body movement can begin abruptly, and patient may turn to the prone position during frontal lobe seizures. This is not typically seen in patients with PNEA. PNEA may occur with epileptic seizures though this only occurs in about 10–15% of patients. Injuries can occur in both PNEA and epileptic seizures though serious injury should raise the suspicion of epilepsy. Reliance on clinical features may result in diagnostic error requiring video-EEG monitoring for a definitive diagnosis. Video-EEG with capture of the typical event is the diagnostic gold standard to differentiate PNEA from epileptic seizures. A typical event must be recorded during prolonged video EEG to differentiate between epileptic seizures and PNEA.

6. Carbamazepine has been used as the first-line treatment for sleep-related hypermotor epilepsy. Patients who continue to have focal seizures despite more than two appropriately chosen anti-seizure medications at adequate doses should be referred to a comprehensive epilepsy centers for a multidisciplinary epilepsy surgery evaluation. Frontal lobe epilepsy accounts for 6–30% of all epilepsy surgery. In patient with lesional MRI, one stage surgery might be recommended when all the diagnostic data and seizure semiology are concordant. When the MRI appears normal, multiple modalities including neurophysiology findings and anatomic and functional imaging are used to refine the epileptogenic network hypothesis and augment the chances of post-surgical seizure outcome. Functional imaging provides supportive localizing data in patients whose seizure onset cannot be clearly delineated by noninvasive evaluations. Digitally subtracted ictal-interictal SPECT images co-registered to MRI improve localization of focal seizure, which can be further refined by statistical processing of the SPECT peri-ictal images. Flourodeoxyglucose-positive emssion tomography (FDG-PET) shows hypometabolic abnormalities related to the area or network of seizure onset. The use of multimodal functional imaging can guide pre-implantation strategies of invasive monitoring and maximize detection of seizure onset zone and improve post-surgical seizure outcome. When noninvasive data are discordant or in near proximity to eloquent cortex, more precise delineation of the epileptogenic zone is needed. When sampling of bilateral hemispheres is needed or if the regions of interest are in deep locations such as the insula or in the periventricular regions, SEEG provides better access than subdural grid-and-strip methodology. Favorable seizure outcome in frontal lobe epilepsy can be more variable and ranges from 20% to 78% depending on series, with better long-term outcome in patients with lesional MRI compared to patients with MRI-negative findings [5].

Pearls of Wisdom

1. Frontal lobe seizures are characteristically brief, tend to cluster, occur during sleep, and manifest with hypermotor semiologies that appear bizarre. Classic semiologies of specific frontal lobe regions include symmetric or asymmetric tonic seizures and fencer's posturing seen in supplementary motor area seizures. Orbitofrontal seizures can mimic focal seizures that emanate from the mesial temporal region.

2. A normal interictal and even ictal EEG does not exclude the possibility of epilepsy especially when it involves the frontal lobe. Video EEG with recorded event is the diagnostic gold standard to differentiate nonepileptic from epileptic events.

3. Sleep-related hypermotor epilepsy is a distinct electroclinical syndrome where seizures are brief <2 min, usually clusters, and occur primarily in non-REM sleep and therefore more likely nocturnal but can occur in daytime or nighttime sleep. Seizures may originate from the frontal lobe or from extrafrontal areas, such as the insulo-opercular, temporal, and parietal lobes. Etiology is unknown for majority of patients. Structural etiology may be due to focal cortical dysplasia, anatomic abnormalities from acquired injuries, or genetic causes including pathogenic mutations in *CHRNA4*, *CHRNB2*, and *CHRNA2* genes encoding subunits of nicotinic acetylcholine receptor.

4. Paroxysmal events can be nonepileptic and psychogenic, nonepileptic and physiologic, or reflect epileptic seizures. Relying solely on the clinical semiology may result in diagnostic error. Epilepsy and psychiatric illness may co-exist, making the diagnosis of epileptic seizures challenging. Paroxysmal nonepileptic behavioral events lack consistency in contrast to epileptic seizures which are stereotypic. However, patients with nonepileptic events may atypically also have concurrent epileptic seizures.

5. Frontal lobe epilepsy accounts for 6–30% of all epilepsy surgery. In patients with MRI-negative findings, the use of multimodal functional imaging can guide pre-implantation strategies of invasive monitoring and maximize detection of seizure onset zone and improve post-surgical seizure outcome.

References

1. Bonini F, McGonigal A, Trebuchon A, Gavaret M, Bartolomei F, Giusiano B, Chauvel P. Frontal lobe seizures: from clinical semiology to localization. Epilepsia. 2014;55(2):264–77.
2. Lee RW, Worrell GA. Dorsolateral frontal lobe epilepsy. J Clin Neurophysiol. 2012;29(5):379–84.
3. Tinuper P, Bisulli F, Cross JH, et al. Definition and diagnostic criteria for sleep-related hypermotor epilepsy. Neurology. 2016;86:1834–42.
4. Dickinson P, Looper KJ. Psychogenic nonepileptic seizures: a current overview. Epilepsia. 2012;53(10):1679–89.
5. Jeha LE, Najm I, Bingaman W, Dinner D, Widdess-Walsh P, Luders H. Surgical outcome and prognostic factors of frontal lobe epilepsy surgery. Brain. 2007;130(Pt 2):574–84.

Pregnancy and Epilepsy

26

Katherine Noe

Case Presentation

A 32-year-old woman with a history of juvenile myoclonic epilepsy presents with questions about pregnancy. Her epilepsy first manifested at age 13 with sporadic early morning myoclonus on awakening. She had her first generalized tonic-clonic seizure at age 16 provoked by a significant sleep deprivation. She was evaluated with MRI of the brain that was normal and a routine EEG that showed generalized spike and wave discharges during sleep. At that time she was started on lamotrigine. Over the next several years, she continued to have generalized tonic-clonic seizures on awakening typically preceded by myoclonus on average every 3–4 months. These were usually associated with sleep deprivation and binge alcohol use. Seizures persisted despite progressive escalation of lamotrigine dosage up to 200 mg twice daily. At age 25, 500 mg of extended-release sodium valproate was added to her regimen. She has subsequently been free of convulsive seizures, with only rare myoclonus on awakening always associated with significant sleep deprivation. She reports that she has tolerated this combination of medication well without adverse side effect. She is employed full-time, is driving, and lives with her spouse of 1 year. She currently has an intrauterine device for contraception, but she would like to have it removed and begin to actively try for pregnancy as she is ready to start a family.

Questions

1. What is the likelihood that her epilepsy medications will adversely impact pregnancy outcome?
2. What steps can be taken to minimize the risk of birth defects in her baby?

K. Noe (✉)
Mayo Clinic Arizona, Phoenix, AZ, USA
e-mail: Noe.katherine@mayo.edu

© Springer Nature Switzerland AG 2021
W. O. Tatum et al. (eds.), *Epilepsy Case Studies*,
https://doi.org/10.1007/978-3-030-59078-9_26

3. What is the likelihood that her seizures will worsen during her pregnancy?
4. Sleep deprivation is a known seizure trigger for this patient. Is this a cause for concern around pregnancy?
5. Can she safely breastfeed her baby?

Discussion

1. Infants exposed to antiseizure drugs in the first trimester pregnancy are observed to have major malformations in about 4–6% of cases, representing a 2–3-fold increase above the rate of malformation seen in the general population [1–6]. The risk appears to be related to pharmacotherapy and not to the underlying epilepsy, as women with epilepsy who ARE off seizure medication during the first trimester of pregnancy outcomes no different than that of the general population. Teratogenic risk varies depending upon the specific antiepileptic drug as well as the dose. In international pregnancy registry observational studies of women with epilepsy, the highest rate of birth defects for monotherapy antiseizure drug exposure is in infants exposed to valproate (Table 26.1 [1]). Between 10% and 15% of these babies have major birth defects, with greater risk at increasing doses of valproate. In contrast, lamotrigine- and levetiracetam-exposed infants do not show significantly different malformation rates compared to controls. Infants exposed to polytherapy antiseizure drug regimens containing valproate or topiramate are at highest risk. Use of valproate in the first trimester has also been linked to adverse neurodevelopmental outcomes, including lower than expected IQ an increased risk of behavioral problems including autistic spectrum disorder [4]. For these reasons use of valproate is no longer recommended in women of childbearing potential, except in unique circumstances where it is shown to be the only medication that provides adequate seizure control.

2. Teratogenic risk can be lowered by adjusting seizure drugs prior to conception. For women where there is a reasonable expectation of adequate seizure control off all seizure drugs during pregnancy, elimination of all medications may be

Table 26.1 Observed rates of major malformations in infants with first trimester monotherapy antiepileptic drug exposure from international observational pregnancy registries

Drug	European Registry of AED and Pregnancy	North American AED Pregnancy Registry	Australian Pregnancy Register
Valproate	10.3% (8.8–12.0%)	9.3% (6.4–13%)	14.8% (2.1–19.5%)
Topiramate	3.9% (1.5–8.4%)	4.2% (2.4–6.8%)	1.9% (0.1–6%)
Phenobarbital	6.5% (4.2–9.9%)	5.5% (2.8–9.7%)	n/a
Phenytoin	6.4% (2.8–12.2%)	2.9% (1.5–5%)	2.3% (0.1–6.6%)
Carbamazepine	5.5% (4.5–6.6%)	3.0% (2.1–4.2%)	5.9% (0.1–5.3%)
Oxcarbazepine	3.0% (1.4–5.4%)	2.2% (0.6–5.5%)	5.3% (0.2–15%)
Levetiracetam	2.8% (1.7–4.5%)	2.4% (1.2–4.3%)	3.6% (0.4–4.3%)
Lamotrigine	2.9% (2.3–3.7%)	2.0% (1.4–2.8%)	4.9% (0.7–4.6%)

Abbreviation: *AED* antiepileptic drug

considered. For those who require ongoing therapy, goals are to use the lowest number and dose of medication that will maintain good seizure control and to avoid higher-risk drugs. In this case, with a diagnosis of juvenile myoclonic epilepsy with still active myoclonus, it is unlikely that the patient would be adequately seizure-free without ongoing therapy. However given that she has been seizure-free for many years, and that previous triggers including routine use of alcohol and irregular sleep habits that were problematic when she was younger are no longer active, it may be feasible to consider getting her down to a monotherapy drug regimen. The most important thing that can be done to lower the risk to her infant would be to get her off valproate. She should also be placed on a prenatal vitamin with at least 0.4 mg of folic acid. Supplementation with folic acid has been shown to lower the risk of malformations particularly neural tube defects in the general population, although not necessarily to counteract teratogenic risk in women exposed to anticonvulsant medications. Use of adequate folic acid supplementation prior to and during pregnancy in women with epilepsy has however been shown to decrease the likelihood of lower than expected IQ, including in infants exposed to valproate [4]. Optimally, she would allow sufficient time to stabilize her medications before she begins to actively pursue pregnancy.

3. Observational pregnancy registry data has demonstrated that over 90% of women who have been seizure-free for 9–12 months prior to conception will remain seizure-free throughout pregnancy. One of the most common factors leading to breakthrough seizures during pregnancy is failure to adequately adjust anticonvulsant medications to compensate for significant physiologic changes that can result in lowering of serum drug level. Lamotrigine is prone to such changes and may require significant dose adjustment throughout pregnancy. Although there is no consensus on absolute recommendations for frequency of drug monitoring, many providers will check serum drug levels at baseline and then anywhere from once a month to once a trimester. In contrast, valproate levels tend to be relatively unaffected by pregnancy, however as noted above it is desirable to eliminate this medication whenever possible prior to conception. Women with generalized epilepsy where valproate is eliminated prior to conception have been shown to be particularly high risk for breakthrough generalized tonic-clonic seizures during pregnancy. This patient therefore would warrant close monitoring.

4. Many women may experience disruption of sleep during pregnancy, and in women with epilepsy who are sensitive to sleep deprivation, this could be a factor contributing to breakthrough seizures. Sleep deprivation is also expected in the initial months of caring for a newborn. It is advisable to have a conversation with this patient about strategies to optimize sleep postpartum, including consideration of help with nighttime feeding. Because it is possible that myoclonic seizures could result in unintentional harm to a newborn if they are not adequately restrained, potential precautions for the new mother could include using a carrier safety harness particularly when sleep deprived rather than holding the baby in arms alone, having assistance with bathing the child, and changing diapers on a low surface or floor.

5. All antiseizure drugs are lipophilic and can be excreted in breast milk [6]. Available studies however indicate that exposure via breast milk tends to result in very low serum drug levels in the child and that associated harm to the infant is very rare. In contrast, there is strong evidence of benefit from breastfeeding to the short- and long-term health outcomes in both the child and the mother. Neurobehavioral studies of children exposed to valproate during pregnancy found that those who were subsequently breastfed had better outcomes, again suggesting that additional exposure via breast milk should not be considered harmful. Women with epilepsy who are able to breastfeed can be encouraged to do so.

Pearls
1. Infants exposed to antiseizure drugs in the first trimester are at 2–3 times increased risk for major birth defects.
2. Valproate should be avoided in women of childbearing potential when possible, as it is highly correlated with increased risk of birth defects and is associated with lower than expected IQ in infants exposed during pregnancy.
3. Women who are seizure-free for 9–12 months prior to pregnancy will usually be seizure-free during pregnancy.
4. Use of an antiseizure drug is not a contraindication to breastfeeding for women with epilepsy.
5. Given that sleep is often disrupted in women during pregnancy, special attention must be paid to this issue so as to make certain that adequate sleep hygiene is maintained.

References

1. Hernandez-Diaz S, Mittendorf R, Smith CR, Hauser WA, et al. Comparative safety of antiepileptic drugs during pregnancy. Neurology. 2012;78(21):1692–9.
2. Tomson T, Battino D, Bonizzani E, et al. Comparative risk of binge or congenital malformations with 8 different antiepileptic drugs: a prospective cohort study of the EURAP registry. Lancet Neurol. 2018;17:530–8.
3. Vajda FJ, Graham JE, Hitchcock AA, et al. Antiepileptic drugs and foetal malformation: analysis of 20 years of data in a pregnancy register. Seizure. 2019;65:6–11.
4. Meador KJ, Baker GA, Browning N, et al. Fetal antiepileptic drug exposure and cognitive outcomes at age 6 years (NEAD study): the prospective observational study. Lancet Neurol. 2013;12:244–52.
5. Vajda FJ, Hitchcock A, Graham J, O'Brien T, Lander C, Eadie M. Seizure control in antiepileptic drug treated pregnancy. Epilepsia. 2008;49:172–6.
6. Birnbaum AK, Meador KJ, Karanam A, Brown C, et al. Antiepileptic drug exposure in infants of breastfeeding mothers with epilepsy. JAMA Neurol. 2020;77(4):441–50.

Epilepsy in Women

27

Katherine Noe

Case Presentation

A 32-year-old woman wants to explore additional options for management of drug-resistant focal epilepsy. Her stereotypic seizure begins with a paroxysmal feeling of anxiety and rising epigastric sensation followed by a stare and unresponsiveness and repetitive lip-smacking. Despite trials of multiple antiseizure drugs over the last 15 years, she continues to have focal impaired awareness seizures on average every month. She was previously evaluated for epilepsy surgery but was found to be a poor candidate due to seizures of independent bi-temporal onset and normal MRI brain. She is currently treated with lamotrigine, carbamazepine, and vagus nerve stimulator. She is otherwise healthy and takes no medications other than her those for epilepsy. She brings a diary in which she has charted her seizures and her menstrual periods (Fig. 27.1). She has observed that her seizures usually occur with menses and would like to know if stopping her periods would help control her epilepsy.

Questions

1. Does the diary contain information valuable to the management of this patient?
2. Could hormonal therapy be used to help control seizures in this patient?
3. Does the diagnosis of catamenial epilepsy expand options for treatment with conventional antiseizure drugs?

K. Noe (✉)
Mayo Clinic Arizona, Phoenix, AZ, USA
e-mail: Noe.katherine@mayo.edu

© Springer Nature Switzerland AG 2021
W. O. Tatum et al. (eds.), *Epilepsy Case Studies*,
https://doi.org/10.1007/978-3-030-59078-9_27

149

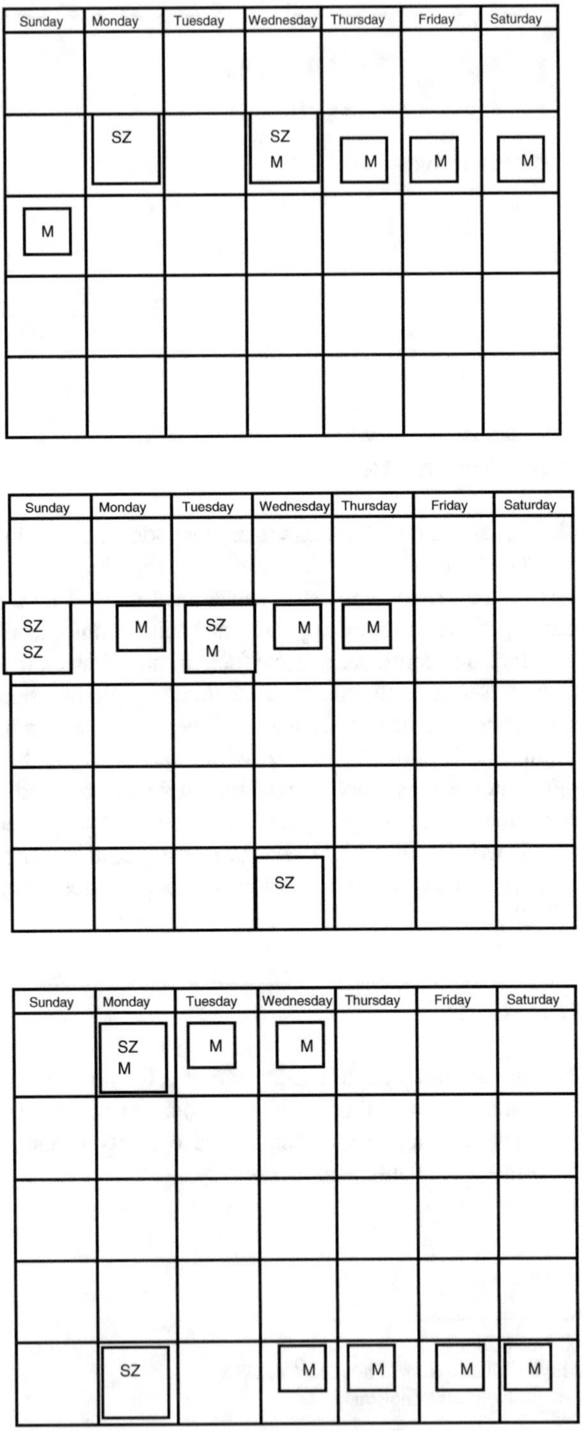

Fig. 27.1 Seizure calendars for 3 months demonstrating a catamenial pattern of breakthrough seizures in relationship to the menstrual cycle. *SZ* seizure, *M* menses

4. Are there other treatments (non-hormonal, not standard antiepileptic drugs) that could be used to treat catamenial epilepsy?
5. In the future as this patient enters perimenopause and menopause, is it likely that her seizure activity will change?

Discussion

1. The diary (Fig. 27.1) documents a pattern of consistent seizure exacerbation related to the menstrual cycle known as catamenial epilepsy. 30–40% of women with drug-resistant focal epilepsy have catamenial epilepsy when strictly defined as a doubling of seizure frequency during a specific phase of the menstrual cycle relative to other phases [1–5]. Three patterns of catamenial epilepsy have been defined: perimenstrual, periovulatory, and anovulatory [1, 2]. The most common, as demonstrated in this patient's diary, is the perimenstrual pattern with increased seizures in the days immediately before or after the onset of menses. The influence of the menstrual cycle on seizure threshold is attributed to the proconvulsant effects of estrogen via enhancement of neuronal sensitivity to glutamate and to the anticonvulsant effect of progesterone mediated primarily through central nervous system gamma-aminobutyric acid (GABA) receptors. Seizures are more likely to occur at any time in the cycle where estrogen levels are high relative to progesterone or when progesterone levels are rapidly declining such as occurs around menses.

2. First-line treatment for women with catamenial epilepsy should be standard anti-seizure drugs prescribed with a conventional dosing regimen. However, when standard treatment is ineffective, such as in this case, it may be reasonable to consider alternative options including hormonal manipulation [2, 4, 5]. It is important to note that the clinical evidence supporting the effectiveness of such treatment is limited. The underlying rationale would be to try to maintain a relatively high and/or stable level of progesterone to estrogen, this attempting to decrease the likelihood of seizure. A standard oral contraceptive might have some efficacy for women with periovulatory seizures, but as these also work with withdrawal of estrogen and progesterone on the 4th week to induce withdrawal bleeding, they are not an appropriate treatment for the perimenstrual pattern. Extended cycle monophasic oral contraceptive pills, avoiding the standard 7 days of placebo tablets, could be an option for perimenstrual seizures. Another alternative is supplemental progesterone, either with sustained release injection therapy (Depo-Provera) or as an oral therapy. Supplemental progesterone provided as a three-times-daily lozenge was shown in a small open-label study to be effective in reducing both focal and secondarily generalized seizures in women with catamenial epilepsy; however, a subsequent randomized placebo-controlled trial showed no benefit [5]. As with any medical therapy, it is important to carefully consider the risks and benefits of hormonal therapy before proceeding. Furthermore, consider that the effectiveness of hormonal contraceptives is

decreased by antiseizure drugs that induce the cytochrome P 450 system, including carbamazepine.

3. Some women may choose to increase the dose of their conventional antiseizure drug intermittently over the course of the month to provide extra coverage during the menstrual phase of risk. For example, for woman with a perimenstrual pattern of seizure exacerbation, seizure medication could be increased in the days prior and during menses. For this strategy to be effective, it is critical to carefully consider the pharmacokinetic profile of the antiseizure drug to be sure that meaningful elevation in serum drug levels can be achieved with short-term changes in dosing. For some women benzodiazepines are also utilized in this way, although side effects including sedation can be limiting. Intermittent drug supplementation will also only be an effective treatment for women whose menstrual cycles are very regular and who are willing to consistently track, and plan 1 supplemental treatments must be started and stopped.

4. Acetazolamide, a carbonic anhydrase inhibitor, is another option that can be considered as adjunctive treatment for catamenial epilepsy that is refractory to standard antiepileptic drug therapy. Anecdotally, this drug has been used as both a daily and cyclical treatment starting 5–7 days prior to expected onset of menses in women with a perimenstrual pattern of seizure exacerbation [3]. Evidence for use is limited. However, in a small retrospective study, use of either continuous or intermittent acetazolamide resulted in a 50% or greater reduction in seizure frequency in 40% of subjects. Tolerance to this medication with loss of impact against seizure can develop with both short- and long-term use.

5. Menopause is defined as cessation of menstrual periods for more than 1 year. This is preceded by perimenopause, several years during which the menstrual cycle becomes increasingly irregular and fertility decreases reflecting fluctuations in the secretion of estrogen and progesterone. During perimenopause there is also an increase in anovulatory cycles. Many women with catamenial epilepsy will report worsen seizure control during perimenopause. Although cessation of a very in production of estrogen and progesterone might be expected to improve epilepsy post-menopause, changes in seizure control during this phase of life are unpredictable.

Pearls
1. Catamenial exacerbation of seizures, a pattern of reproducible seizure exacerbation related to a specific phase of the menstrual cycle, is common among women with epilepsy.
2. Seizures may be more likely to occur when estrogen levels are high relative to progesterone or when progesterone levels are rapidly dropping.
3. Catamenial seizures refractory to conventional antiseizure drugs may be treated adjunctively with cyclical supplementation of standard seizure medications, hormonal therapies, or acetazolamide though the clinical evidence for efficacy of all these therapies is limited.

4. Women with catamenial epilepsy may experience increased seizure frequency during perimenopause.
5. From menarche through menopause, gender-specific management is required and involves careful selection of antiseizure medication to provide optimal treatment to women with epilepsy.

References

1. Herzog AG, Harden CL, Liporace J, et al. Frequency of catamenial seizure exacerbation in women with localization-related epilepsy. Ann Neurol. 2004;56(3):431–4.
2. Hezog AG. Catamenial epilepsy: update on prevalence, pathophysiology and treatment from the findings of the NIH progesterone treatment trial. Seizure. 2015;28:18–25.
3. Lim LL, Foldvary N, Mascha E, Lee J. Acetazolamide in women with catamenial epilepsy. Epilepsia. 2001;42(6):746–9.
4. Herzog AG. Progesterone therapy in women with complex partial and secondary generalized seizures. Neurology. 1995;45:1660–2.
5. Herzog AG, Fowler KM, Smithson SD, et al. Progesterone vs. placebo therapy for women with epilepsy: a randomized clinical trial. Neurology. 2012;78(24):1959–66.

Convulsive Syncope

28

William P. Cheshire and William O. Tatum

Case Presentation

A 16-year-old female presented with a 1-year history of recurrent spells in which she would collapse to the ground and was found to be limp and unarousable. Each event lasted about half a minute. Witnesses reported that she appeared as pale as a ghost. Her skin felt clammy, her pulse felt weak, and on several occasions, she exhibited repetitive jerking of her arms and legs. One event was followed by urinary incontinence. The events occurred sporadically, many of them on hot days while she was standing outdoors during school band practice. She knew when an event was about to happen, because she would feel warm, queasy, and dizzy; her thoughts became unfocused, her vision blurry, and her hearing muffled.

The most recent event, which occurred immediately following phlebotomy when her pediatrician checked a complete blood count to rule out anemia, was prolonged, lasting about 3 min as the phlebotomist and her family held her upright to keep her from falling out of the chair. Unlike previous events, from which she recovered rapidly, this time she appeared drowsy, and her speech was muddled for another 10 min. She was diagnosed with epilepsy and treated with topiramate, but the events continued despite dose increases to 200 mg daily.

Neurologic examination was unremarkable. Routine electrolytes, blood counts, 12-lead EKG, and CT brain were normal. Standard EEG was normal as well, although no clinical events occurred during the recording.

W. P. Cheshire (✉) · W. O. Tatum
Mayo Clinic, Department of Neurology, Jacksonville, FL, USA
e-mail: cheshire@mayo.edu; tatum.william@mayo.edu

© Springer Nature Switzerland AG 2021
W. O. Tatum et al. (eds.), *Epilepsy Case Studies*,
https://doi.org/10.1007/978-3-030-59078-9_28

Clinical Questions

1. Does this history suggest a most likely clinical diagnosis?
2. What is the clinical significance of the rhythmic jerking limb movements? And the postictal state?
3. Would further diagnostic testing be of value?
4. What treatment should be recommended at this point?
5. What is the anticipated prognosis?

Diagnostic Discussion

1. This patient presents with episodes that suggest vasovagal syncope. The equivalent terms neurally mediated syncope and neurocardiogenic syncope, which signify that the origin is in the brain rather than the heart, are used interchangeably to describe this common syndrome [1]. Syncope is defined as sudden transient loss of postural tone resulting from global cerebral hypoperfusion with spontaneous and complete recovery without neurologic sequelae [1, 2]. Loss of consciousness is brief, on average 12 s [3].

   Vasovagal syncope may occur spontaneously, often when the patient is in an upright posture which causes relative pooling of blood volume in the abdomen and lower extremities, or in response to specific situations. These include medical instrumentation including intravenous catheter insertion or phlebotomy, blood donation, the sight of blood, heat exposure, pain, or emotional distress [1].

   The mechanism of syncope is complex, the final common pathway being withdrawal of sympathetic cardiovascular tone, which reduces arterial pressure and cerebral perfusion. In parallel, parasympathetic vagal tone increases, slowing heart rate. Once mean arterial pressure falls below about 50 mmHg, decreased perfusion of the reticular activating system leads to loss of consciousness within 7 s [4].

   Paramount to accurate diagnosis is a careful clinical history, which includes asking the patient about prodromal symptoms and interviewing witnesses about the patient's appearance and behavior during the event [5, 6]. In most cases, patients will recall a prodrome beginning gradually from 30 s to several minutes prior to loss of consciousness. This prodrome may include any combination of dizziness, difficulty focusing thoughts, general weakness, nausea, feeling warm or cold, blurry or dim vision, muffled hearing, tinnitus, clammy skin, fecal urgency, neck ache, or restlessness [2, 4]. Witnesses will report that the patient then goes limp and collapses like a rag doll. Facial pallor is highly characteristic of vasovagal syncope. The eyes usually remain open initially. Hyperventilation may precede an event and during unresponsiveness breathing continues and may appear shallow. The pulse pressure decreases [2, 4]. The patient recovers rapidly without postictal confusion but may report fatigue, headache, or diaphoresis.

2. Myoclonic jerks frequently accompany vasovagal syncope and may lead to a misdiagnosis of epilepsy. This "convulsive syncope" has been reported in between 12% and 90% of syncopal events and consists of multifocal arrhythmic jerks involving bilateral proximal and distal muscles and, with a duration of 1 to

15 s, is more brief than epileptic clonic contractions [3–5]. In contrast to epilepsy, which originates in the cerebral cortex, syncopal myoclonic jerks are caused by hypoperfusion of the brainstem [7]. Loss of consciousness precedes the myoclonus of syncope. A videorecording of a typical example of convulsive syncope may be viewed at the educational website Syncopedia [8].

Another feature of vasovagal syncope that is sometimes mistaken to be a clue to epilepsy is urinary incontinence, which occurs in 10–25% of cases and is of no diagnostic value in distinguishing syncope from a seizure [4].

Key diagnostic features that can occur specifically in epilepsy but do not occur in syncope include oral automatisms, neuroanatomical march, amnesia, lateral tongue-biting, and prolonged postictal confusion [9]. Also to be considered in the differential diagnosis is the more rare condition of epilepsy with ictal bradycardia.

Prolonged unresponsiveness (beyond 1 min) or prolonged postictal confusion (beyond 1–2 min) generally indicates a diagnosis other than vasovagal syncope, with one important exception. If the unconscious patient is restrained and allowed to remain in an upright position, the restoration of cerebral perfusion, and hence recovery of full consciousness, may be delayed [2]. The patient who faints should be assisted to a recumbent position to allow cerebral perfusion to return.

3. When the diagnosis by history is uncertain, prolonged video-EEG monitoring with the goal of capturing a typical event can lead to a definitive diagnosis. During syncope the EEG typically demonstrates a "slow-flat-slow" profile, in which attenuation of alpha rhythm progresses to slow activity of increasing amplitude, and then disappearance of slow wave activity leading to a flat tracing (Fig. 28.1) [10].

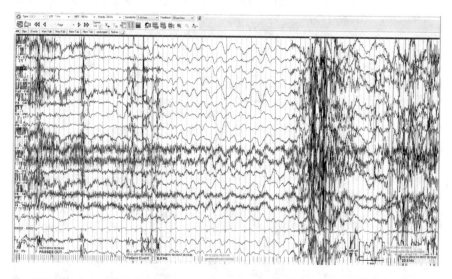

Fig. 28.1 21-channel EEG demonstrating increase in generalized theta and delta associated with syncope that occurred during intermittent photic stimulation. Note the progressive increase in amplitude and slowing of the background activity during the episode of convulsive syncope. Prominent myogenic artifact is seen during the time the patient "passed out"

Head-up tilt-table testing is a useful provocative diagnostic maneuver in the evaluation of unexplained syncope with the goal of reproducing an event under monitored conditions [11].

4. The most effective preventative measure for vasovagal syncope is for the patient to learn to recognize premonitory symptoms that indicate impending loss of consciousness and respond by sitting down or lying down and waiting for them to pass. Triggering factors, if they are known, may be avoided or encountered with caution. Increasing dietary salt intake or drinking sports beverages to ensure adequate intravascular volume are also helpful. Additionally, physical counter-pressure maneuvers that activate leg and abdominal muscles and improve venous return have been shown to be effective [12].

Regarding pharmacologic interventions, there is limited evidence of efficacy for midodrine, beta blockers, and fludrocortisone in some patients [2].

The antiseizure medication topiramate, which did not prevent syncope in this patient, could potentially aggravate heat intolerance and make matters worse. Topiramate, which inhibits carbonic anhydrase, can cause anhidrosis in susceptible patients [13]. Under conditions of heat stress, a patient who lacks the ability to sweat will become flushed as a second mechanism to liberate body heat. Thermoregulatory blood shunting to the skin can contribute to the reduction in blood pressure that leads to syncope.

5. Syncope is extremely common with a lifetime prevalence of 30–40% [14]. Approximately two-thirds of patients will go on to experience a second or third event, and a small proportion will experience recurrent events [14]. For patients with a positive tilt-table test and three or more lifetime syncopal events, the probability of recurrence during the succeeding year for those with no events, fewer than 2 events, or more than six events during the previous year was 7%, 22%, and 69%, respectively [15].

Clinical Pearls

1. Vasovagal syncope is quite common in the general population and is sometimes mistaken for epilepsy when myoclonic jerks or tonic posturing are reported.

2. "Convulsive syncope" refers to the myoclonic jerks that accompany syncope and is caused by insufficient perfusion of the brainstem during conditions of transient arterial hypotension. This consists of multifocal, arrhythmic jerks involving bilateral proximal and distal muscles with a duration of 1–15 s.

3. Vasovagal syncope, in contrast to epilepsy, is brief in duration, often occurs during prolonged standing or in response to specific stimuli, typically is preceded by a recognizable prodrome, and is manifested by facial pallor, open eyes, and sweating, proceeding to collapse with loss of postural tone, followed by rapid recovery and no postictal state.

4. Antiseizure medication is of no value in preventing vasovagal syncope and may be detrimental in terms of producing side effects. The most effective

preventive measure for convulsive syncope is recognizing it as a physiologic nonepileptic condition by recognizing premonitory symptoms and response to position by sitting down. Treatment is with adequate hydration including added salt and physical countermaneuvers to improve venous return.

5. The prognosis for convulsive syncope is excellent, although a minority of patients will proceed to have recurrent events.

References

1. Freeman R, Wieling W, Axelrod FB, et al. Consensus statement on the definition of orthostatic hypotension, neurally mediated syncope and the postural tachycardia syndrome. Clin Auton Res. 2011;21:69–72.
2. Cheshire WP. Syncope. Continuum (Minneap Minn). 2017;23(2):335–58.
3. Lempert T, Bauer M, Schmidt D. Syncope: a videometric analysis of 56 episodes of transient cerebral hypoxia. Ann Neurol. 1994;36(2):233–7.
4. Wieling W, Thijs RD, van Vijk N, et al. Symptoms and signs of syncope: a review of the link between physiology and clinical clues. Brain. 2009;132(pt 2):2630–42.
5. Sheldon RS, Rose S, Connolly S, et al. Diagnostic criteria for vasovagal syncope based on a quantitative history. Eur Heart J. 2006;27(3):344–50.
6. Sheldon R. Syncope diagnostic scores. Progr Cardiovas Dis. 2013;55(4):390–5.
7. Crompton DE, Berkovic SF. The borderland of epilepsy: clinical and molecular features of phenomena that mimic epileptic seizures. Lancet Neurol. 2009;8(4):370–81.
8. Syncopedia.org. Accessed. at: https://www.syncopedia.org/straining-induced-syncope/.
9. Sheldon R. How to differentiate syncope from seizure. Cardiol Clin. 2015;33:377–85.
10. Gastaut H, Fischer-Williams M. Electroencephalographic study of syncope; its differentiation from epilepsy. Lancet. 1957;273(7004):1018–25.
11. Cheshire WP, Goldstein DS. Autonomic uprising: the tilt table test in autonomic medicine. Clin Auton Res. 2019;29(2):215–30.
12. Wieling W, van Dijk N, Thijs RD, et al. Physical countermaneuvers to increase orthostatic tolerance. J Intern Med. 2014;277(1):69–82.
13. Karachristianou S, Papamichalis E, Sarantopoulos A, et al. Hypohidrosis induced by topiramate in an adult patient. Epileptic Disord. 2013;15(2):203–6. https://doi.org/10.1684/epd.2013.0568.
14. Ganzeboom KS, Mairuhu G, Reitsma JB, et al. Lifetime cumulative incidence of syncope in the general population: a study of 549 Dutch subjects aged 35-60 years. J Cardiovasc Electrophysiol. 2006;17(11):1172–6.
15. Sumner GL, Rose MS, Koshman ML, et al. Recent history of vasovagal syncope in a young, referral-based population is a stronger predictor of recurrent syncope than lifetime syncope burden. J Cardiovas Electrophysiol. 2010;21(12):1373–80.

Psychogenic Nonepileptic Attacks

29

William O. Tatum

Case Presentation

A 45-year-old right-handed female nurse had mitral valve prolapse, fibromyalgia, obstructive sleep apnea, and depression and was being evaluated by neurology for "brain fog." She previously underwent hospitalization for a suicide attempt following a rape when she was 20 years old. She was, otherwise in her state of usual health until she was confronted by her husband with the fact that he had been having an affair with her best friend and wanted a divorce. She did not have a history of seizures and had no early risk factors for epilepsy. She did have a minor closed head injury and brief loss of consciousness when she fell off a skateboard at 9 years old but was otherwise normal. She was distressed about the realization that her life was about to change. Two weeks after receiving the information from her husband, she was involved in a minor car accident. She had accidentally driven over a curb at slow speeds in a grocery store parking lot and hit a tree. She did not hit her head, recalled the accident, and did not lose consciousness. Later that day, she was watching TV with a friend having just attempted to talk about the divorce when suddenly her friend witnessed the patient fall over on the couch, eyes roll backwards, before she "shook all over". She was unresponsive during the event which lasted for "5–10 minutes" and was tired and sore all over her body after the event. Her friend dialed 911, and she was transported to the local emergency department where she was loaded with levetiracetam (LEV). A CT brain, a 12-lead EKG, and electrolytes were normal. Recurrent episodes occurred within the week, and she was seen by a neurologist who increased the levetiracetam from 500 mg twice daily to 1000 mg twice daily. An

W. O. Tatum (✉)
Mayo Clinic, Department of Neurology, Jacksonville, FL, USA
e-mail: tatum.william@mayo.edu

© Springer Nature Switzerland AG 2021
W. O. Tatum et al. (eds.), *Epilepsy Case Studies*,
https://doi.org/10.1007/978-3-030-59078-9_29

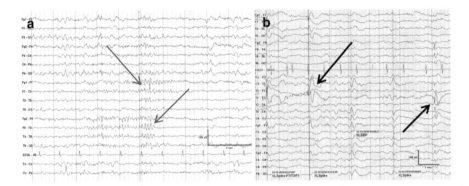

Fig. 29.1 (**a**) EEG demonstrating the patient's "abnormality" of bilateral wicket spikes which are a benign variant of uncertain significance unrelated to epilepsy (*red arrows*). Compare the patient's EEG in (**a**) with another EEG taken from a patient with focal epilepsy (**b**) revealing pathological bilateral independent spike-and-slow wave discharges in the temporal regions (*black arrows*). Note the differences between the EEGs shown demonstrating bitemporal bursts of wicket spikes in (**a**) and isolated spike-and-slow waves in (**b**)

EEG was performed in the office and was abnormal due to "temporal spikes that are potentially epileptogenic" (Fig. 29.1). On LEV, the episodes continued, but she became very depressed and contemplated "not wanting to live." When she was evaluated at Mayo Clinic, her father provided an outpatient smart phone video of one of the events that was clearly a nonepileptic event.

Clinical Questions

1. What does the clinical history suggest as a diagnosis?
2. What are the EEG findings that help support the diagnosis?
3. What is the prevalence of episodes that mimic epileptic seizures?
4. What is the approach to treatment for patients with psychogenic nonepileptic attacks (PNEA)?
5. What is the overall prognosis for remission of in people with PNEA?

Diagnostic Discussion

1. The history of paroxysmal events with loss of consciousness and post-event fatigue is suspicious for the diagnosis of epilepsy especially when they are associated with an abnormal epileptiform EEG. However, the history of depression, fibromyalgia, and mitral valve prolapse have been associated with psychological conditions including anxiety and disordered mood. Minor head injuries without loss of consciousness are a minimal risk factor for post-traumatic epilepsy in the context of this patient's clinical history. The episodes themselves are frequent and daily without any response to antiseizure medication. The principal difference between PNEA and epileptic seizures (ES) are listed in the Table 29.1

Table 29.1 The clinical features of psychogenic nonepileptic attacks and epilepsy

Feature	PNEA	Epilepsy
Age involved	15–35 years	All ages
Seizure onset	Gradual	Abrupt
Population	80% female	Male = female
Semiology	Non-stereotyped	Stereotyped
	Head side to side	Head fixed unilateral
	Eyes closed	Eyes open
	Limbs out of phase	Limb in phase
	Opisthotonus	Body straight
	On and off	Evolution
	Variable	Stereotyped
Duration	Prolonged >2–3 min	Usually <1–2 min
Post-ictal	Rare and variable	Yes (confused)
Injury	Infrequent usually mild	Tongue biting and injury/burns
Suggestion	Reliable	Rare
EEG	Normal	Abnormal
Witnessed	Usually	Not always

2. While the sensitivity of an EEG in patients with epilepsy is low to moderate, the specificity of an epileptiform EEG in patients with epilepsy is high. Only about 1–2% of adult patients with abnormal interictal epileptiform discharges do not have clinical evidence of epilepsy. However, there are many variations of normal and benign variants of uncertain significance that may mimic pathological epileptiform discharges leading to misdiagnosis from a misinterpreted EEG. In this case, the EEG contained wicket waves that were present and misinterpreted as "abnormal." These benign waveforms are the most common misinterpreted "normal" variant [2]. They consist of intermittent bursts or sporadic monophasic arciform "spiky" waveforms located in the temporal regions maximal during drowsiness that may be mistaken for an abnormal temporal epileptiform discharge. However, wickets are typically not associated with after-going slow waves, do not distort the background activity, and have a similar frequency within the bursts though they may be bilaterally independent and asyncrhonoous similar to patients with epilepsy yet are benign.

3. Approximately 20–30% of patients (range 10–50%) will have a different diagnosis other than epilepsy when evaluated for spells with video-EEG monitoring [3, 4]. Video-EEG monitoring is the gold standard for the diagnosis of PNEA [1–4]. Ninety percent of these nonepileptic events will be due to a psychogenic cause [3]. Induction or activation using a placebo has been used to demonstrate suggestibility associated with psychogenic etiologies. Ten percent of the time physiologic episodes (predominately syncope) will be present [1, 3]. The diagnosis hinges on recording the typical event with a normal or unchanged "ictal" EEG. When consciousness is impaired, the EEG will exhibit abnormal electrocerebral activity that reflects loss of cerebral blood flow with slowing and attenuation of the background rhythms to the end point of a "flat" recording. Convulsive syncope is a common physiologic nonepileptic event manifest as multifocal myoclonic jerks or less often tonic stiffening that can mimic epileptic seizures.

4. The treatment of psychogenic nonepileptic attacks begins with the delivery of the diagnosis. Patient reactions to accepting a psychological cause portend the response to follow through with recommendations and the overall benefit of realizing the diagnosis. It is important to present the diagnosis with a strong and positive attitude to introduce the new diagnosis. PNEA reflects a conversion disorder with seizures that are mimics of epileptic seizures in people with epilepsy. Many patients are "disabled" by their "seizures" given their unpredictability and lack of ability to control them [5, 6]. Pseudostatus epilepticus may occur in approximately one-third of individuals. Identifying a mental health practitioner experienced in the treatment of PNEA to providing a bridge between neurology and psychiatric management. Antidepressants such as the selective serotonin reuptake inhibitors are helpful for depression but may have less impact on resolution of the episodic behavior. Cognitive behavioral therapy tailored to the individual needs by psychology is a treatment of choice that may lead to reduction of the events [6].

5. The prognosis for patients with PNEA is variable. Children have a much better likelihood of remission than adults. Like adolescents they have different stressors than adults and may have their episodes for a shorter period of time. Most PNEA diagnoses are delayed by 1–7 years from onset. Overall prognosis for remission of in people with the attacks is limited by the relatively limited number of people following through and completing treatment with Psychiatry and/or Psychology as many patients are lost to follow-up or do not attend sessions to undergo cognitive behavioral therapy. Long-term outcomes suggest that after years of PNEA, nearly 50% of patients continue to have the attacks despite a definitive diagnosis [5]. Many patients are not working and are reliant on social security disability. Outcome may be better for those people with higher levels of education, less severe motor involvement (one-third of patients), and short times to diagnosis in addition to those individuals with limited somatoform complaints and those who lack significant psychiatric diagnoses [5].

Pearls of Wisdom
1. PNEA is most common in women. They account for approximately 20–30% of patient hospitalizations for diagnostic video-EEG evaluation of uncontrolled paroxysmal attacks. Notable delays (years) are often present prior to arriving at a definitive diagnosis.
2. Abnormal EEGs should be reviewed when the clinical diagnosis of epilepsy is suspect to ensure over-interpretation of an abnormality is absent.
3. When waveforms on EEG are reviewed in patients with PNEA, variations of normal features in the EEG and benign variants of uncertain significance account for majority of misinterpreted EEGs that resulted in treatment.

4. The attacks in patients with PNEA represent a conversion disorder, and a history of abuse is common. Treatment with antiseizure medication is ineffective and should be discontinue when no psychiatric or neurological comorbidity is present. No psychological "intent" exists in people with PNEA, and patients do not "fake" seizure-like activity in the vast majority of cases. The opportunity for remission starts at delivery of the diagnosis though is guarded for long-term remission.

5. Always screen for psychiatric comorbidity in people with PNEA to identify a primary diagnosis and stressors with the purpose of considering medical treatment. An Axis 1 diagnosis is commonly anxiety-depression in patients with PNEA yet it is also a frequent comorbidity in patients with epilepsy. Cognitive behavioral therapy in conjunction with medication used to treat a comorbid psychological disorder can improve daily function and may lead to reduction in the attacks when the patient accepts the diagnosis of PNEA and complies with treatment recommendations.

References

1. Devinsky O, Gazzola D, LaFrance WC. Differentiating between nonepileptic and epileptic seizures. Nature reviews. Neurology. 2011;7(4):210–20.
2. Krauss G, Abdallah A, Lesser R, et al. Clinical and EEG features of patients with EEG wicket rhythms misdiagnosed with epilepsy. Neurology. 2005;64:1879–83.
3. Benbadis SR, O'Neill E, Tatum WO, Heriaud L. Outcome of prolonged video-EEG monitoring at a typical referral epilepsy center. Epilepsia. 2004;45(9):1150–3.
4. Martin RC, Gilliam FG, Kilgore M, et al. Improved health care resource utilization following video-EEG-confirmed diagnosis of nonepileptic psychogenic seizures. Seizure. 1998;7(5):385–90.
5. Brown RJ, Reuber M. Psychological and psychiatric aspects of psychogenic non-epileptic seizures (PNES): a systematic review. Clin Psychol Rev. 2016;45:157–82.
6. Baslet G, Dworetzky B, Perez DL, Oser M. Treatment of psychogenic nonepileptic seizures: updated review and findings from a mindfulness-based intervention case series. Clin EEG Neurosci. 2015;46(1):54–64.

Neuropsychological Assessment in Temporal Lobe Epilepsy Surgery

David Sabsevitz and Karen Blackmon

Case Presentation

This is a 59-year-old, right-handed, high school educated male with drug-resistant focal epilepsy. The patient began experiencing seizures at 2 years of age. His initial semiology was consistent with focal to bilateral tonic-clonic seizures. No precipitating events were identified, and there was no family history of epilepsy. He was started on phenobarbital but continued to have breakthrough seizures over the years whenever his anti seizure medication was tapered. He began experiencing focal impaired awareness seizures at age 54. These were described as staring, inability to talk or respond, lip-smacking, and flexion posturing of the left upper extremity. He failed several anti-seizure medication (ASM) trials, including phenobarbital, phenytoin, oxcarbazepine, gabapentin, and levetiracetam. MRI of the brain showed volume loss of the left hippocampus with increased T2-weighted signal in the cornu ammonis as well as the dentate gyrus, consistent with left hippocampal sclerosis. FDG-PET showed bitemporal hypometabolism (left greater than right). Long-term video-EEG monitoring revealed strong evidence for left mesial temporal lobe epilepsy with interictal occasional left temporal intermittent rhythmic delta activity (TIRDA), frequent left 2–3 Hz polymorphic slowing, and eight captured electrographic seizures of left anterior temporal onset. Left ATL versus LITT was considered for treatment.

The patient underwent a comprehensive pre-surgical neuropsychological evaluation to help assess risk for cognitive morbidity with surgical intervention. Testing

D. Sabsevitz (✉)
Mayo Clinic, Department of Psychology and Psychiatry, Jacksonville, FL, USA

Mayo Clinic, Department of Neurological Surgery, Jacksonville, FL, USA
e-mail: Sabsevitz.David@mayo.edu

K. Blackmon
Mayo Clinic, Department of Psychology and Psychiatry, Jacksonville, FL, USA
e-mail: Blackmon.karen@mayo.edu

© Springer Nature Switzerland AG 2021
W. O. Tatum et al. (eds.), *Epilepsy Case Studies*,
https://doi.org/10.1007/978-3-030-59078-9_30

revealed largely average performances with no clear lateralizing or localizing features aside from mild weakness in rote verbal memory (i.e., word list-learning) functions, thought to perhaps reflect mild left medial temporal lobe involvement. Verbal memory for contextually organized information (i.e., stories), object naming, and semantic word generation abilities were notably intact and within the average range for his age. The patient underwent the intracarotid amobarbital procedure (i.e., Wada test), which indicated strong left dominance for speech and language functions and bilaterally adequate memory functions (Wada memory asymmetry = 0, recognized 8/8 objects with 1 false-positive error in both left and right injection conditions).

Considering his left hemisphere dominance for language functions and bilaterally intact memory functions, the patient underwent left medial temporal lobe LITT, with the aim of minimizing cognitive decrements, while still achieving a successful seizure outcome. MRI of the brain acquired 6-months post-surgery showed postoperative left anterior hippocampal and adjacent inferolateral amygdala ablative lesion from LITT with expected secondary reduction in the size of the left mammillary body (Fig. 30.1).

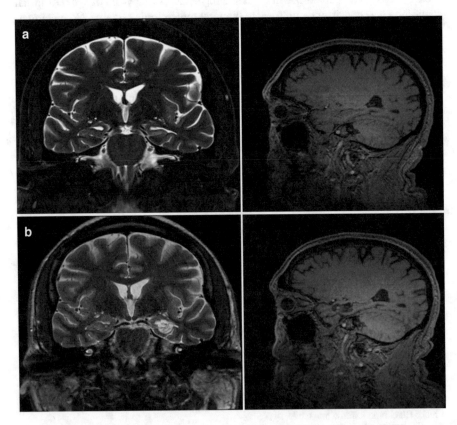

Fig. 30.1 (a) Preoperative and (b) 6 months post-LiTT coronal T2 and T1 sagittal MRI

Postoperative neuropsychological evaluation revealed only very mild cognitive decrements in episodic memory, naming, and verbal fluency functions but otherwise stable cognitive performance. The patient has remained seizure-free since undergoing LITT. There was no evidence of epileptiform discharges or subclinical seizures during a 48-hour ambulatory EEG study completed 6 months post-surgery.

Clinical Questions

1. What clinical variables predict neuropsychological outcome following dominant ATL?
2. What is known about the cognitive outcomes following LITT versus standard ATL?
3. What would the predicted risk of cognitive decline be for the patient in this case report? Would this predicted risk favor one treatment over the other?
4. What role does pre-surgical imaging play in predicting cognitive decline?
5. What is the role of extra-hippocampal regions in verbal memory and why might a more targeted resection preserve memory functions?

Discussion

1. It is estimated that between 30% and 60% of patients undergoing dominant ATL experience decline in verbal memory functions [1–3], while 25–60% experience decline in object naming abilities [4–6]. Side of surgery is the strongest predictor of memory and naming decline with surgery in the dominant hemisphere associated with more decline. Better preoperative memory and naming performance and later age at epilepsy onset have also been identified as risk factors for decline in these domains [6, 7].
2. LITT appears to have an advantage over standard ATL in preserving language functions. Drane and colleagues first reported on this advantage and showed a significant difference between the rate of decline on a picture naming and/or famous person naming task in patients undergoing dominant LITT of the amygdala hippocampal region versus standard ATL; no LITT patients showed decline (0–9 declined), whereas 95% (21/22) of ATL patients declined, as defined by reliable change indices [8]. Findings on whether there is an advantage of LITT over ATL in preserving episodic memory functions are more mixed. Several case reports and small case series show lower rates of decline on episodic memory tests (e.g., story memory, list learning) in patients undergoing LITT compared to historically reported rates of decline following ATL, while other studies show decline in this domain [9].
3. Given the patient's strong left hemisphere dominance for language on Wada testing and intact naming abilities on neuropsychological testing, he would be considered at risk for naming decline following a standard left temporal lobectomy. Despite evidence of left mesial temporal sclerosis (MTS) on MRI, he showed

good left hemisphere memory capacity on the Wada test and intact verbal memory performance on neuropsychological testing, which would indicate a high risk for some degree of verbal memory decline with left ATL. He would not, however, be considered at risk for a global amnestic syndrome as he showed good contralateral (i.e., right hemisphere) memory on the Wada test. In contrast, laser ablation of the hippocampus would likely reduce risk of naming decline via sparing temporal neocortical language systems, although risk for verbal memory decline would be less clear. In this case, LITT might be favored over ATL given the high risk for naming decline.

4. Patients with pre-surgical MRI evidence of left MTS show higher rates of seizure freedom following LITT than patients without MTS [10]. However, the presence of MTS as a predictor of verbal memory outcomes following LITT is unclear. In two patients with left temporal lobe epilepsy who were MRI-/PET+ (i.e., no MTS), LITT resulted in preserved naming and verbal fluency but decline in verbal and visual memory [11]. Patients with a normal hippocampus on MRI demonstrate an approximate decrease of 35% in verbal memory following ATL, whereas those with significant MTS show minimal change [7]. This may be in part related to their general level of pre-surgical memory functioning, given that a structurally intact left hippocampus is also associated with better pre-surgical verbal memory performance [12, 13]. However, it is possible that the presence of MTS may be associated with some degree of functional reorganization and a greater reliance on extra-hippocampal regions to support memory functions. A sclerotic left hippocampus is less likely to show fMRI activation during a verbal encoding task than a healthy, non-sclerotic hippocampus. Intact ipsilateral Wada test memory scores may reflect extra-hippocampal contributions, given limited perfusion of amytal to the hippocampus in many cases [14]. Thus, it is possible that targeted ablation of sclerotic hippocampal tissue and preservation of peri-hippocampal regions might optimize verbal memory outcomes, although the presence/absence of MTS has yet to be formally investigated as a predictor of post LITT cognitive outcomes.

5. Examination of the patient's post-surgical MRI shows preservation of the left posterior hippocampus, as well as parahippocampal and entorhinal regions. The critical role of these regions in supporting verbal memory functions has long been appreciated. Lesions to peri-hippocampal regions, even in the absence of hippocampal lesions, can lead to severe memory impairment [15]. In general, the larger the extent of left ATL, the greater the decline in verbal memory [16, 17]. More specifically, after accounting for baseline memory performance, the extent of left parahippocampal and entorhinal resection accounts for 27% and 37% of the variance in rote verbal memory decline, respectively [18]. Functional imaging of post-ATL patients shows that activation of the left posterior hippocampal remnant was associated with better postoperative verbal fluency and naming [19], suggesting that this region may not only be an important component of associative learning and memory networks, as previously appreciated, but also in broader language networks. Regarding this patient, it is likely that preservation of these regions contributed to his relatively good memory and language outcomes in the context of postsurgical seizure freedom.

Pearls

- Dominant hemisphere surgery, higher preoperative performance, and younger age at epilepsy onset are risk factors for language and verbal memory decline following ATL.
- LITT is associated with more optimal naming outcomes in patients with left TLE, whereas verbal memory outcomes are mixed.
- The presence of left lateralized language functions and intact language abilities in a patient with left temporal lobe epilepsy favors a more targeted and less invasive approach with LITT over ATL.
- Mesial temporal sclerosis may be an important predictor of post-surgical seizure and memory outcomes in LITT.
- Parahippocampal, entorhinal, and posterior hippocampal regions play a critical role in language and memory networks and preservation of these regions with LITT may contribute to better cognitive outcomes.

References

1. Baxendale S. Amnesia in temporal lobectomy patients: historical perspective and review. Seizure. 1998;7:15–24.
2. Bell BD, Davies KG. Anterior temporal lobectomy, hippocampal sclerosis, and memory: recent neuropsychological findings. Neuropsychol Rev. 1998;8:25–41.
3. Rausch R, Kraemer S, Pietras CJ, Le M, Vickrey BG, Passaro EA. Early and late cognitive changes following temporal lobe surgery for epilepsy. Neurology. 2003;60(6):951–9.
4. Busch RM, Floden DP, Prayson B, Chapin JS, Kim KH, Ferguson L, et al. Estimating risk of word-finding problems in adults undergoing epilepsy surgery. Neurology. 2016;87(22):2363–9.
5. Ives-Deliperi VL, Butler JT. Naming outcomes of anterior temporal lobectomy in epilepsy patients: a systematic review of the literature. Epilepsy Behav. 2012;24(2):194–8.
6. Sherman EM, Wiebe S, Fay-McClymont TB, Tellez-Zenteno J, Metcalfe A, Hernandez-Ronquillo L, et al. Neuropsychological outcomes after epilepsy surgery: systematic review and pooled estimates. Epilepsia. 2011;52(5):857–69.
7. Bell B, Lin JJ, Seidenberg M, Hermann B. The neurobiology of cognitive disorders in temporal lobe epilepsy. Nat Rev Neurol. 2011;7(3):154–64.
8. Drane DL, Loring DW, Voets NL, et al. Better object recognition and naming outcome with MRI-guided stereotactic laser amygdalo-hippocampotomy for temporal lobe epilepsy. Epilepsia. 2015;56:101–13.
9. Drane DL. MRI-guided stereotactic laser ablation for epilepsy surgery: promising preliminary results for cognitive outcome. Epilepsy Res. 2018;142:170–5.
10. Willie JT, Laxpati NG, Drane DL, et al. Real-time magnetic resonance guided stereotactic laser amygdalohippocampotomy for mesial temporal lobe epilepsy. Neurosurgery. 2014;74:569–84.
11. Dredla BK, Lucas JA, Wharen RE, Tatum WO. Neurocognitive outcome following stereotactic laser ablation in two patients with MRI-/PET+ mTLE. Epilepsy Behav. 2016;56:44–7.
12. Lencz T, et al. Quantitative magnetic resonance imaging in temporal lobe epilepsy: relationship to neuropathology and neuropsychological function. Ann Neurol. 1992;31:629–37.
13. Trenerry MR, et al. MRI hippocampal volumes and memory function before and after temporal lobectomy. Neurology. 1993;43:1800–5.
14. de Silva R, Duncan R, Patterson J, Gillham R, Hadley D. Regional cerebral perfusion and amytal distribution during the Wada test. J Nucl Med. 1999;40:747–52.

15. Zola-Morgan S, Squire LR, Amaral DG, Suzuki WA. Lesions of perirhinal and parahippo-campal cortex that spare the amygdala and hippocampal formation produce severe memory impairment. J Neurosci. 1989;9(12):4355–70.
16. Helmstaedter C, Petzold I, Bien CG. The cognitive consequence of resecting nonlesional tis-sues in epilepsy surgery—results from MRI- and histopathology negative patients with tempo-ral lobe epilepsy. Epilepsia. 2011;52(8):1402–8.
17. Helmstaedter C, Roeske S, Kaaden S, Elger CE, Schramm J. Hippocampal resection length and memory outcome in selective epilepsy surgery. Neurol Neurosurg Psychiatry. 2011;82(12):1375–81.
18. Liu A, Thesen T, Barr W, Morrison C, Dugan P, Wang X, et al. Parahippocampal and ento-rhinal resection extent predicts verbal memory decline in an epilepsy surgery cohort. J Cogn Neurosci. 2017;29(5):869–80.
19. Bonelli SB, Thompson PJ, Yogarajah M, et al. Imaging language networks before and after anterior temporal lobe resection: results of a longitudinal fMRI study. Epilepsia. 2012;53(4):639–50.

Reflex Epilepsies

31

Anthony Ritaccio

Case

A 23-year-old right-handed man was evaluated for a history of epilepsy over many years. Four years previously, he had suffered a left frontal hemorrhage associated with the sudden onset of expressive aphasia. Four days after presentation, a left frontal arteriovenous malformation was removed. Two months postoperatively, he began to experience habitual episodes of "electrical or clicking sensations" in his head/jaw associated with a brief forced expiration. These occurred only when he was reading; on three occasions, when he continuing to read despite clusters of recurrent spells, witnessed convulsions resulted. There was no family history of epilepsy. The patient's medical history was otherwise unremarkable. There was no history of developmental learning disability or traumatic head injury. Neither the patient nor family members noted any personality or behavioral changes associated with the frontal-lobe lesion and its removal. There were no obvious expressive or receptive speech difficulties on initial evaluation. Previous computed tomographic scans as well magnetic resonance (MR) image revealed a 2-cm region of encephalomalacia in the left frontal lobe, presumably the site of previous arteriovenous malformation removal (Fig. 31.1). Reading activation tests involving material of varied complexity were administered during continuous video-EEG monitoring. These reading activation tests reliably reproduced jaw myoclonus with associated audible stuttering, accompanied by ictal EEG correlates. All seizures were consistently associated with a 0.2- to 0.4-second ictal discharge in the left frontocentral region (Fig. 31.2). The paroxysmal abnormality consisted of sharp or spike transients with associated slow waves. Thirty-four clinical seizures with characteristic EEG features were provoked during the testing time of 3 h 41 min.

A. Ritaccio (✉)
Mayo Clinic, Department of Neurology, Jacksonville, FL, USA
e-mail: ritaccio.anthony@mayo.edu

© Springer Nature Switzerland AG 2021
W. O. Tatum et al. (eds.), *Epilepsy Case Studies*,
https://doi.org/10.1007/978-3-030-59078-9_31

Fig. 31.1 T2-weighted (repetition time, 2800 milliseconds; echo time, 80 milliseconds) axial cut. A 2-cm region of high signal abnormality is seen anterior to the left precentral gyrus. (Reproduced with permission from reference [1])

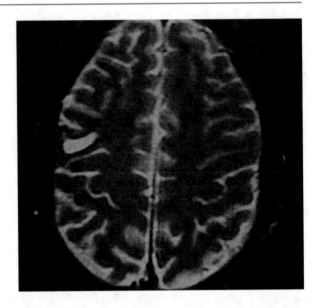

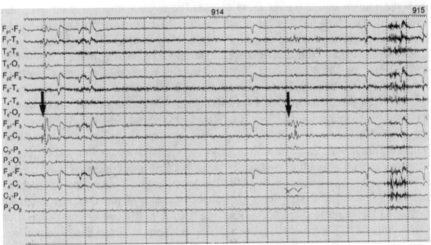

Fig. 31.2 Two electroclinical seizures during reading activation (*arrows*) demonstrate maximum electronegativity in the left frontocentral region. Both discharges were synchronous with brief jaw myoclonus. (Reproduced with permission from reference [1])

Questions

1. What is a working definition of reflex epilepsy?
2. How is reflex epilepsy categorized?
3. Can seizures be precipitated by higher cognitive tasks such as reading?
4. How is reflex epilepsy diagnosed?
5. How is reflex epilepsy treated?

Discussion

1. Reflex epilepsy refers to seizures that are regularly precipitated by a specific identifiable stimulus. It is not a syndrome but rather a collection of common seizure types (e.g., myoclonic, focal, and tonic-clonic) whose initiation has both a consistent and specific provoking stimulus. Common precipitating factors include somatosensory stimuli, visual stimuli, auditory, vestibular, olfactory stimuli, and high-level processes such as cognitive, emotional, decision-making tasks, and other complex stimuli. The majority of patients have spontaneous seizures as well. Stimulus-evocation of seizures may occur in 5–6% of all new epilepsy patients encountered by the clinical neurologist [2].

2. The common reflex syndromes encountered and currently classified suggest that neural networks subserving the provoking task promote seizures on either a topographic basis (shared with the seizure onset zone) or on a functional/connective basis. We commonly associate seizures with state-dependent triggers. State-dependent pathways profoundly influence seizure susceptibility illustrated by the increased seizure frequency around transition out of or into sleep (e.g., generalized tonic-clonic seizures-alone, juvenile myoclonic epilepsy, and benign childhood epilepsy with centrotemporal spikes; a.k.a Rolandic epilepsy).

   Similarly, channel-dependent pathways rely on specific interneuronal connections determining language, complex visuoperceptual and spatial processing, and explicit memory. Channel-dependent cognitive tasks are well-described seizure triggers. Linguistic tasks, both verbal and nonverbal, can provoke reflex seizures. The recent observation that spatial and episodic memory tasks promote temporal lobe interictal spikes implicates that precipitation of seizures by the stimulation of unique networks and may be operant in commonly encountered forms of temporal epilepsies [3].

   An organized complete classification of the reflex epilepsies does not exist [4]. Reviewers have historically categorized reflex epilepsies into a myriad of novel categories according to the triggering stimulus, (e.g., "chess-playing epilepsy," photo-sensitive epilepsy, etc.). It must clearly be stated that the majority of patients experience these uniquely precipitated seizures imbedded in established generalized and focal epilepsy syndromes (Table 31.1). Photosensitive epilepsy

Table 31.1 Summary of reflex seizures

Reflex epilepsy	
(As defined by the commonly encountered syndromes that seizures occur within)	
Generalized syndromes	Focal syndromes
Induced by light or pattern stimuli	Induced by somatosensory stimulation
Induced by thinking and decision-making	Induced by music, sound, or voice
	Induced by eating
	Induced by hot water immersion
	Induced by reading or other language functions
	Induced by startle
	Induced by proprioception

Reproduced with permission from reference [2]

is the most prevalent reflex epilepsy and the best known example of stimulus-induced seizures. Seizures induced by light as well as those initiated by higher cognitive tasks are most frequently the result of activating broadly distributed and bilateral networks in patients with various forms of genetic generalized epilepsies such as childhood absence epilepsy and juvenile myoclonic epilepsy. The majority of encountered patients have seizures precipitated by functional activation of cortex embedded in their seizure onset zone (SOZ), seizures triggered by music/voice in patients with their SOZ in temporal neocortex subserving auditory function, and seizures triggered by stimulating an extremity in patients with their SOZ in parietal/primary sensory cortex.

3. Linguistic operations involving both verbal and nonverbal tasks can provoke seizures reflexively. Although reading is the most frequent linguistic stimulus, writing and speaking can also induce seizures [5].

   Processes involving strategy and decision making such as calculating math, playing chess or backgammon, or playing card and video games may induce seizures. Reading epilepsy is characterized by myoclonic movements of oropharyngeal facial musculature (or sensations of movements in the jaw or throat) during reading [2]. Reading epilepsy occurs as both an unknown focal epilepsy with autosomal dominant inheritance and infrequently as a symptomatic or lesional process. Continuing the reading task can increase the movement frequency, culminating in a generalized tonic-clonic seizure (GTCS). The jaw movements may be unilateral or bilateral. The myoclonic seizures may be misdiagnosed as stuttering or a motor tic. During oral reading there may be hesitation, stuttering, or speech arrest.

   Multiple factors influence the seizure threshold in people with reflex epilepsy. When reading triggers seizures the level of attention, visual patterns, proprioceptive impulses from jaw and ocular muscles, or complexity of the reading material may influence seizure genesis. A potential neuroanatomic basis for one type of reading epilepsy is suggested by this case. Lesional analysis identified a 2-cm region of postsurgical encephalomalacia in dominant premotor cortex on brain MRI (Fig. 31.1). Jaw myoclonus was associated with brief left frontocentral epileptiform discharges and developed after resection of a left frontal arteriovenous malformation (Fig. 31.2). Dominant premotor cortex may activate motor sequences that generate graphic and phonetic (motor linguistic) output. Video-EEG with activation testing revealed phonological reading-evoked seizures.

4. The principal diagnostic tool for identifying reflex epilepsy remains a heightened awareness of these phenomena by clinicians as defined by a probing history with respect to commonly encountered precipitants (Table 31.1). Universally, stroboscopic photic stimulation is, pro forma, performed as a screening tool in routine EEGs to determine the presence of pathologic photosensitivity. Where indicated, prolonged video-EEG monitoring is invaluable to attempt provocation that is able to and repetitively demonstrate a patient's unique response to a specific stimulus and establish a consistent relationship to electrographic seizures, as in this case of reading epilepsy.

5. Control of reflex epilepsies involves antiseizure medication and, in selected cases, epilepsy surgery, neuromodulation, and less conventional methodologies of stimulus alteration, threshold alteration, and avoidance conditioning. For example, valproate is the most effective antiseizure medication for photosensitive seizures (e.g., absence, myoclonic, and tonic-clonic) in a patient with juvenile myoclonic epilepsy. If a patient has focal seizures arising from the right temporal lobe and a history of music-triggered episodes, antiseizure medication commonly utilized to treat focal seizures should be selected. (Patients with drug-resistant focal seizures provoked by specific stimuli are candidates for neuromodulatory and surgical strategies that are guided by the results obtained from a typical presurgical assessment (i.e., anatomic and functional neuroimaging, interictal and ictal EEG, and neuropsychological assessment).

Pearls
1. Reflex epilepsy refers to a loosely tied assortment of syndromes that have very specific simple sensory or cognitive triggers.
2. Seizures precipitated by unique stimuli are typically associated with generalized and focal epilepsy syndromes. Classification of seizure types and epilepsy syndromes has a well-established system and applies to patients with reflex epilepsies.
3. The identification of reflex epilepsy relies primarily on the history and the physician's high level of suspicion. The use of video-EEG monitoring to demonstrate consistent stimulus-specific seizure provocation that defines one of the reflex epilepsies is invaluable.
4. Pharmacologic, neuromodulatory, and surgical therapies are employed in the treatment of commonly encountered epilepsies also applies to those with reflex epilepsies.
5. Precipitation of seizures by specific stimuli is probably more common than currently appreciated.

References

1. Ritaccio AL, Hickling EJ, Ramani V. The role of dominant premotor cortex and grapheme to phoneme transformation in reading epilepsy. A neuroanatomic, neurophysiologic, and neuropsychological study. Arch Neurol. 1992;49(9):933–9.
2. Ritaccio AL. Reflex seizures. Neurol Clin. 1994;12(1):57–83.
3. Vivekananda U, Bush D, Bisby JA, et al. Spatial and episodic memory tasks promote temporal lobe interictal spikes. Ann Neurol. 2019;86:304–9.
4. Xue LY, Ritaccio AL. Reflex seizures and reflex epilepsy. Am J Electroneurodiagnostic Technol. 2006;46(1):39–48.
5. Ritaccio AL, Singh A, Devinsky O. Cognition-induced epilepsy. Epilepsy Behav. 2002;3(6):496–501.

Infrequent Seizures (Oligoepilepsy)

Gregory D. Cascino and William O. Tatum

Case Presentation

A 52-year-old man with probable focal epilepsy presents for consideration of anti-seizure medication (ASM) withdrawal. The patient had three unprovoked nocturnal tonic-clonic seizures in the past 10 years. All seizures occurred during sleep lasting approximately 1–2 min. During the seizures, there was tongue biting, loss of awareness, and postictal headache and myalgias. The patient was not on an ASM at the time of any seizure. The last seizure reportedly occurred approximately 5 years ago. There is a history of probable "concussion" as a child on two occasions but no other history of risk factors for epilepsy or remote symptomatic neurological disease. However, there is a family history of childhood absence. There is a history of epilepsy in a younger sibling who is in remission on ethosuximide. The patient currently is on carbamazepine (CBZ) 200 mg twice daily which was started after the third seizure. Compliance with ASM is excellent. The patient is quite self-confident for a successful trial of ASM because he has been seizure-free on CBZ. The patient complains of "mild sedation" and mild "forgetfulness with names" that he attributes to CBZ. The patient works for an investment company, operates a motor vehicle, and is married with two children. He enjoys running, golf, and hiking.

Neurological examination has been normal. The most recent trough CBZ level is 5.7 mcg/mL (range, 4–12 mcg/mL). MRI shows very mild, scattered small nonspecific T2 hyperintensities consistent with "small vessel disease or migraine." No

G. D. Cascino (✉)
Mayo Clinic, Department of Neurology, Rochester, MN, USA
e-mail: gcascino@mayo.edu

W. O. Tatum
Mayo Clinic, Department of Neurology, Jacksonville, FL, USA
e-mail: tatum.william@mayo.edu

© Springer Nature Switzerland AG 2021
W. O. Tatum et al. (eds.), *Epilepsy Case Studies*,
https://doi.org/10.1007/978-3-030-59078-9_32

definite epileptogenic lesion is present. EEG studies have shown sleep-activation of bitemporal, independent sharp waves. The most recent EEG (6 months ago) is "essentially normal"; the patient did not adequately fall asleep during the recording.

The patient has two questions: What are the risks of continued antiseizure medication vs. drug discontinuance for him? Why should he take ASM?

Clinical Questions

1. What is oligoepilepsy?
2. What are the potential challenges of treatment to consider in this patient with infrequent seizures?
3. What are the goals of treatment in patients with infrequent seizures?
4. What is the consequence of chronic ASM administration vs no treatment?
5. What is the natural history of patients who take no ASM with infrequent seizures?

Diagnostic Discussion

1. Some patients with epilepsy have a relatively benign course with infrequent seizures [1]. Oligoepilepsy is an obscure term used to describe the rare condition of a relatively benign seizure disorder. It is not a distinct syndrome but instead refers to a condition of infrequent seizures. Infrequent seizures pose a treatment challenge. Some patients maintain a stable pattern involving infrequent seizures for years using no ASM. Patients with frequent seizures are usually readily amenable to treatment, and two-thirds are well-controlled with ASM. Our patient had no seizures since medical treatment with ASM was initiated 5 years ago. Considerations of ASM withdrawal need to be balance the long inter-seizure interval and risk and implications of experiencing a breakthrough seizure (i.e., driving restrictions reimposed).
2. Challenges in the treatment of patients with infrequent seizures lie in attempting to balance seizures and side effects due to ASM especially when the natural history is unknown at the onset [2, 3]. In our patient, it is difficult to know with certainty whether CBZ at his current dose is producing "mild sedation" and "forgetfulness with names" given the low dosage utilized. There are other potential causes for tiredness and fatigue to be considered including occupation, lifestyle, family commitments, or any recognized medical disorder, e.g., obstructive sleep apnea or depression. Word finding difficulties and cognitive deficits can occur with selected ASDs such as topiramate. Individuals may have trouble with remembering names unrelated to ASM, e.g., developmental disorder and normal aging. However, even at low dosages, CBZ may produce clinical neurotoxicity with associated sedation and cognitive impairment.
3. The goals of ASM therapy are no seizures and no side effects. This patient may be a candidate for ASM taper and withdrawal because he has been

Table 32.1   Features suggesting high- and low-risk epilepsies for seizure recurrence.

May suggest increased risk	May suggest decreased risk
Remote symptomatic disease	No etiology
Developmental delay; focal neurological deficit(s)	Normal examination
History of drug-resistant epilepsy	Seizure remission with initial ASD
MRI-identified structural pathology	Normal or indeterminate MRI brain
Long history of epilepsy, i.e., "years"	Isolated or few seizure episodes
Prior ASM taper or withdrawal was unsuccessful, i.e., recurrent seizures	Seizure remission on low ASD dose and "modest" drug level
Selected genetic generalized epileptic syndromes (e.g., juvenile myoclonic epilepsy) and EEG-identified generalized epileptiform discharges	EEG shows no activation or rare-infrequent focal interictal epileptiform discharges
In adults: seizure-free <2 years	In adults: seizure-free >2–5 years
History of tonic/atonic seizures (drop attacks) and atypical absence seizures	Seizure-free following epilepsy surgery for focal epilepsy

seizure-free 5 years and does not have a history of remote symptomatic neu-rological disease, has a normal neurological examination, and has no definite structural imaging abnormality that would account for his seizures (Table 32.1). Spontaneous remission of epilepsy may occur in a substantial proportion of untreated patients affected by chronic epilepsy when a known cause is not identified in individuals who experience infrequent seizures. In one study, mortality was increased in patients with a remote symptomatic etiology.

4. Chronic ASM administration may lead to cognitive impairment, metabolic bone disease, falling and gait unsteadiness, potential drug interactions, and teratogen-esis which are important chronic side effects to consider when treating patients with infrequent seizures. In general, three times the inter-seizure interval is nec-essary to determine a treatment effect [4]. Unfortunately, all ASM has idiosyn-cratic and dose-dependent treatment emergent adverse effects that may undermine the effectiveness of therapy. The "newer" ASMs may also prove less effective than CBZ. A very rare concern with electing to not treat with ASM or recommending ASM withdrawal in a patient with seizures in apparent remission is the development of prolonged seizures and sudden unexplained death in epilepsy.

5. In some countries and in tropical areas, untreated epilepsy is not uncommon, especially when seizures are infrequent [3, 5]. The success of any treatment strategy is to render the patient seizure-free and avoid adverse effects. Educating the patient regarding the multiple therapeutic options is critical for any success of treatment. The individual's current occupation, lifestyle, and recreational activities govern the potential impact from infrequent seizures to compromise their overall quality of life. Driving status requires him to be seizure-free. One option in this patient is to consider a reduction in CBZ dosing to see if this improves the alleged adverse effects of treatment though there is uncertainty as to the potential for failing a trial of taper when ASM is lowered or withdrawn [6]. The role of the EEG prior to withdrawal of ASM when patients present with

treatment yields conflicting results. In generalized epilepsy, the presence of generalized epileptiform discharges indicates a high risk of seizure recurrence (Table 32.1).

Clinical Pearls

1. Some patients have a relatively benign form of epilepsy with recurrent but infrequent seizures.
2. Adult patients who are seizure-free 2 years or longer should be considered candidates for ASM withdrawal normally though the goals of treatment in patients with infrequent seizures are complex.
3. The goals of therapy should be no seizures and no side effects. Issues such as driving status, employment, and living situation may need to be considered.
4. Patients receiving chronic ASM may have acute, idiosyncratic, and chronic adverse effects that undermine the effectiveness of treatment.
5. The natural history of epilepsy varies. There is limited evidence in the literature on the natural history and mortality of epilepsy in an untreated population though in tropical countries up to 80–85% of patients with epilepsy are not treated [3]. Some individuals in developing countries forego treatment when they have experienced infrequent seizures (oligoepilepsy) over years without consequence.

References

1. Labate A, Gambardella A, Andermann E, Aguglia U, Cendes F, Berkovic S, et al. Benign mesial temporal lobe epilepsy. Nat Rev Neurol. 2011;7:237–40.
2. Kwan P, Sander JWAS. The natural history of epilepsy: an epidemiological view. Neurol Neurosurg Psychiatry. 2004;75:1376–81.
3. Nicoletti A, Sofia V, Vitale G, Bonelli S, Bejarano V, Bartalesi F, et al. Natural history and mortality of chronic epilepsy in an untreated population of rural Bolivia: a follow-up after 10 years. Epilepsia. 2009;50:2199–206.
4. Kwan P, Brodie MJ. Early identification of refractory epilepsy. N Engl J Med. 2000;342(5):314–9.
5. Placencia M, Sander JW, Roman M, Madera A, Crespo F, Cascante S, Shorvon SD. The characteristics of epilepsy in a largely untreated population in rural Ecuador. J Neurol Neurosurg Psychiatry. 1994;57:320–5.
6. Bartolini L, Majidi S, Koubeissi MZ. Uncertainties from a worldwide survey on antiepileptic drug withdrawal after seizure remission. Neurol Clin Pract. 2018;8(2):108–15.

Epilepsy, Mood, and Disability

33

Joseph I. Sirven

Case Presentation

A 26-year-old man presents with the chief complaint of recurrent "events." The episodes began approximately 2 years ago after he had been involved in an automobile accident and suffered a closed head injury. The spells were characterized by a sensation of "zoning out" that was preceded by a fearful sense of panic. They occurred at least twice a week and lasted between 50 and 90 s. After the event he felt tired and had difficulty focusing on his work or during his activities of daily living. He worked as a window installer, which requires driving, carpentry work, and use of tools.

No past family history of similar events was present. He would notice that after his spells that he was able to return to his work but always felt that his cognition and especially his word-finding ability were compromised. On one occasion when he had an event at work, a coworker took him to the ER where he was prescribed levetiracetam. His family also notes that the patient has had changes in his mood and seems more emotional and irritable lately. His girlfriend broke up with him recently because he is so easily irritated as well and found him impossible to live alongside. He presented for a definitive diagnosis and also counseling as to what he should tell his employer. Imaging studies of the brain were normal. A routine scalp EEG (Fig. 33.1) was performed and demonstrated the following;

Questions

1. What does the EEG show?
2. What are the implications for the individual's work?

J. I. Sirven (✉)
Mayo Clinic, Department of Neurology, Jacksonville, FL, USA
e-mail: Sirven.Joseph@mayo.edu

© Springer Nature Switzerland AG 2021
W. O. Tatum et al. (eds.), *Epilepsy Case Studies*,
https://doi.org/10.1007/978-3-030-59078-9_33

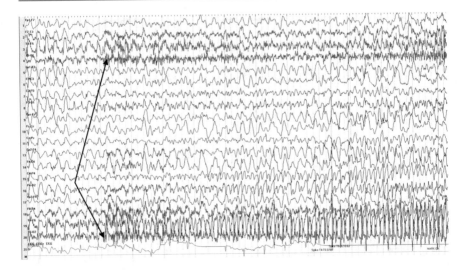

Fig. 33.1 EEG demonstrating an electrographic seizure involving the right hemisphere during which he complained of feeling panicky (note the superimposed temporal-occipital myogenic artifact (*arrows*))

3. What can be done for the irritability and mood issues?
4. Can his employer fire him because of seizures and will federal law prevent discrimination of epilepsy?
5. Will this individual be eligible for Social Security Disability?

Discussion

1. The EEG demonstrates an electroclinical seizure that involves the right hemisphere though is only associated with a subjective sensation of panic. With the patient history of recurrent episodes and an ictal EEG, the recording is therefore diagnostic of focal epilepsy. Antiseizure medication should be recommended and be the first line of therapy.
2. Unprovoked focal seizures are often associated with cognitive dysfunction as comorbidity. Short-term memory and language difficulties are not uncommon when the temporal lobe is involved. The symptoms produced by recurrent seizures however depend upon the anatomic localization of seizure onset zone. Therefore, if the seizures were not controlled, there could be significant implications for a patient's career. Given that this patient is driving, operating complex machinery and tools, there are some concerns about his safety. If his seizures are controlled without side effects, he should be able to continue gainful employment.
3. Like cognitive issues, psychiatric comorbid conditions are extremely common with seizures. Depression and anxiety are often reported with persistent seizures and must be managed along with the seizures. It is important to note that many antiseizure medications can impact psychiatric comorbidities (Table 33.1).

Table 33.1 Antiseizure drugs and mood

Mood stabilizing antiseizure drug	Neutral effect	Mood antagonizing antiseizure drug
Carbamazepine	Brivaracetam	Benzodiazepines
Eslicarbazepine	Cannabidiol	Clobazam
Oxcarbazepine	Felbamate	Levetiracetam
Lamotrigine	Gabapentin	Perampanel
Valproic acid	Lacosamide	Phenobarbital
	Pregabalin	Primidone
	Topiramate	Tiagabine
	Zonisamide	

Levetiracetam is particularly noteworthy in that it can magnify underlying mood issues and irritability, which is what happened in this particular patient. When this occurs, it is important to consider alternative antiseizure medications. If changing the medication does not help, then treating the underlying psychiatric condition is essential. Other antiseizure medications that augment comorbid psychiatric issues include perampanel, phenobarbital, and benzodiazepines such as clobazam (Table 33.1) and potentially topiramate and zonisamide despite a tendency for cognitive dysfunction [1].

4. According to the American with Disabilities Act (ADA) passed in 1990, the US law ensures equality of opportunity, full participation, independent living, and economic self-sufficiency for individuals with disabilities [2]. Civil rights are addressed across several domains and include employment discrimination. Discrimination includes both public services and those involving public accommodations. Title I of the ADA specifically protects people with disabilities from being discriminated against in the workplace. Any discrimination involved in hiring, the advancement or discharge of employees, compensation involving job training and job execution, and equal conditions and privileges of employment are subject to the ADA. Titles II and III prohibit discrimination based on disability by public entity. This includes limiting access to public transportation at both the local and state level and require public accommodations be available if needed. An individual cannot legally be fired because of seizures or a diagnosis of epilepsy. In 2008 the ADA provided protection for patients with disabilities that included epilepsy by adopting an amendment to the ADA. This amendment specifically addressed epilepsy even though seizures are episodic in nature; their occurrence (despite remission) could disable one's life style. Therefore, our patient has protection by US law. In addition, reasonable accommodations should be made to prevent undue hardship. These include carpeting to cushion falls, a private area to rest after a seizure, day shift working hours, waive non-essential tasks, or reassignment to an alternate job (i.e., a non-driving position). Additionally, eligible employees may utilize the Family and Medical Leave Act to take up to 12 weeks of unpaid leave within a 12-month time period [3].

5. With regard to qualifying for Social Security Disability, the Social Security Administration does consider epilepsy a condition that may lead to disability. There are two inclusions for epilepsy. The first involves epilepsy that is

manifested as convulsions, and another exists for those who have seizures that are non-convulsive. To qualify for benefits with convulsive epilepsy, at least one seizure a month must be present with at least 3 months of antiseizure medication. The seizures must be daytime seizures and involve convulsions that involve a loss of consciousness or be nighttime seizures that result in symptoms that result in impairment of daytime activities. To qualify with non-convulsive epilepsy, one must prove that there is at least one seizure per week despite at least 3 months of compliance with a prescription antiepileptic medication. In addition, the seizures must significantly interfere with daily activities or create abnormal postictal behavior. Lastly, if one does not meet the criteria spelled out above, one can qualify for disabilities under the medical vocational guidelines. This means that the symptoms of epilepsy must interfere with daily activities such that there are no jobs available that one could consistently perform. However, this involves a more rigorous review prior to receiving disability. The claims examiner will address the individual's age, level of education, transferable work skills, and other medical and psychiatric conditions. He will take note of the individual's ability to work as well as any restrictions that the treating physician has placed on the person including driving restrictions and avoidance of work around machinery. In general, one must show that you are unable to perform any work-related activities on a full-time basis. Simply voicing that you are unable to do your job is insufficient. Older individuals and those that have less education and fewer transferable employment skill sets increase the chances of being awarded disability benefits [4, 5].

Clinical Pearls
1. The American with Disabilities Act and the 2008 ADA amendment protects individuals with epilepsy with or without a psychiatric illness.
2. One can qualify for Social Security Administration Disability with epilepsy and either convulsive or non-convulsive seizures.
3. Seizures alone are not required to be the only issue impairing the ability to work. Cognitive and psychiatric issues including those associated with treatment may also be associated with employment disability.
4. One should refer patients to advocacy organization when discrimination or disability occurs such as the Epilepsy Foundation of America (https://www.epilepsy.com).
5. It is important to note that epilepsy and treatments for epilepsy are often associated with initiating or aggravating of psychiatric comorbidities. It is essential to assess whether psychiatric symptoms occurring from seizures, from treatment, or alongside epilepsy management render appropriate treatment in order to improve quality of life.

References

1. Sirven JI. Management of epilepsy comorbidities. Continuum 2016;22(1 Epilepsy): 191–203.
2. http://www.ssa.gov/disability/professionals/bluebook/11.00-Neurological-Adult.htm. Accessed 6 June 2020.
3. http://www.iom.edu/Activities/Disease/Epilepsy.aspx. Accessed 6 June 2020.
4. Chaplin JE, Wester A, Tomson R. Factors associated with the employment problems of people with established epilepsy. Seizure. 1998;7:299–30.
5. Drazkowski JF. Management of the social consequences of seizures. Mayo Clin Proc. 2003;78:641–9.

Neuroimaging and Epilepsy

34

Vivek Gupta, Erik H. Middlebrooks,
and Prasanna G. Vibhute

Case Presentation

A 28-year-old, right-handed white man was referred for evaluation of long-standing, drug-resistant focal epilepsy beginning in the fourth year of life. No early risk factors were present. The developmental milestones were normal, and he completed college education at age 22.

His typical seizures were preceded by a prodrome of dizziness and were described as stereotypical episodes of head and eye deviation to the right lasting up to 20 seconds with reduced postictal cognitive processing speed. Lack of sleep, acute illness, and over exertion triggered his seizures. His mother also reported altered awareness, lip smacking, and right arm posturing.

MRI at seizure onset at age 4 was reported as normal. Initial treatment with carbamazepine failed, prompting unsuccessful trials of divalproex sodium, lamotrigine, and levetiracetam. At the time of the referral, seizures were occurring 1–2 times per month, forcing him off work 1–3 days per month. He also had occasional generalized tonic-clonic seizures and was hospitalized twice for status epilepticus. He also complained of frequent headaches and depressed mood due to antiepileptic medication.

His neurological examination was normal. Neuropsychological evaluation suggested mild compromise of frontal lobe function, greater in the left hemisphere including lateralized slowing in right-hand motor skills and impaired cognitive organization in copying a complex figure. No other focal or lateralized findings were evident.

Video-EEG monitoring revealed interictal midline and central spike-and-wave discharges. Two habitual seizures were captured that were characterized by

V. Gupta (✉) · E. H. Middlebrooks · P. G. Vibhute
Mayo Clinic, Department of Radiology, Division of Neuroradiology, Jacksonville, FL, USA
e-mail: Gupta.Vivek@mayo.edu; middlebrooks.erik@mayo.edu;
Vibhute.prasanna@mayo.edu

© Springer Nature Switzerland AG 2021
W. O. Tatum et al. (eds.), *Epilepsy Case Studies*,
https://doi.org/10.1007/978-3-030-59078-9_34

generalized ictal fast activity for 3–4 s evolving to generalized voltage attenuation immediately followed by 6 Hz focal left posterior centrotemporal rhythmic activity. All of these electrographic changes preceded head deviation to the right. The electroclinical correlation was consistent with left frontal seizure onset.

Brain MRI performed with a dedicated 3 T, high-resolution epilepsy protocol was reported as normal. The FDG-PET did not reveal focal hypometabolism on quantitative analysis. Subtracted ictal SPECT co-registered to MRI (SISCOM) showed bilateral post-central ictal hyperperfusion. A magnetoencephalogram (MEG) was noncontributory, revealing questionable epileptiform disturbances in the left parietal region without concomitant EEG changes.

A review of the brain MRI prompted by electroclinical findings revealed a subtle focal cortical dysplasia (FCD) at the depth of the left superior frontal sulcus (Fig. 34.1).

Intracranial EEG was performed with intraoperative MR guidance, with placement of two depth electrodes targeting the FCD and the second depth electrode along a parallel trajectory 4 mm anteromedial to the first electrode (Fig. 34.2). In addition, a 1 × 6 subdural strip along the superior temporal gyrus, an 8 × 8 grid over the frontotemporoparietal region, and a 4 × 4 grid over the prefrontal cortex were placed (Fig. 34.2). Frequent interictal spiking was present in the deep contact points of both the anterior and posterior stereotactic depth electrodes, and occasional spikes were also seen on the posterior border of the 8 × 8 grid, approximating the anterior parietal lobe and those overlying the motor cortex.

Four provoked seizures and two spontaneous seizures were captured. Provoked seizures occurred during electrocortical stimulation localized to the posterior stereotactic depth electrode at the distal contact points adjacent to the suspected FCD. The aura and ictal behaviors characterized by tonic extension of the right arm, splaying of the right fingers, head and eye deviation to the right (Fig. 34.3), and a

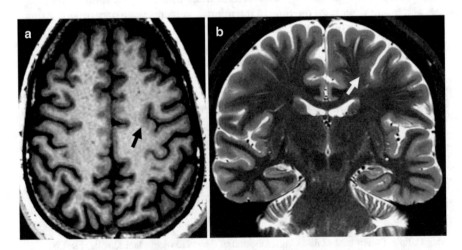

Fig. 34.1 Subtle focal cortical thickening and blurring of the *gray-white* matter interface, suggesting focal cortical dysplasia (**a** and **b**, *arrows*) along the medial aspect in the depth of an unusually deep left superior frontal sulcus (**b**)

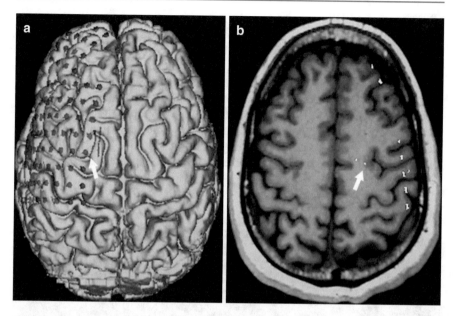

Fig. 34.2 Coregistration of the MPRAGE MRI with post-grid placement CT showing the location of subdural grids and depth electrodes in the left hemisphere on a 3D-shaded surface display (**a**) and axial section (**b**). Note the proximity of the distal contact of the posterolateral depth electrode to the FCD (*arrows*)

Fig. 34.3 Tonic extension of the right arm, splaying of the right fingers, and right head deviation during a typical seizure captured during video-EEG monitoring

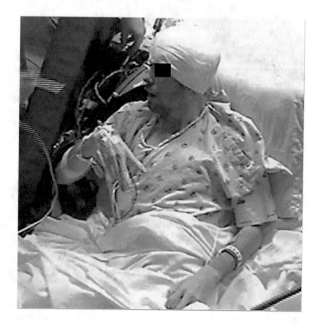

brief period of verbal unresponsiveness and altered awareness during these pro-voked seizures were typical of his habitual events. The patient also had two sponta-neous focal seizures and one focal to bilateral tonic-clonic seizure, all with an electroclinical pattern like that of the provoked seizures.

Two months later, an MR-guided stereotactic ablation of left frontal FCD was performed with laser interstitial thermal therapy (LiTT), reproducing the trajectory used for placement of the depth electrode (Fig. 34.4). Intraoperative MRI confirmed technically successful ablation. No post-operative neurological deficit occurred, and the patient has remained seizure-free (Engel Class 1) since the ablation. He is cur-rently working and continues to take levetiracetam 1500 mg BID and lamotrigine 200 mg TID.

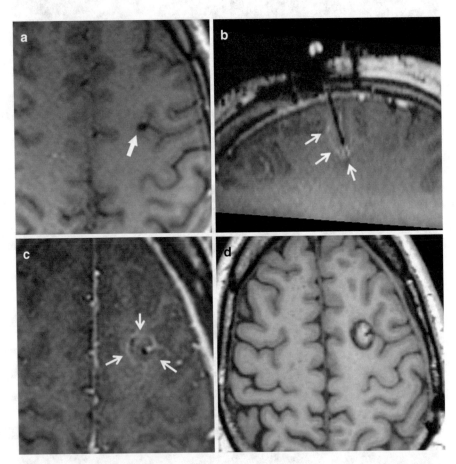

Fig. 34.4 Laser ablation of the FCD: intraoperative MR showing laser fiber targeting the lesion (**a**, *arrow*); peripheral enhancement of the zone of thermocoagulation surrounding the fiber (**b** and **c**, *arrows*); and 8-month MR follow-up (**d**) showing ablation of the FCD with high degree of precision

Clinical Questions

1. What is the role of MR imaging in localization of seizure onset?
2. What is the optimal MR technique or protocol in evaluation of seizures?
3. What is the role of imaging in planning and successful localization with intracranial EEG monitoring?
4. How does the location of this FCD explain the clinical and EEG features?
5. What is the role of imaging in minimally invasive techniques used in the surgical treatment of patients with epilepsy?

Answers

1. Detection of a cortical or juxtacortical structural abnormality by neuroimaging provides a reliable noninvasive means of localization. MRI is the modality of choice owing to its highest sensitivity and specificity among all neuroimaging techniques in identifying the epileptogenic focus [1–3]. Abnormalities detected on MRI when concordant with ictal electrographic recordings from scalp electrodes are often sufficient for surgical decision-making in patients with drug-resistant focal epilepsy, obviating the need for intracranial EEG monitoring [4]. Normal MRI (nonlesional epilepsy) remains a predictor of poorer seizure outcome from surgery compared to patients undergoing lesional epilepsy surgery [5].
2. The MRI is best obtained with 3T magnet and must include high-resolution and high gray-white matter contrast sequences [3, 6]. The MR imaging of medial temporal structures including the hippocampus and amygdala is best performed with 2 mm FSE T2 perpendicular to the long axis of the hippocampus with in-plane resolution of 0.4×0.4 mm [6]. Isotropic 1.0 mm resolution MPRAGE or MP2RAGE sequences provide optimal gray-white matter contrast and resolution for imaging of the neocortical lesions [6]. Volumetric T2 FLAIR is also valuable in detection of mesial temporal and neocortical lesions [6]. High-resolution susceptibility-weighted imaging (SWI) is also highly recommended for detection of small cavernomas, calcifications, and posttraumatic lesions of the cortex [1, 2]. Incremental gain in detection of epileptogenic lesions has also been shown at ultra-high field MRI (7T), but clinical implementation is currently limited due to lack of widespread availability.
3. In contrast to temporal lobe epilepsy, electroclinical findings are frequently unreliable for surgical decision-making in extratemporal epilepsy, and localization is vastly improved by the presence of a structural lesion on MRI [7, 8]. In this patient, the scalp EEG suggested a rather broad left frontal onset, and the localizing evidence from ictal SPECT was conflicting. The semiology was concordant with the location of the FCD (see Answer 4 for explanation) but not specific. Presence of a structural abnormality on MRI not only predicts favorable postsurgical seizure outcome but also plays a critical role in planning and success of icEEG for localizing the seizure onset [1, 2, 7]. In this patient, identification of

the cortical lesion (FCD) provided the key information for the placement of the depth electrodes for icEEG monitoring.

4. Seizures arising from the frontal lobe can have highly variable semiology, and electrographic characteristics are typically poorly localizing as the ictal activity can rapidly and unpredictably propagate after seizure onset due to the rich and variable connectivity of the frontal cortex to other brain regions in epilepsy patients [8, 9]. Contralateral tonic version of the eyes and head deviation in this patient is consistent with seizure origin near the frontal eye fields (Brodmann area 8) where this FCD was located.

5. Laser interstitial thermal therapy (LITT) or stereotactic laser ablation is rapidly becoming an effective minimally invasive alternative to open resection [10]. MRI plays a critical role in planning, intraoperative guidance, and confirmation of the location and adequacy of the surgical ablation. Multiplanar reformatting of the volumetric sequences such as MPRAGE allows identification of the target landmarks and safe trajectory of approach avoiding cortical veins, deep arteries, ventricles, and choroid plexus. The size, anatomic location, availability of a safe surgical corridor, and the proximity of the lesion to eloquent cortices were critical to surgical decision-making and in selecting LITT as opposed to an open resection. Real-time MR thermography increases the efficacy and safety of LITT by monitoring both target and collateral tissue temperatures. Immediate post-ablation MRI is performed with gadolinium-enhanced T1, FLAIR, or DWI before removing the probe to confirm the location and technical adequacy of ablation. The acute ablation zone is ovoid in shape and shows peripheral T2/FLAIR hyperintense signal and gadolinium enhancement (Fig. 34.4).

Clinical Pearls

1. Imaging is a critical component of the multimodality approach required for localization of drug-resistant epilepsy.

2. MRI is the imaging modality of choice for presurgical localization in patients with chronic drug-resistant focal epilepsy. The MRI should be obtained with 3T magnet with a dedicated epilepsy protocol comprising of high-resolution and high gray-white matter contrast sequences.

3. Abnormalities detected on MRI when concordant with ictal electrographic recordings from scalp electrodes are often sufficient for surgical decision-making in patients with drug-resistant focal epilepsy.

4. Knowledge of electroclinical features leads not only to improved detection of lesions on imaging studies but also in determining their epileptogenic potential.

5. Detection of the epileptogenic lesion by MRI is critical to planning and success of epilepsy surgery and intracranial EEG monitoring. A careful review and re-review of the MRI is always warranted in all nonlesional (normal or "negative" MRI) epilepsy before proceeding to intracranial EEG monitoring (phase 2).

References

1. Zucconi WB, Gupta V, Bronen RA. Epilepsy. In: Atlas SW, editor. Magnetic resonance imaging of the brain and spine. Philadelphia: Wolters Kluwer; 2017. p. 277–303.
2. Gupta V, Bronen RA. Overview of MR techniques for epilepsy. In: Chugani HT, editor. Neuroimaging in epilepsy. New York: Oxford University Press; 2011. p. 8–36.
3. Middlebrooks EH, Ver Hoef L, Szaflarski JP. Neuroimaging in epilepsy. Curr Neurol Neurosci Rep. 2017;17:32.
4. Engel JJ, Shewon D. Who should be considered a surgical candidate? In: Engel JJ, editor. Surgical treatment of the epilepsies. 2nd ed. New York: Raven Press; 1993. p. 23–34.
5. Téllez-Zenteno JF, Hernández Ronquillo L, Moien-Afshari F, Wiebe S. Surgical outcomes in lesional and non-lesional epilepsy: a systematic review and meta-analysis. Epilepsy Res. 2010 May;89(2–3):310–8. https://doi.org/10.1016/j.eplepsyres.2010.02.007.
6. Bernasconi A, Cendes F, Theodore WH, et al. Recommendations for the use of structural magnetic resonance imaging in the care of patients with epilepsy: a consensus report from the international league against epilepsy neuroimaging task force. Epilepsia. 2019;60:1054–68. https://doi.org/10.1111/epi.15612.
7. Spencer SS. Selection of candidate for invasive monitoring. In: Cascino GD, Jack Jr CR, editors. Neuroimaging in epilepsy: principles & practice. Newton: Butterworth-Heinemann; 1996. p. 219–34.
8. Wieser HG, Hajek M. Frontal lobe epilepsy: compartmentalization, presurgical evaluation, and operative results. In: Jasper HH, Riggio S, Golsman-Rakie PS, editors. Epilepsy and functional anatomy of the frontal lobe. New York: Raven Press; 1995. p. 297–353.
9. Luo C, An D, Yao D, Gotman J. Patient-specific connectivity pattern of epileptic network in frontal lobe epilepsy. NeuroImage Clin. 2014;4:668–75. https://doi.org/10.1016/j.nicl.2014.04.006.
10. LaRiviere MJ, Gross RE. Stereotactic laser ablation for medically intractable epilepsy: the next generation of minimally invasive epilepsy surgery. Front Surg. 2016;3:64. https://doi.org/10.3389/fsurg.2016.00064.

Stroke and Epilepsy

35

Scott D. Spritzer

Case

An 87-year-old female with distant history of ischemic cardiomyopathy, sick sinus syndrome, and chronic atrial fibrillation presented to the emergency department after waking up at 7 am with observed "garbled" speech and difficulty with language comprehension. She had gone to bed in her normal health the night prior at 9 pm. Two weeks prior to presentation, she had stopped therapeutic anticoagulation due to recurrent falls and presumed risk of major hemorrhage.

On initial presentation in the emergency department, she was noted to have a moderate mixed aphasia and mild right hemiparesis, with an initial NIHSS score of 8. Head CT showed no intracranial hemorrhage or early ischemic changes (Fig. 35.1), and CT angiogram of the head showed no large vessel occlusion. She was admitted to the hospital with a presumptive diagnosis of stroke. She was unable to get an MRI due to the pacemaker. Over the course of the following 4 days, she had gradual improvement of the right-sided weakness, with ongoing fluctuating mixed aphasia. Two additional head CTs were obtained over the next 36 h, without clear evidence of evolving infarct. An EEG was obtained 24 h after admission, showing left temporal lateralized periodic discharges and mild bitemporal slowing. Due to clinical symptoms and EEG findings, a lumbar puncture was performed, with unremarkable spinal fluid testing. After 4 days, a repeat EEG showed resolution of the left temporal

S. D. Spritzer (✉)
Mayo Clinic Health System, Department of Neurology, Eau Claire, WI, USA
e-mail: spritzer.scott@mayo.edu

© Springer Nature Switzerland AG 2021
W. O. Tatum et al. (eds.), *Epilepsy Case Studies*,
https://doi.org/10.1007/978-3-030-59078-9_35

Fig. 35.1 CT head
obtained on initial
presentation,
demonstrating no clear
early ischemic change or
evidence of cerebral
infarction

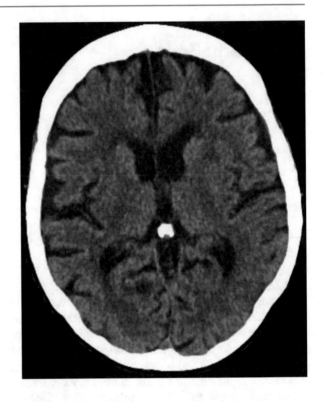

discharges with ongoing mild focal left temporal slowing. Due to findings on
EEG and clinical presentation, she was discharged from the hospital on levetiracetam with a diagnosis of new-onset focal seizure with prolonged postictal
state. One day after hospital discharge, her husband noticed progressively
worsening language deficits and right-sided weakness, prompting reevaluation
in the emergency department, at which time a follow-up head CT (obtained
6 days after her initial presentation) demonstrated an evolving infarct in the left
insula (Fig. 35.2). She was admitted to the hospital, and levetiracetam was
discontinued after an additional EEG demonstrated ongoing resolution of left
temporal lateralized periodic discharges. Anticoagulation was resumed for secondary stroke prevention, and she was discharged for ongoing rehabilitation.
She was seen in the neurology clinic 1 month after her initial presentation, with
moderate residual aphasia and a mild spastic right hemiparesis, without reports
of clinical seizures. CT head obtained prior to her clinic follow-up demonstrated a completed infarct involving the middle M2 branch of the left MCA
territory (Fig. 35.3).

Fig. 35.2 CT head
obtained 5 days after
symptoms onset,
demonstrating an evolving
ischemic infarct in the
left insula

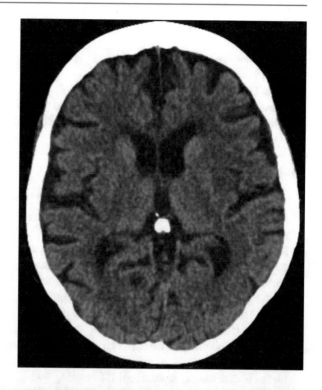

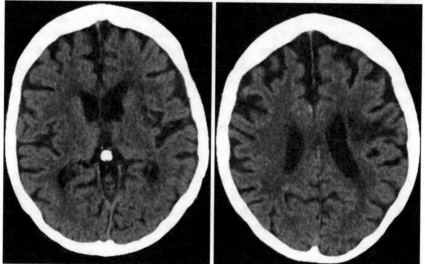

Fig. 35.3 CT head obtained 2 months after initial presentation, demonstrating a chronic ischemic
infarct involving the middle (M2) branch of the left MCA territory

Clinical Questions

1. What does the clinical history suggest? What did the EEG demonstrate?
2. What is the epidemiology of stroke?
3. What EEG abnormalities are most commonly associated with acute stroke?
4. What is the clinical significance of lateralized periodic discharges?
5. What is the association between seizures and stroke?

Diagnostic Discussion

1. The clinical history of abrupt-onset aphasia and right-sided weakness that persists for several days, in a patient with known cerebrovascular risk factors, is most suggestive of an acute left hemispheric stroke. The history of known atrial fibrillation with a recent discontinuation of anticoagulation would further favor cerebrovascular cause. Although strokes commonly cause new-onset focal seizures, the clinical history would not support this primarily due to the persistence of symptoms despite resolution of epileptiform abnormalities on follow-up EEG. Advanced age and lack of headache history, in addition to prolonged duration and lack of associated headache, suggest a non-migrainous etiology. The inability to obtain brain MRI with diffusion-weighted sequences further confounded her diagnosis, as this likely would have confirmed a cerebral infarct. In these circumstances, multimodal CT imaging with CT perfusion and CT angiography may have provided diagnostic clarity earlier on [1]. Although the patient's initial EEG demonstrated an epileptiform pattern (left temporal lateralized periodic discharges), these EEG abnormalities resolved at the conclusion of the patients initial hospitalization, despite ongoing clinical symptoms. A seizure of left temporal lobe origin could explain the patient's initial clinical symptoms. If clinical suspicion for focal seizure was high, video EEG for 24–48 h would have been helpful in clarifying whether ongoing subclinical seizures would possibly explain the persistent symptoms [2].
2. Stroke is the fifth leading cause of death in the United States [3]. Most strokes are ischemic in origin (~85%), with the remainder being hemorrhagic. With the advancement of primary prevention strategies focusing on optimal recognition and treatment of vascular risk factors, along with the advent of acute stroke therapies, the overall mortality rate of stroke has declined significantly in the past 30 years. In addition, with evolving knowledge regarding risk factor management and secondary stroke prevention, the rate of recurrent stroke has declined significantly.
3. EEG abnormalities are commonly seen in association with acute ischemic stroke. Infarcts involving the cerebral cortex frequently have associated ipsilateral focal slowing in the theta and delta range. In contrast, smaller subcortical infarcts rarely cause EEG abnormalities. Certain EEG changes have been associated with unfavorable stroke outcomes, including background activity slowing, asymmetry, suppression, lateralized rhythmic slowing, and lateralized periodic

discharges [4]. Lateralized epileptiform discharges are often seen when EEG is obtained early on after an acute stroke; however, not all patients with lateralized periodic discharges on EEG have seizures [5].

4. Lateralized periodic discharges, (f.k.a periodic lateralized epileptiform discharges (PLEDS)) are most commonly caused by stroke [6]. Additional causes include encephalitis (viral, autoimmune), tumor, etc. The general mechanism relates to an underlying severe focal cerebral injury or insult. Studies report between 58% and 100% of patients with lateralized periodic discharges on EEG have clinical seizures. In contrast, the presence of lateralized periodic discharges without a clear clinical correlate worrisome for seizure is not felt to represent an ictal pattern and would not warrant antiseizure medication. Regardless of underlying etiology, lateralized periodic discharges on emergent EEG have been associated with increased morbidity and mortality [7].

5. Approximately 50% of new-onset seizures in patients over the age of 60 are due to stroke [8]. Early post-stroke seizures, defined by occurrence within 7 days of acute stroke, are a result of the cytotoxic cascade induced by disruption of the blood-brain barrier causing localized cerebral irritability [9]. Late post-stroke epilepsy, or seizures developing outside of 7 days after the acute stroke, is caused by gliosis, neuronal loss, chronic inflammation, and altered synaptic plasticity. Those at increased risk of early post-stroke seizures include patients less than 65 years of age and patients with hemorrhagic stroke, ischemic stroke with hemorrhagic transformation, high stroke severity (defined by Barthel Index score 0–4), and alcoholism. Post-stroke epilepsy occurs more often in patients with high stroke severity and ischemic stroke with cortical involvement, with additional data suggesting patients with early post-stroke seizures having increased risk of developing post-stroke epilepsy. Overall, the prognosis in patients with stroke-related epilepsy is good, with less than 5% of reported patients being drug resistant. Drug-resistant post-stroke epilepsy has been associated with greater disability and reduced functional outcomes.

Clinical Pearls

1. An acute ischemic stroke presents as abrupt-onset persistent neurological deficit(s) localizing to a focal region of the brain. Emergent CT head is less sensitive than brain MRI in detecting small acute infarcts or subtle early ischemic change. More obvious changes are seen on head CT in subacute to chronic ischemic stroke.

2. The diagnosis of seizure is clinical, and overreliance on EEG results can obscure a more obvious clinical diagnosis.

3. A broad range of EEG abnormalities have been described in association with acute ischemic stroke, including lateralized periodic discharges. If clinical suspicion for seizure is high, continuous EEG monitoring is a useful tool to evaluate for the potential for ongoing electrogaphic seizures.

4. Strokes are commonly associated with seizures, with distinct mechanisms causing early post-stroke seizures and late-onset post-stroke epilepsy.
5. Although empiric antiseizure medication is not recommended in patients presenting with acute ischemic stroke, recognition and treatment of seizures in patients hospitalized with acute stroke may help optimize stroke recovery. Poorly controlled post-stroke epilepsy has been associated with poorer functional outcome and greater disability following stroke.

References

1. Lin MP, Liebesking DS. Imaging of ischemic stroke. Continuum. 2016;22(5):1399–423.
2. Herman ST, Abend NS, Hirsch LJ, et al. Consensus statement on continuous EEG in critically ill adults and children, part 1: indications. J Clin Neurophysiol. 2015;32:87–95.
3. Guzik A, Bushnell C. Stroke epidemiology and risk factor management. Continuum. 2017;23(1):15–39.
4. Bentes C, Peralta AR, Ferro JM, et al. Seizures, electroencephalographic abnormalities, and outcome of ischemic stroke patients. Epilepsia Open. 2017;2(4):441–52.
5. Charlin C, Tiberge M, Larrue V. The clinical significance of periodic lateralized epileptiform discharges in acute ischemic stroke. J Stroke Cerebrovasc Dis. 2000;9(6):298–302.
6. Lin L, Drislane FW. Lateralized periodic discharges: a literature review. J Clin Neurophysiol. 2018;35:189–98.
7. Kate MP, Dash GK, Radhakrishnan A. Long-term outcome and prognosis of patients with emergent periodic lateralized epileptiform discharges. Seizure. 2012;21:450–6.
8. Feyissa AM, Hasan TF, Meschia JF. Stroke-related epilepsy. Eur J Neurol. 2019;26:18–26.
9. Zhang C, Wang X, Shao X, et al. Risk factors for post-stroke seizures: a systematic review and meta-analysis. Epilepsy Res. 2014;108:1806–16.

Status Epilepticus Convulsive

36

Joseph I. Sirven

Case Presentation

A 23-year-old male with a history of focal epilepsy manifest as recurrent focal impaired awareness seizures and intermittent focal to bilateral tonic-clonic seizures was taking levetiracetam 500 mg twice a day. He was seizure-free as long as he remained compliant with his antiseizure medication (ASM). He was reported to have recently been away on a camping trip with several of his friends. While he was away, he was sleep deprived due to the long period of time he remained awake often staying up until late hours of the early morning. Shortly after midnight he developed a generalized tonic-clonic seizure. This was repeated two more times, and his friends called 911 for help. He was transported to the nearest hospital and had persistent impairment of his consciousness. In the emergency department (ED), he did not answer questions and was "just staring at the nurses." A CT of the brain was unrevealing. Laboratory evaluation did not demonstrate any abnormalities in his electrolytes or complete blood count with differential. A toxicology screen was negative for illicit substances as well as for alcohol. A carbamazepine level was undetectable.

An EEG was obtained in the ED (Fig. 36.1) due to persistent alteration of consciousness.

Clinical Questions

1. What is the definition of status epilepticus?
2. How does the EEG help in making the diagnosis?
3. What should comprise the initial evaluation of status?

J. I. Sirven (✉)
Mayo Clinic, Department of Neurology, Jacksonville, FL, USA
e-mail: Sirven.Joseph@mayo.edu

© Springer Nature Switzerland AG 2021
W. O. Tatum et al. (eds.), *Epilepsy Case Studies*,
https://doi.org/10.1007/978-3-030-59078-9_36

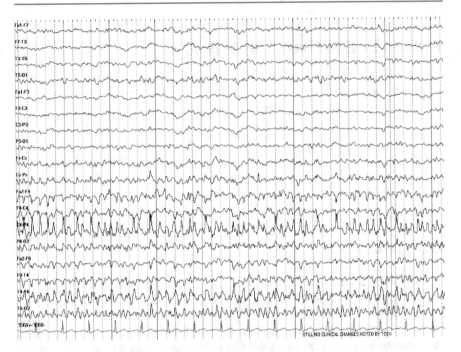

Fig. 36.1 Focal electrographic status epilepticus confined to the right hemisphere

4. What is the initial approach to treatment?
5. What role does the EEG have in the management of this condition?

Diagnostic Discussion

1. Status epilepticus has been defined as 30 min or more of a prolonged seizure or the patient does not return to their baseline state between recurrent seizures. Operational definitions now include any seizure that is greater than 5 min. Status epilepticus is a medical emergency, and newer definitions reflect the move toward earlier treatment [1–6].

2. This EEG shows ongoing status epilepticus with ongoing seizure activity emanating from the right hemisphere (see arrow on Fig. 36.1). This patient initially had convulsive status epilepticus that evolved to nonconvulsive seizures to explain the impaired consciousness in the emergency department (ED).

3. Status epilepticus is a serious life-threatening condition with a risk of significant morbidity and mortality. The initial evaluation includes neuroimaging studies of the brain to identify a potential structural basis of status and the need for treatment of the cause. Laboratory evaluation should include a complete metabolic profile and blood count. Addressing electrolyte imbalance and evidence of infection are especially important. Toxicology for therapeutic and illicit substance use and abuse is essential in the primary search for the etiology of status.

4. Figure 36.2 [6] demonstrates the protocol for status epilepticus management. It is essential that first responders ensure a patent airway and adequate respiration. Circulation also is addressed and maintained for primary life support. The initial approach to treatment should include administration of 1 ampule of D50W (glucose) to limit potential consequences from hypoglycemia. Especially in diabetics, this common cause of status epilepticus can lead to permanent damage if not

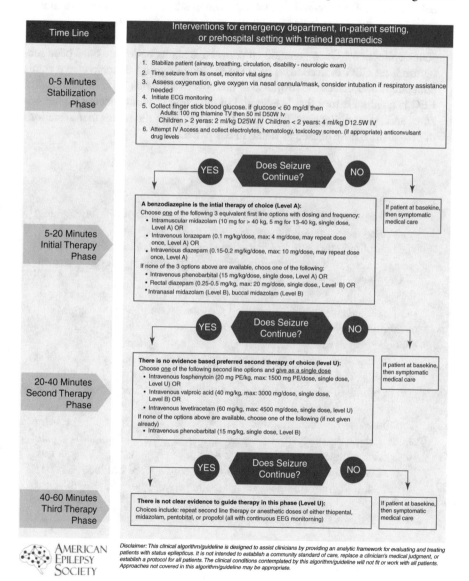

Fig. 36.2 American Epilepsy Society Protocol for Status Epilepticus, fig taken from ref. [6])

treated aggressively. Similarly, folic acid and thiamine are administered (especially in chronic alcohol abusers) to off-set nutritional deficits. The initial drug treatment should include a benzodiazepine. 2–4 mg of IM midazolam, 2–4 mg of IV lorazepam, or 5–10 mg of IV diazepam should be given. This should then immediately be followed by maintenance ASM. Twenty mg/kg of IV fosphenytoin or 40 mg/kg of valproic acid or 60 mg/kg of levetiracetam are all acceptable choices and has been the usual approach in adults with focal seizures unless there are extenuating circumstances that mitigate against its use.

5. The EEG has one of the most important roles in the management of convulsive status epilepticus. Once generalized convulsive status epilepticus has been recognized, an EEG is needed in order to exclude ongoing nonconvulsive status epilepticus and assess the response to therapy. Continuous EEG or quantitative EEG is a valuable tool that is essential in detecting ongoing electrographic seizures and status epilepticus that may often occur after the motor manifestations of convulsions have ceased as noted in our patient.

Clinical Pearls
1. Convulsive status epilepticus is serious and a potentially life-threatening neurological emergency.
2. The operational definition of status epilepticus applies to seizures that are greater than 5 min in duration reflecting the emergent need for treatment due to the likelihood of continued seizure.
3. The evaluation of patients presenting with convulsive status epilepticus should include assessments for illicit substance, complete blood count and metabolic profile, urinalysis, chest X-ray, EKG, brain imaging, and antiepileptic drug levels if the patient has a history of epilepsy.
4. All clinicians who manage people with status epilepticus should have a clear well-delineated protocol. This is essential so that an established course of action exists for patients who present with status to ensure that no time is lost.
5. The three most crucial prognostic factors determining the outcome from status epilepticus reflects the underlying etiology, the speed of anti-seizure treatment, and the age of the individual. Older-aged individuals frequently have a symptomatic cause as well as possessing a more limited reserve to recover due to comorbidities and have a higher mortality rate with status epilepticus.

References

1. Trinka E, Cock H, Hesdorffer D, Rossetti AO, Scheffer IE, Shinnar S, et al. A definition and classification of status epilepticus—report of the ILAE task force on classification of status epilepticus. Epilepsia. 2015;56(10):1515–23.
2. Silbergleit R, Durkalski V, Lowenstein D, Conwit R, Pancioli A, Palesch Y, Barsan W. NETT investigators. Intramuscular versus intravenous therapy for prehospital status epilepticus. N Engl J Med. 2012;366(7):591–600.
3. Lowenstein DH, Cloyd J. Out-of-hospital treatment of status epilepticus and prolonged seizures. Epilepsia. 2007;48(Suppl 8):96–8.
4. Treiman DM, Meyers PD, Walton NY, et al. A comparison of four treatments for generalized convulsive status epilepticus. Veterans affairs status epilepticus cooperative study group. N Engl J Med. 1998;339(12):792–8.
5. Kaplan PW. The EEG of status epilepticus. J Clin Neurophysiol. 2006;23(3):221–9.
6. Glauser T, Shinnar S, et al. Treatment of convulsive status Epilepticus in children and adults: report of the guideline Committee of the American Epilepsy Society. Epilepsy Curr. 2016;16(1):48–61.

Comorbidities and Seizures: Bone Health

37

Gregory D. Cascino

Case Presentation

A 73-year-old man with focal epilepsy presents for reevaluation following a recent breakthrough focal impaired awareness seizure. The patient has a history of recurrent focal seizures for 30 years of unknown etiology. He has intermittent "petit mal" seizures each month beginning with an abdominal aura and evolving to behavioral arrest, staring, and impaired awareness. Prior EEG recordings have shown bitemporal, independent interictal epileptiform discharges. A recent head CT revealed mild generalized atrophy. The patient has been on phenobarbital 90 mg nightly with phenytoin 100 mg three times daily for "years." The patient has observed increased fatigue and "tiredness" which he attributed to his ASM. During a recent focal seizure, the patient fell and now has pain in the right hip. The neurological examination is essentially unremarkable. EEG shows mild diffuse background slowing without definite epileptiform discharges. MRI of the brain using a dedicated seizure protocol revealed mild to moderate generalized cortical atrophy without a definite causal anatomical substrate for focal seizures. Phenobarbital level was 18 mcg/ml (range: 10–40 mcg/ml), and total phenytoin level was 9 mcg/ml (range: 10–20 mcg/ml). Selected chemistry and hematology studies were normal. X-ray of the pelvis and hips shows no evidence for fracture but identified degenerative arthritis and diffuse osteopenia. A total 25-hydroxyvitamin D (D2 + D3) level was 13 ng/mL (optimal levels 20–50 ng/ml). Dual-energy X-ray absorptiometry (DXA) showed bone density scores indicating osteoporosis (Table 37.1).

G. D. Cascino (✉)
Mayo Clinic, Department of Neurology, Rochester, MN, USA
e-mail: gcascino@mayo.edu

© Springer Nature Switzerland AG 2021
W. O. Tatum et al. (eds.), *Epilepsy Case Studies*,
https://doi.org/10.1007/978-3-030-59078-9_37

Table 37.1 Bone density study of the spine and hips

Left hip [single scan]
  Femur neck: BMD = 0.659 g/cm (sq)
    T-score = −3.2   Z-score = −2.0
  Total hip: BMD = 0.693 g/cm (sq)
    T-score = −2.8   Z-score = −2.2
Right hip [single scan]
  Femur neck: BMD = 0.706 g/cm (sq)
    T-score = −2.8   Z-score = −1.6
  Total hip: BMD = 0.712 g/cm (sq)
    T-score = −2.7   Z-score = −2.1
Lumbar spine [single scan]
  L1: BMD = 0.823 g/cm (sq), T-score = −2.8, Z-score = −2.4
  L2: BMD = 0.991 g/cm (sq), T-score = −2.1, Z-score = −1.7
  L3: BMD = 0.978 g/cm (sq), T-score = −2.2, Z-score = −1.8
  L4: BMD = 1.071 g/cm (sq), T-score = −1.5, Z-score = −1.0
  Total lumbar spine: BMD = 0.972 g/cm (sq)
    T-score = −2.1   Z-score = −1.6

Note: Osteoporosis may be diagnosed in postmenopausal Caucasian women when the T-score is at or below −2.5 as defined by the WHO. Osteopenia is present at T-scores between −1 and − 2.5 and normal BMD when T-score is at or above −1.0. The diagnosis in premenopausal women and men can be based on low bone mass or evidence of skeletal fragility in the appropriate clinical setting

Clinical Questions

1. Why is the vitamin D total level low?
2. Why is this patient at risk for osteoporosis and possible fracture(s)?
3. What treatment strategies could be used to reduce metabolic bone disease in this patient?
4. Should the phenytoin dose be increased with the recent seizure and the "low" level of ASM?
5. Should an alternative ASM be used to replace phenobarbital and phenytoin? If so, which drug should be considered?

Diagnostic Discussion

1. This patient has hypovitaminosis D that may have several causes including poor dietary intake, lack of sun exposure, obesity, gastrointestinal disorders, renal and hepatic diseases, and selected medications [1–3]. An important potential etiology for this patient's low vitamin D level is chronic exposure to enzyme-inducing ASM [1–4]. Both phenobarbital and phenytoin may increase the hepatic metabolism of vitamin D. Vitamin D plays a pivotal role in calcium deposition in bone by increasing intestinal absorption of calcium [2–5]. Vitamin D is necessary to regulate serum calcium and phosphate. Supplemental calcium and vitamin D

should be administered to patients receiving ASMs, especially enzyme-inducing drugs such as carbamazepine products, phenytoin, and phenobarbital. Supplements of both vitamin D (approximately 1000 IU/day) and calcium (approximately 1000–1200 mg/day) have been shown to reduce the risk of bone loss and fractures.

2. Patients with epilepsy and those receiving chronic ASM are at risk for metabolic bone disease [1–4]. There are multiple potential etiologies for bone health issues in these patients. The pathogenesis may be complex and not limited to hypovitaminosis D alone. Metabolic bone disease may occur with several ASM, especially enzyme-inducing agents [1]. Periodic vitamin D levels and DXA scan are appropriate as nearly one-third of patients with epilepsy receiving ASM may be at risk for this disorder [1, 2]. It is appropriate in higher risk-patients receiving ASM (elderly, postmenopausal women, patients with low vitamin D levels, and patients with osteoporosis) to screen patients annually with vitamin D, fasting calcium, and phosphate levels; bone densitometry (DXA study) should be performed every 2–5 years depending on the findings [1, 2]. Unfortunately, the initial clinical symptom may be a disabling hip fracture that can occur spontaneously or after a fall.

3. Patients with osteopenia and osteoporosis may require an evaluation by a metabolic bone disorder specialist (rheumatologist or endocrinology) for further assessment and treatment [1]. This patient should receive adequate supplementation with calcium and vitamin D. Other potential factors to improve bone health in people with epilepsy include adequate exercise, avoid excess alcohol intake, avoid smoking, and maintain an appropriate body weight. Bisphosphonate therapy may be effective in selected patients. The patient is also at risk for possible fractures because phenobarbital and phenytoin may produce gait and balance difficulties that may result in falls [1, 5].

4. Increasing the phenytoin dose in this patient may improve seizure control but carries a greater risk of potential adverse effects especially in the elderly population. The patient's observed drowsiness may be related to her combination therapy with two sedating ASMs. Increasing phenytoin may also further reduce the vitamin D levels and increase his risk of fracture.

5. Use of monotherapy ASM may be more efficacious and safer for this individual [5]. This patient has focal epilepsy with focal impaired awareness seizures. The interictal EEG discharges and abdominal aura suggests temporal lobe epilepsy. Additional medication trials may be appropriate with non-enzyme-inducing ASM such as lamotrigine or levetiracetam that do not depress vitamin D levels and may be less likely to be associated with metabolic bone disease [5]. There is limited information regarding bone density studies in patients receiving newer ASM [5]. Phenobarbital or phenytoin can be gradually tapered and withdrawn as the new ASM is added. Depending on response to the new medication, the patient may ultimately be a candidate for monotherapy treatment which is likely to have less dose-related adverse effects and drug interactions.

Clinical Pearls
1. Low vitamin D levels are common in people with epilepsy and may indicate an increased risk for bone fractures and metabolic bone disease. Adequate supplementation with vitamin D and calcium is often necessary, especially in patients with hepatically metabolized enzyme-inducing ASM.
2. Metabolic bone disease in patients receiving ASM has multiple potential etiological factors and cannot be explained by hypovitaminosis D alone in most individuals. Preventative and treatment strategies include adequate intake of vitamin D and calcium as well as appropriate lifestyle and diet.
3. In general, patients receiving ASM (especially the elderly) are at particular risk for falls and fractures related to impaired gait and balance. Phenytoin and phenobarbital are poor choices in this age group with total serum concentrations not always representative of the free fraction that is bioactive.
4. The issues related to metabolic bone disease with use of ASM is almost certainly not limited to the diagnosis of epilepsy. Individuals receiving these drugs for psychiatric disease, fibromyalgia, and chronic pain may have similar issues and concerns.
5. Periodic screening of patients for metabolic bone disease with vitamin D, fasting calcium, and phosphate levels and bone densitometry (DXA study) should be performed.

References

1. Carbone LD, Johnson KC, Robbins J, et al. Antiepileptic drug use, falls, fractures, and BMD in postmenopausal women: findings from the women's health initiative (WHI). J Bone Miner Res. 2010;25:873.
2. Vestergaard P. Epilepsy, osteoporosis and fracture risk-a meta-analysis. Acta Neurol Scand. 2005;112:277.
3. Pack AM, Morrell MJ, Randall A, et al. Bone health in young women with epilepsy after one year of antiepileptic drug monotherapy. Neurology. 2008;70:1586.
4. Kim SH, Lee JW, Choi KG, et al. A 6-month longitudinal study of bone mineral density with antiepileptic drug monotherapy. Epilepsy Behav. 2007;10:291.
5. Pack AM. Falls and fractures in patients with epilepsy: is there an increased risk? If so, why? Neurology. 2012;79:119.

SUDEP and Cardiac Arrhythmia

Joseph I. Sirven

Case Presentation

A 25-year-old female had drug-resistant epilepsy characterized by recurrent generalized tonic-clonic seizures. She had a history of a mosquito-borne encephalitis at the age of 12 years and subsequently developed epilepsy. Daily nocturnally predominant recurrent generalized tonic-clonic seizures became noted that were proved to be resistant to multiple antiseizure medications (ASM). Her interictal EEGs demonstrated diffuse slowing of the background activity. Video-EEG monitoring was ultimately performed as part of a comprehensive presurgical evaluation. During video-EEG monitoring, poorly localized seizures were captured though her EKG was abnormal during her seizures (Fig. 38.1).

During her course of evaluation and management, a call was received from her grandparents reporting that they were unable to awaken the patient from sleep. The emergency medical system was subsequently activated and dispatched to her home. Upon arrival, the patient was found unresponsive and face down in the prone position. Upon further examination, no clinical response to verbal or tactile stimulation was present, and vital signs were unable to be obtained. An EKG revealed asystole prompting unsuccessful treatment following evidence of nocturnal cardiopulmonary arrest. She was pronounced dead at the scene while still in her bedroom. Retrospectively, she had always been adherent to her ASM regimen of clobazam, levetiracetam, and lacosamide. At autopsy, no underlying cause of death was evident overtly and seizure was not suspected. Toxicology revealed therapeutic antiseizure drug levels and no illicit substances were recovered to explain her demise.

J. I. Sirven (✉)
Mayo Clinic, Department of Neurology, Jacksonville, FL, USA
e-mail: Sirven.Joseph@mayo.edu

© Springer Nature Switzerland AG 2021
W. O. Tatum et al. (eds.), *Epilepsy Case Studies*,
https://doi.org/10.1007/978-3-030-59078-9_38

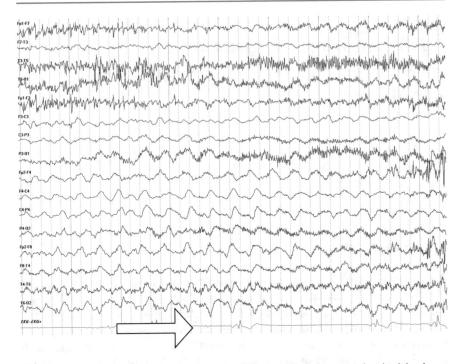

Fig. 38.1 Ictal EEG during diagnostic video-EEG monitoring demonstrating ictal bradycardia (*arrow*)

Clinical Questions

1. What is the most likely cause of death?
2. What does the ictal EEG from previous epilepsy monitoring suggest as the possible etiology?
3. What pathological mechanisms underlie sudden unexpected death in epilepsy?
4. What are risk factors for SUDEP in this patient?
5. How should other individuals with seizures and epilepsies be counseled regarding their risk of death in epilepsy?

Diagnostic Discussion

1. The likely cause of death in this case is sudden unexpected death in epilepsy (SUDEP). SUDEP is the most common cause of atraumatic epilepsy-related death. The risk of death in people with epilepsy is more than 20 times greater than that of the general population [1–5].
2. The ictal EEG suggests that the patient has previously demonstrated ictal bradycardia and a propensity to cardiac arrhythmias during seizures. This suggests a

cardiac mechanism may be implicated as the principal cause of death. Cardiac arrhythmias are well known to occur with seizures and can present in a number of variations, including ictal tachycardia (frequently present in 80% of patients) and rarely ictal bradycardia or asystole (in <1% of cases). In addition, more malignant ventricular dysrhythmias may occur peri-ictally and exist as an important component of SUDEP [1–5].

3. The mechanisms that underlie SUDEP include the possibility of a fatal cardiac arrhythmia, suffocation, and neurogenic pulmonary edema. The exact cause of death in these cases is still yet to be fully elucidated, but a number of cardiorespiratory mechanisms may be responsible independent of clinical seizures or status epilepticus at the time of death.

4. Table 38.1 lists the most important risk factors for SUDEP. The most commonly recognized and predictable risk factor for SUDEP is the presence of uncontrolled seizures. Seizure-related risk factors also include the onset of epilepsy at an early age, ongoing frequent seizures, frequent generalized tonic-clonic seizures, nocturnal occurrence, and a long duration of epilepsy. Neurological features that are risks for SUDEP include an IQ less than 70 and the presence of a significant neurological abnormality, illicit substance abuse, and noncompliance. Clinical studies have found an increased risk with fluctuation in ASM administration, subtherapeutic ASM levels, ASM polytherapy, nocturnal seizures, and patients with drug-resistant epilepsies such as those failing epilepsy surgery or requiring neurostimulators [3–5].

5. Numerous advocacy groups and consensus opinion recognize that individuals with epilepsy and their caregivers want to know about the risk of death in epilepsy. It is important to present the information in an appropriate light given the lack of unpredictability that limits control over preventing a death in people with epilepsy. However, it is important information that may serve to help reinforce the seriousness of the condition relative to encouraging adherence to medical and surgical treatment while avoiding unnecessary anxiety or coercing patients into a specific form of therapy such as surgical treatments. Rather, it should be noted from the initial visit that uncontrolled seizures carry a real yet small risk of morbidity and even mortality that are associated with uncontrolled seizures.

Table 38.1   Factors associated with risk of SUDEP

Factor	Odds ratio (CI)
Presence of generalized tonic-clonic seizures (GTCs)	10 (7–14)
Frequency of GTCs	5.07 for 1–2 GTCs per year (2.94–8.76) 15.46 for >3 GTCs per year (9.92–24.10)
Not being seizure-free 1–5 years	4.7 (1.4–16)
Not adding an ASD when patients are medically refractory	6 (2–20)
Nocturnal supervision (risk reduction)	0.4 (0.2–0.8)
Use of nocturnal listening device	0.1 (0.0–0.3)

Clinical Pearls
1. Seizures, especially when they are drug resistant, can result in sudden unexplained death in epilepsy.
2. Recurrent uncontrolled seizures including nocturnal convulsions are the most important risk factor for SUDEP.
3. Patients with epilepsy may experience serious cardiac rhythm disturbances during seizures. Cardiac pacemakers may therefore be required for cardiac stabilization during arrhythmia when seizures are unable to be controlled.
4. All patients and their families have the right and deserve to be informed about the risk of SUDEP to ensure that they are aware of the seriousness that is associated with seizures and its treatment.
5. Epilepsy surgery should be considered when seizures are uncontrolled since if patients achieve seizure freedom, then this has a greater likelihood of averting the risk of SUDEP.

References

1. Institute of Medicine. Epilepsy across the Spectrum. Washington, DC: National Academies Press; 2012. p. 96–9.
2. Nashef L, So E, Ryvlin P, Tomson T. Unifying the definitions of sudden unexpected death in epilepsy. Epilepsia. 2012;53(2):227–33.
3. Tomson T, Nashef L, Ryvlin P. Sudden unexpected death in epilepsy: current knowledge and future directions. Lancet Neurol. 2008;7(11):1021–31.
4. Devinsky O. Sudden unexpected death in epilepsy. NEJM. 2011;365:1801–11.
5. Harden C, et al. Sudden unexpected death in epilepsy: incidence rates and risk factors. Neurology. 2017;88(17):1674–80.

Investigational Devices for Epilepsy

39

Gregory A. Worrell, Ben Brinkmann,
and Jamie J. Van Gompel

Case Presentation

A 32-year-old employed female working in an insurance claims office has 10-year history of drug-resistant epilepsy. She has previously tried five antiseizure drugs at appropriate doses and has continued to have multiple focal seizures involving impaired each month. She denies risk factors for epilepsy. She does not use alcohol or illicit drugs. She works full time and uses public transportation.

The options for this patient include continued ASM trials. There are more than 30 ASMs available, with more in the drug development pipeline. However, data support the chance of seizure freedom after trials of two ASM are low [1]. The patient can also consider a trial of the low glycemic diet as an alternative, which has shown comparable efficacy to adding additional ASMs. In addition to further trials of ASM and the option of a low glycemic diet, the patient and physician should consider an evaluation for epilepsy surgery or a neuromodulation device when disabling seizures are drug resistant. The patient elected to proceed with evaluation for epilepsy surgery.

Phase I evaluation (scalp-based seizure monitoring): The semiology of her seizures was consistent with temporal lobe seizures with an epigastric aura, speech arrest, and followed by loss of awareness. Scalp EEG shows interictal epileptiform sharp waves independently occurring over right and left temporal head regions, maximal left. Video-EEG monitoring over the course of 4 days recorded five

G. A. Worrell (✉) · B. Brinkmann
Mayo Clinic, Department of Neurology, Rochester, MN, USA
e-mail: Worrell.Gregory@mayo.edu; Brinkmann.Benjamin@mayo.edu

J. J. Van Gompel
Mayo Clinic, Department of Neurosurgery, Rochester, MN, USA
e-mail: VanGompel.Jamie@mayo.edu

© Springer Nature Switzerland AG 2021
W. O. Tatum et al. (eds.), *Epilepsy Case Studies*,
https://doi.org/10.1007/978-3-030-59078-9_39

seizures originating from the right temporal and rapid spread (<2 s) to left temporal head regions. The MRI (seizure protocol 3T) is normal. PET shows bilateral temporal hypometabolism. Because of normal MRI and indeterminant scalp EEG localization of her seizures, she went on to an invasive diagnostic evaluation (phase II) with stereo-EEG (sEEG).

Phase II evaluation: Stereo-EEG (sEEG) was performed with electrodes implanted into bilateral mesial temporal lobe and additional limbic network targets. The sEEG demonstrated seizures independently originating from right mesial temporal and left mesial temporal lobes. Because of bilateral independent seizures, a trial of hippocampal stimulation was performed with the externalized sEEG electrodes. Continuous electrical stimulation using a low frequency (7 Hz, 90 μs pulse width, 4 mA) and high frequency (140 Hz, 90 μs, 4 mA) was trialed as part of a clinical practice assessment to evaluate if chronic subthreshold cortical stimulation (CSCS) [2] would reduce her seizures, given recent reports in the literature [3]. The trials of low- and high-frequency electrical stimulation during chronic subthreshold cortical stimulation (CSCS) did not appreciably reduce interictal or ictal activity.

Clinical Discussion

Unfortunately, given the bilateral independent temporal lobe seizures, she is not a resective epilepsy surgery candidate. She is a candidate for a neuromodulation device. Current FDA-approved options are vagus nerve stimulation (VNS), responsive neurostimulation (RNS), and deep brain stimulation (DBS) targeting the anterior nucleus of the thalamus. All of these are palliative options, but with a good chance of reducing seizures [4]. In this patient we performed a trial of CSCS that did not show evidence for potential efficacy.

For multiple reasons she elected to enroll in an investigational device exemption (IDE) study. The FDA-approved human investigational device exemption study (IDE: G180224) is investigating the safety and feasibility of electrical stimulation and continuous tracking of electrophysiology from bilateral limbic network with the goals of (1) quantitative tracking of seizures and interictal activity, (2) seizure forecasting, and (3) adaptive electrical brain stimulation (EBS) to prevent seizures. The IDE study uses an investigational Medtronic Inc. Summit System (Fridley, Minnesota USA) includes an RC + S implantable neural stimulator and 4 leads with 4 contacts each. Our patient had bilateral mesial temporal and anterior nucleus of thalamus leads implanted (Fig. 39.1). The Medtronic Summit System was integrated with the Mayo Epilepsy Patient Assistant Device (EPAD) enabling off-the-body local and distributed computing for artificial intelligence applications to detect and predict seizures and adjust therapy [5].

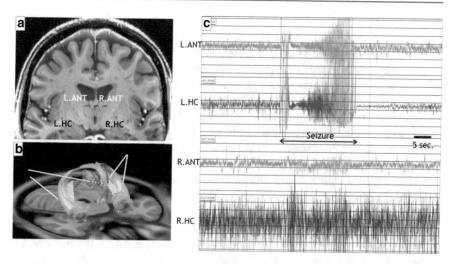

Fig. 39.1 Bilateral anterior nucleus of thalamus (ANT) and hippocampus (HC) implant. (**a**) MRI with ANT and HC electrodes labeled. (**b**) Papez circuit and implanted electrodes. (**c**) Spontaneous focal seizure with simultaneous left ANT and HC involvement automatically detected in patient natural environment. The data was telemetered off the implant to the EPAD device and to the cloud store ge for review. Clinically the patient reported intense fear (Figure courtesy of Nicholas Gregg, MD and Vaclav Kremen, PhD)

Clinical Questions

1. What were the FDA-approved device options for this patient?
2. What is a FDA premarket approval (PMA)?
3. What is an FDA IDE study?
4. What is off-label use of FDA-approved device?
5. Can physicians use devices without FDA approval?

1. The patient is a candidate for a neuromodulatory device. The FDA-approved neuromodulatory therapies are currently VNS, RNS, and DBS targeting the anterior nucleus of the thalamus. These are palliative options with a good chance to reduce seizures [4]. The long-term data are encouraging with all forms of available neuromodulation showing improved efficacy over time [6, 7].
2. The VNS, RNS, and DBS are FDA-approved class III devices. The classification of a device as class III denotes the greatest potential risk to patients and determines, among other things, the type of premarketing submission/application required for FDA clearance to market. For class III devices, a premarket approval application (PMA) will be required unless the device is a preamendment device (on the market prior to the passage of the medical device amendments in 1976, or substantially equivalent to such a device) and PMA not required by FDA. The PMA studies leading to FDA approval for the RNS and DBS for epilepsy were multicenter, randomized, controlled trials that demonstrated efficacy.

3. An investigational device exemption (IDE) allows the use of an investigational device in a clinical study to be used in order to collect safety, feasibility, and effectiveness data. An IDE is required to support a premarket approval application or a premarket notification [510(k)] submission to the US Food and Drug Administration (FDA). All clinical evaluations of investigational devices must have an approved IDE before a clinical research study is initiated.

4. In addition to FDA-approved devices, her physician performed an evaluation of electrical stimulation during intracranial EEG monitoring (phase 2) using an external Medtronic stimulator. This stimulator is already FDA approved for use in patients with Parkinson's disease for DBS therapy. This is an off-label device use in a patient with epilepsy. Off-label use of a drug or device is legally permitted in the practice of medicine with justification.

5. The off-label use of FDA-approved devices is allowed within the practice of medicine. Such a use for research would require FDA and institutional research board (IRB) approvals. This is similar to the off-label use of medications for treatments if the drugs are FDA approved for a different disease indication.

Clinical Pearls

1. Presenting the complexity and range of neuromodulation devices and safety and efficacy data to patients is challenging, but critical to ensure appropriate informed consent.

2. It is important for patients to understand the current device options are palliative therapies and the chance for long-term seizure freedom is modest, but not zero. Patients generally remain on ASM but may potentially be managed on lower doses and with fewer medications.

3. The difference between FDA-approved devices and those that are used off-label is the former have undergone a premarket approval (PMA) study and have the best evidence for safety and efficacy. Physicians can practice medicine and use devices off-label, but it is imperative that physicians understand this is for clinical use and not research and applicable when it is determined to be in patients' best interest.

4. IDE device trials are FDA-approved studies that are designed to show safety and feasibility.

5. The current evidence of efficacy for VNS, RNS, and DBS neuromodulation outcomes is remarkably similar, and selecting the appropriate therapy involves careful discussion with the patient and family. Some patients may not be interested in a device that involves electrode implantation in the brain (RNS and DBS). The VNS is certainly a reasonable option in this case and has proven efficacy.

References

1. Kwan P, Brodie MJ. Early identification of refractory epilepsy. N Engl J Med. 2000;342:314–9.
2. Lundstrom BN, van Gompel J, Khadjevand F, Worrell G, Stead M. Chronic subthreshold cortical stimulation and stimulation-related EEG biomarkers for focal epilepsy. Brain Commun. 2019; https://doi.org/10.1093/braincomms/fcz010.
3. Cukiert A, Cukiert CM, Burattini JA, Mariani PP, Bezerra DF. Seizure outcome after hippocampal deep brain stimulation in patients with refractory temporal lobe epilepsy: a prospective, controlled, randomized, double-blind study. Epilepsia. 2017;58:1728–33.
4. Fisher RS, Velasco AL. Electrical brain stimulation for epilepsy. Nat Rev Neurol. 2014;10:261–70.
5. Kremen V, Brinkmann BH, Kim I, Guragain H, Nasseri M, Magee AL, et al. Integrating brain implants with local and distributed computing devices: A next generation epilepsy management system. IEEE J Transl Eng Heal Med. 2018;6:1–12.
6. Bergey GK, Morrell MJ, Mizrahi EM, et al. Long-term treatment with responsive brain stimulation in adults with refractory partial seizures. Neurology. 2015;84:810–7.
7. Salanova V, Witt T, Worth R, et al. Long-term efficacy and safety of thalamic stimulation for drug-resistant partial epilepsy. Neurology. 2015;84:1017–25.

Alternative Medicines in Epilepsy

40

Joseph I. Sirven

Case Presentation

A 24-year-old male lawyer had a known diagnosis of focal epilepsy from a traumatic brain injury. His focal seizures were ultimately controlled using an antiseizure medication (ASM) with combined lamotrigine and carbamazepine. His mother brought the patient to the emergency department (ED) 1 day when she noted her son had "not been himself" after receiving a phone call from his girlfriend. On examination, the patient was confused and did not answer questions appropriately. He appeared to be awake, and his neurological examination was without focal or lateralizing features. When asked questions, he parroted the words in the questions back to the examiner. According to his mother, he was compliant with ASM. There had been no other recent major changes in his activities other than imbibing several energy drinks (at least 6 a day) in order to help his concentration and focus. In addition, he had obtained cannabis from a local dispensary because he thought that it might help improve control of his epilepsy. When he arrived in the emergency department, laboratory testing revealed no significant abnormalities of his complete blood count and comprehensive metabolic profile. The ASM concentrations were found to reflect levels that were in the low normal range for lamotrigine, and the carbamazepine level was low at 2 mg/dL. Neuroimaging studies were unremarkable. A urine drug toxicology screen was positive for cannabis. Subsequently, an EEG was obtained.

J. I. Sirven (✉)
Mayo Clinic, Department of Neurology, Jacksonville, FL, USA
e-mail: Sirven.Joseph@mayo.edu

© Springer Nature Switzerland AG 2021
W. O. Tatum et al. (eds.), *Epilepsy Case Studies*,
https://doi.org/10.1007/978-3-030-59078-9_40

Questions for Discussion

1. What does the EEG demonstrate?
2. What is a complementary and alternative medicine (CAM)?
3. Is there any medical evidence to suggest using CAM for epilepsy?
4. Are there any concerns with CAM use?
5. What is the role of cannabis in epilepsy management?

Discussion

1. The EEG figure demonstrates lateralized periodic discharges emanating from the posterior quadrant in the left hemisphere. This was clinically associated with nonconvulsive status epilepticus manifest as confusion. During this EEG, both carbamazepine and lamotrigine levels were low and suspected to be the primary explanation (Fig. 40.1).
2. Complementary and alternative medicine (CAM) is defined as a group of diverse medical and health care systems, practices, and products not generally considered part of traditional western medicine by the National Center on Complementary and Alternative Medicine (NCCAM; aka the Office of

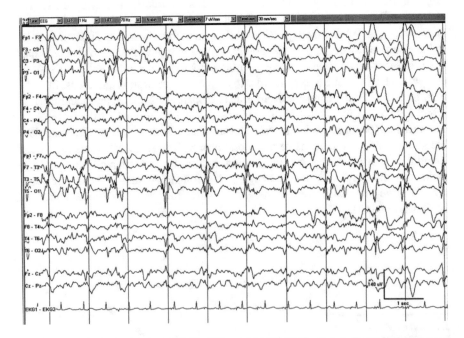

Fig. 40.1 EEG obtained during confusion demonstrating lateralized periodic discharges emanating from the posterior quadrant of the left hemisphere associated with a diffusely slow background activity

Table 40.1 CAM treatments

CAM treatments
Herbals/botanicals
Ayurvedic care
Chiropractic care
Biofeedback
Yoga
Homeopathy
Spirituality

Alternative Medicine) [4]. The NCCAM is a US governmental agency that evaluates CAM and is one of the many centers and institutes that comprise the NIH within the Department of Health and Human Services. Many individuals with epilepsy may seek out the use of "complementary" or "alternative" treatments to improve their outcomes. CAM treatment can include a number of different compounds and approaches (Table 40.1). Treatment with hormones, oxygen therapy, nutrition, and vitamins may be encountered in addition to Asian and traditional Chinese medicine and herbal and botanical treatments, and other homeopathic compounds may be used by patients. Stress relief practices such as exercise, reiki, chiropractic, meditation, Ayurvedic care, and acupuncture may be used among others that carry ramifications to treatment [1–5].

3. There have been no clear randomized control studies that have evaluated the usefulness of CAM for epilepsy. However, a Cochrane review has found that stress relief through either yoga or acupuncture may have theoretical implications for benefit yet lack studies that are sufficient to establish definitive proof of benefit [1, 2].

4. Some CAMs can be concerning for people with epilepsy. Some individuals may harbor the commonly held, false belief that if they take CAM that they can stop their ASM in lieu of using alternative therapies. In the case above, the individual stopped carbamazepine and his lamotrigine with the goal of using cannabidiol supplements as a "natural" treatment. Unfortunately, this resulted in a seizure emergency not uncommonly seen with nonadherence to the treatment regimens prescribed by one's physician. Moreover, some alternative therapies can be proconvulsants or possess drug-drug interactions. For instance, some compounds may act as proconvulsants. Curiously, different extracts from the same plant may result to be seizure protective.

Additionally, this patient was also imbibing energy drinks. These beverages have large amounts of caffeine, guarana, and taurine. Each of these compounds ingested in low amounts may be safe. However, when combined and their dose is increased as seen in high consumption of energy drinks, seizures may result. There are several anecdotal reports linking energy drink consumption to either new-onset seizures or increased seizures in people with epilepsy. In this case, counseling the patient about avoiding use of energy drinks and potential risks of CAM is essential.

Physicians need to ask patients about these drinks and other supplements that are often not disclosed or checked in urine to screen.

5. Although epilepsy is frequently cited as one of the conditions that cannabis use may benefit, evidence from randomized controlled trials demonstrating evidence to support this is present only when use of highly purified cannabidiol (CBD) (99% pure) for seizures is used in people with Lennox-Gastaut syndrome and Dravet syndrome [6–8]. There is no evidence showing that the psychoactive ingredient of the marijuana tetrahydrocannabinol (THC) helps improve seizures. Moreover, dispensary-based cannabidiol is not purified CBD and is not regulated for purity or quality. Therefore, ingesting these compounds could be problematic as they often have multiple drug-drug interactions. Furthermore, case reports of patients with epilepsy who switched from standard ASM to cannabis therapy have been linked to fatal outcomes suggesting that there is a risk for death in patients who rely only on cannabis to manage their seizures.

Clinical Pearls
1. It is important that one be supportive of the concept of alternative and complementary medicine techniques especially if it poses little risk to the therapies that are being prescribed.
2. Stress reduction is always beneficial for individuals with epilepsy and methods in which that stress can be reduced. Biofeedback, yoga, sprituality and similar methods are appropriate choices.
3. Switching from traditional antiseizure drugs to rely upon alternative medicines as a sole treatment for epilepsy is a recipe for problems in lieu of the well-demonstrated benefit from more traditional antiseizure drug treatment.
4. Although energy drinks are incredibly popular, overconsuming this product may produce seizures in susceptible individuals. Physicians should ask about a history of ingesting these beverages in patients who present with new seizures or an increase in seizures.
5. Although cannabis has achieved "grassroots" popularity, there is only evidence to support the use of highly purified CBD for Lennox-Gastaut syndrome and Dravet syndrome [6–8]. Caution must be undertaken when using cannabis as a sole treatment or when obtained from a dispensary, given the limited information on efficacy and the lack of regulation as to how cannabis is distributed and what other ingredients are added. Always disclosing to one's physician the full variety of treatments being utilized is the best means to minimize unexpected complications.

References

1. Cheuk DK, Wong V. Acupuncture for epilepsy. Cochrane Database of Systemic Reviews 2008, Issue 4. Art. No CD005062.
2. Ramaratnam S, Sridharan K. Yoga for epilepsy. Cochrane Database of Systemic Reviews 2000, Issue 2, Art No: CD001524.
3. Devinsky O, Schachter SC, Pacia SV. Alternative therapies for epilepsy. New York: Demos Medical Publishers, Inc; 2012. p. 1–319.
4. http://nccam.nih.gov/health/whatiscam. Accessed 19 Apr 2020.
5. Iyadurai A, Chung S. New onset seizures in adults: possible association of consumption of popular energy drinks. Epilepsy Behav. 2007;10(3):504–8.
6. Devinsky O, Patel A, et al. Effect of cannabidiol on drop seizures in the Lennox–Gastaut Syndrome. NEJM. 2018;378:1888–97.
7. Thomas RH, Cunningham MO. Cannabis and epilepsy. Pract Neurol. 2018;18:465–71.
8. Kollmyer DM, Wright KE, Warner NM, Doherty MJ. Are there mortality risks for patients with epilepsy who use cannabis treatments as monotherapy? Epilepsy Behav Case Rep. 2018;11:52–3.

Surgical Candidate (Skip)

41

William O. Tatum and Sanjeet S. Grewal

Case Presentation

A 47-year-old right-handed Indian-American female was self-referred for uncontrolled seizures. She was healthy other than taking antiseizure medication (ASM) for epilepsy. When she was 2 years of age, she experienced a prolonged febrile convulsion lasting 15 min associated with a fever of 103°. At the time she was told "nothing was wrong" and that is was a benign occurrence. She developed normally throughout childhood with above average scholastic achievement. At 11 years of age, she developed her first afebrile seizure which recurred manifest as a staring spell that she referred to as a "petit mal" seizure. Her seizures involved a warning where she would experience an indescribable feeling just prior to a wide-eyed stare, manifest subtle lip smacking, and impaired responsiveness for 45 seconds in duration. Following this she would be sleepy with transient difficulty "getting the words out." She failed five ASM with ongoing seizures and was maintained on lamotrigine and levetiracetam. Several seizures per month occurred with rare injury mostly involving lacerations, abrasions, and contusions of the head. She never experienced a "grand mal" seizure. Her neurological examination was normal. A high-resolution brain MRI with an epilepsy protocol demonstrated left mesial temporal sclerosis (Fig. 41.1a). EEG revealed left anterior temporal interictal epileptiform discharges (Fig. 41.1b). A surgical evaluation was recommended to her by her neurologist after she fell down a flight of stairs. Subsequent evaluation included a FDG-PET scan of

W. O. Tatum (✉)
Mayo Clinic, Department of Neurology, Jacksonville, FL, USA
e-mail: tatum.william@mayo.edu

S. S. Grewal
Mayo Clinic, Department of Neurosurgery, Jacksonville, FL, USA
e-mail: Grewal.sanjeet@mayo.edu

© Springer Nature Switzerland AG 2021
W. O. Tatum et al. (eds.), *Epilepsy Case Studies*,
https://doi.org/10.1007/978-3-030-59078-9_41

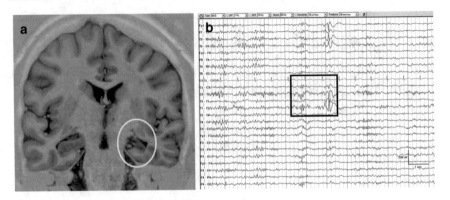

Fig. 41.1 (**a**) Brain MRI with left hippocampal formation atrophy (*yellow circle*) and (**b**) representative interictal EEG showing left temporal spikes (*box*)

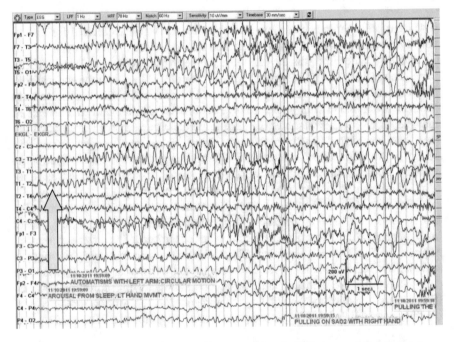

Fig. 41.2 Left temporal onset seizure manifest as evolving rhythmic temporal theta (*arrow*)

the brain that revealed hypometabolism of the left temporal lobe. She was admitted to the hospital's epilepsy monitoring unit and underwent video-EEG monitoring. During this time frequent state-independent left anterior temporal epileptiform discharges were apparent, and three focal seizures typical of her outpatient events were recorded (Fig. 41.2). Neuropsychological testing revealed mild verbal memory deficit. A Wada test was performed. Injection of sodium brevital revealed 8/8 object recall and aphasia upon left hemispheric injection and 0/8 recall and dysarthria upon right injection. A left amygdalohippocampectomy was recommended; however, her son (an anesthesiologist) recommended against it. 10 years elapsed before surgery was performed. Following surgery, she became seizure-free for more than 2 years.

Clinical Questions

1. What parts of the clinical history suggest focal seizures?
2. What is the likelihood that further ASM will result in seizure freedom, and what are the reasons for drug resistance?
3. Why is seizure monitoring needed when the MRI is abnormal?
4. What further testing is required if surgery is to be pursued?
5. What is the prognosis after surgery for seizures, and what about surgical consequences?

Diagnostic Discussion

1. The diagnosis of epilepsy is suggested by the paroxysmal recurrent episodes of impaired consciousness, and a treatment algorithm is practical [1]. Many patients describe their seizures as "petit mal" seizures when they are nonconvulsive, though in 70% of adults, focal seizures rather than generalized seizures predominate. In two-thirds of these individuals, ASM will not result in sustained seizure control. Many adults with focal seizures experience a warning (aura), though it is the post-ictal state that is the characteristic feature of focal seizures to distinguish it from other events associated with transitory loss of consciousness including absence seizures or "petit mal." If uncontrolled seizures are permitted to continue, a greater risk for morbidity with higher accident and injury rates, psychiatric and cognitive deterioration (especially memory), social isolation, stigmatization, and impaired self-esteem, and even mortality from sudden unexplained death accrues.

2. Approximately one-third of patients with focal seizures and 15–20% with generalized epilepsy will remain refractory to ASM despite different treatment options [2]. After the failure of two appropriate ASMs given for an adequate duration, at an effective dose, there is less than a 5–10% likelihood that further ASM changes will result in seizure freedom. It is important to exclude pseudo-resistance as the reason for drug failure. An incorrect diagnosis may result in ongoing seizures because treatment of a nonepileptic seizure mimic is unlikely to respond to ASM. Similarly, treatment with an incorrect ASM choice targeting the wrong seizure or epilepsy type or too low a dose of ASM will result in apparent drug failure. Genetic generalized epilepsies for example may be aggravated by narrow spectrum ASM such as carbamazepine or phenytoin, and the use of ethosuximide to treat "petit mal" seizures will be ineffective in patients with focal

seizures. Patient-related issues are yet another reason for poor results. When noncompliance or an adverse lifestyle is encountered, the ASM may be the correct choice, though efficacy may be compromised due to reasons such as subtherapeutic use from non-compliance or drug and alcohol abuse. Epilepsy surgery is a standard of care [3] and remains a cornerstone of therapy due to efficacy proven in randomized controlled trials as a more effective treatment compared to continued medial therapy when seizures continue despite ASM [4, 5].

3. When the MRI and interictal EEG are concordant, the likelihood of a correct localization is approximately 80%. The demonstration of a "lesion" (mesial temporal sclerosis on MRI in our patient) has the best predictive value as a localizing feature and as a favorable prognosticator for a successful outcome following epilepsy surgery [6–8]. Ictal EEG recordings are recommended to confirm the diagnosis of epilepsy. Approximately 20–30% of patients admitted for epilepsy monitoring will not have epilepsy. The majority of them have psychogenic non-epileptic attacks (PNEA). Even in patients with epileptic seizures (ES), about 10–15% may exhibit both ES and PNES. Excluding incorrect ASM choices will be made possible by accurately classifying the seizures correctly when they are captured during video-EEG monitoring. Recording EEG during seizures will also identify a single semiology and ictal EEG pattern that morphologically is able to support a diagnosis of unifocal epilepsy. Excluding more than one source for generating recurrent seizures may be difficult based solely upon semiology. An example of the latter situation may be seen in patients with bitemporal epilepsy where staring episodes may be caused by focal seizures arising from each hemisphere independently.

4. When all aspects of a "phase 1" evaluation (non-invaive) are concordant (i.e., history and semiology, MRI, PET, video-EEG monitoring, neuropsychological testing), these candidates may "skip" and proceed directly to surgery without the need to undergo further invasive EEG monitoring with intracranial electrodes for further seizure localization. In our patient, Wada testing was used to firmly localize language function and predict memory function after surgery which was robust, demonstrating a significant difference in participation between the hemispheres to predict a favorable outcome with respect to working memory in addition to anticipating seizure freedom. Functional MRI has been used to identify atypical areas subserving language and is increasingly being used in place of Wada testing as a noninvasive alternative. All of the results of the presurgical evaluation are favorable in our patient and provide localizing information to identify impaired hippocampal function within a limbic neural network. Each of the classic aspects of the presurgical evaluation strongly suggest a favorable outcome with respect to eliminating seizures through surgery.

5. This patient illustrates the most common surgically remediable syndrome of drug-resistant temporal lobe epilepsy (TLE). The presurgical evaluation above involving MRI, PET, and interictal and ictal EEG demonstrate concordance to support unifocal localization. Unfortunately, only a small percentage of potential surgical candidates are being referred to surgical epilepsy centers. Lengthy delays of 15–20 years are unfortunately common. However, 50–90% of patients

become seizure-free with limited morbidity postoperatively. Laser interstitial thermal therapy is another option that potentially has less cognitive consequences albeit with a slightly reduced likelihood of resultant seizure-free outcome [9, 10]. Overall, the most favorable predictor to obtain a seizure-free outcome following surgery or ablation exists when a lesion is present on neuroimaging. It has a high rate of success especially if it is due to hippocampal sclerosis as in our patient. Complications are related to the craniotomy and to the site and the extent of resected tissue. Nobody "wants" surgery, but it is important to present surgery as an option in a realistic and objective fashion. After declining epilepsy surgery for years despite experiencing uncontrolled seizures, our patient underwent successful surgery despite the urging of her family to the contrary. Early surgery has proven to be 15–21% more effective than delayed surgery [11]. She had no complications and became seizure-free as expected. She later wished she would have undergone surgery 10 years earlier and not listened to her son who advised against it.

Pearls of Wisdom
1. Epilepsy surgery is a standard of care and should be considered early when a patient with focal seizures has proven to be drug-resistant to ASM.
2. A lesion on neuroimaging is the best predictor for localizing seizure onset and for prognosticating a seizure-free outcome following epilepsy surgery or stereotactic laser interstitial thermal ablation.
3. Video-EEG monitoring is essential to perform before epilepsy surgery. It will verify the diagnosis of epilepsy and exclude the possibility of other seizure mimics as the reason for drug resistance. In addition, it can provide localizing information about the site of seizure onset by demonstrating electrophysiological information that is concordant with the other "phase 1" evaluations to allow the patient to "skip" invasive monitoring and proceed directly to surgical therapy when concordance is identified.
4. Temporal lobe epilepsy is the most common epilepsy surgery performed. TLE is often due to hippocampal sclerosis and the most common adult epilepsy syndrome that is amenable to surgery.
5. Overall, about 70% of patients are seizure-free after surgery, and an additional 20% have a significant reduction in their seizures. Though the ideal surgical candidate has the best predictability for a seizure-free outcome, epilepsy surgery is more likely to result in seizure freedom when patients have failed >2 appropriate trials of ASM.

References

1. Jobst BC. Treatment algorithms in refractory partial epilepsy. Epilepsia. 2009;50(Suppl 8):51–6.
2. Engel J Jr. What can we do for people with drug-resistant epilepsy? The 2016 Wartenberg lecture. Neurology. 2016;87:2483–9.

3. Wiebe S, Blume WT, Girvin JP, Eliasziw M. A randomized, controlled trial of surgery for temporal-lobe epilepsy. N Engl J Med. 2001;345(5):311–8.
4. Engel J Jr, McDermott MP, Wiebe S, Langfitt JT, Stern JM, Dewar S, Sperling MR, Gardiner I, Erba G, Fried I, Jacobs M, Vinters HV, Mintzer S, Kieburtz K. Early surgical therapy for drug-resistant temporal lobe epilepsy: a randomized trial. JAMA. 2012;307:922–30.
5. Engel J Jr, Wiebe S, French J, et al. Practice parameter: temporal lobe and localized neocortical resections for epilepsy: report of the quality standards subcommittee of the American Academy of Neurology, in association with the American Epilepsy Society and the American Association of Neurological Surgeons. Neurology. 2003;60(4):538–47.
6. Spencer SS, Berg AT, Vickrey BG, et al. Initial outcomes in the Multicenter study of epilepsy surgery. Neurology. 2003;61(12):1680–5.
7. Englot DJ, Chang EF. Rates and predictors of seizure freedom in resective epilepsy surgery: an update. Neurosurg Rev. 2014;37:389–404.
8. Capraz IY, Kurt G, Akdemir O, Hirfanoglu T, Oner Y, Sengezer T, Kapucu LO, Serdaroglu A, Bilir E. Surgical outcome in patients with MRI-negative, PET-positive temporal lobe epilepsy. Seizure. 2015;29:63–8.
9. Grewal SS, Tatum WO. Laser thermal ablation in epilepsy. Expert Rev Neurother. 2019;6:1–8.
10. Drane DL, Loring DW, Voets NL, Price M, Ojemann JG, Willie JT, Saindane AM, Phatak V, Ivanisevic M, Millis S, Helmers SL, Miller JW, Meador KJ, Gross RE. Better object recognition and naming outcome with MRI-guided stereotactic laser amygdalohippocampotomy for temporal lobe epilepsy. Epilepsia. 2015;56:101–13.
11. Bjellvi J, Olsson I, Malmgren K, Ramsay KW. Epilepsy duration and seizure outcome in epilepsy surgery. Neurology. 2019;93(2):e159. https://doi.org/10.1212/WNL.0000000000007753.

Epilepsy Surgery: Intracranial EEG (iEEG) Candidate

42

Jamie J. Van Gompel and Gregory D. Cascino

Case Presentation

A 66-year-old right-handed man with no known epilepsy risk factors has a history of drug-resistant focal epilepsy. His first seizure was in 1971 (19 years old) and was a generalized tonic-clonic seizure (GTC). He had yearly seizures until 1974. He remained seizure-free for 12 years between 1974 and 1986. In 1992 he had a new type of seizures described as dream-like state and confusion with intact awareness. These lasted for 30 s and used to occur monthly. These likely progressed into his new and current type of seizures that are characterized by behavioral arrest, staring, face rubbing, and impaired awareness as described in a note by his friend in 2008, and described by the patient in his last admission as being "confused about things" during which he calls his friend and speaks to her, with probable postictal disorientation and confusion. These seizures last between 10 s and 1 min and became refractory to medication. He currently has seven seizures monthly. His last GTC was in 2001. During his admission, he had a focal seizure that was associated with ictal asystole, so cardiac pacemaker was implanted.

His seizures resulted in a motor vehicle accident in 2005 while driving and a fall in 2007 with subdural hematoma. He was previously maintained on phenytoin and pregabalin which failed to control his seizures. Currently he is maintained on lamotrigine 300 mg/day, levetiracetam 4500 mg/day, and lacosamide 500 mg/day.

Overnight video-EEG monitoring of interictal EEG demonstrated abundant right posterior spikes and sharp waves (Pz-P4-P8-P10), with occasional field over the left posterior head regions. In addition, there were right hemispheric polyspikes, highest

J. J. Van Gompel (✉)
Mayo Clinic, Department of Neurosurgery, Rochester, MN, USA
e-mail: Vangompel.jamie@mayo.edu

G. D. Cascino
Mayo Clinic, Department of Neurology, Rochester, MN, USA
e-mail: gcascino@mayo.edu

© Springer Nature Switzerland AG 2021
W. O. Tatum et al. (eds.), *Epilepsy Case Studies*,
https://doi.org/10.1007/978-3-030-59078-9_42

in amplitude over the right temporal areas, along with frequent intermittent diffuse right and midline periodic discharges. He had two diurnal clinical seizures recorded, clinically characterized by transient left head turn, looking around, alteration in awareness, with preserved speech in the second. No postictal speech disturbance was noted. Electrographically the onset was over the right and midline posterior head regions. Radioactive dye injected within 29 s of his second seizure.

His prior EEG showed right temporal spikes and bitemporal sharp waves. MRI demonstrated bitemporal (inferior) left more than right encephalomalacia and mild bifrontal atrophy (Fig. 42.1). Subtraction ictal SPECT co-registered to MRI (SISCOM) showed right lateral temporal lobe/middle temporal gyrus and posterior right parietal lobe with extension to the right occipital lobe but was a relatively late injection in view of the brief duration of the seizure. After review of the imaging and semiology, it was discussed at epilepsy conference, and bilateral stereotactic EEG

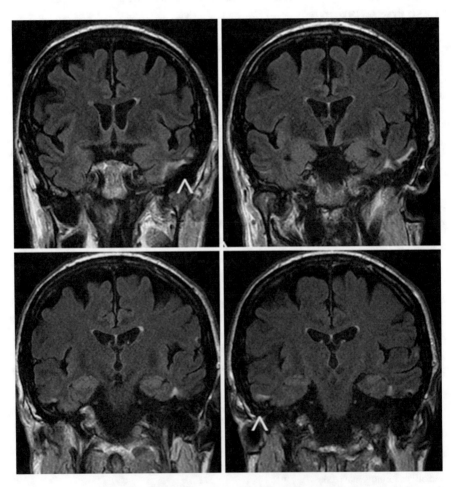

Fig. 42.1 Coronal serial flair MRI images showing bilateral temporal encephalomalacia (*arrows*)

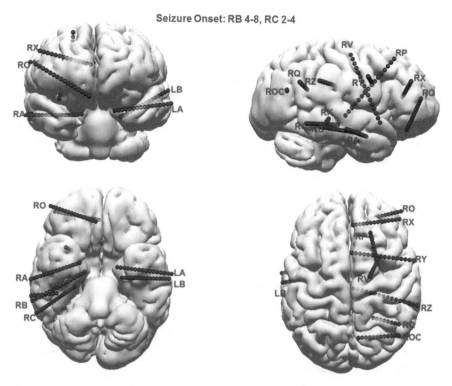

Fig. 42.2 sEEG reconstruction demonstrating scope of implant and onset over the medial temporal lobe at RC and RB (red contacts)

(sEEG) implant was recommended; the implant is demonstrated in Fig. 42.2. sEEG recorded six clinical seizures with right temporal onset, specifically over RC3-4 and RB3-4 contacts, corresponding to the tail and head of the right hippocampus. Five of these seizures were characterized by subtle nonspecific movements of the arms. One seizure was characterized by confusion, nonspecific movements of both feet, with progression into the left head version, and generalized tonic-clonic movements, during which there was significant involvement of the right neocortical temporal lobe very quickly upon seizure onset, along with rapid spread to the left mesial temporal lobe, and the seizure ended over the left mesial temporal structures. Independent mesial bitemporal spikes and right temporal and posterior temporal (RK) superficial neocortical spikes in addition to runs of diffuse right paroxysmal fast activity were seen.

These findings are suggestive of predominantly right mesial temporal lobe epilepsy, with a propensity for independent left mesial temporal seizures. In addition, the significant involvement of the right neocortical temporal/posterior temporal region may suggest involvement in the seizure onset zone. This was discussed again at our multidisciplinary epilepsy conference, and it was the consensus of the conference that further testing is required to better define the function of the patient's left temporal lobe. In regard to treatment options, a modified right temporal lobectomy (with expanded resection region to try and include neocortical regions back to RK) would provide the best chance of seizure freedom, but given the atrophic left hippocampus (hippocampal volume third percentile), cognitive morbidity was a concern. An alternative treatment would be neurostimulation with responsive neurostimulation system (RNS) or chronic subthreshold cortical stimulation, focusing on the right mesial temporal and right neocortical regions involved in the seizure onset, with secondary consideration to cover left mesial temporal structures. After discussion with the patient, he elected for an extended temporal lobectomy. At 18 months he is Engel Class I and appears to have retained neurocognitive function and good quality of life.

Clinical Questions

1. In the evaluation for epilepsy surgery, what factors are considered?
2. What aspects of the presurgical evaluation are predictive of outcome?
3. When are intracranial electrodes used?
4. What types of electrodes and location are implanted?
5. What is the likelihood of a seizure-free outcome following intracranial EEG (iEEG)?

Diagnostic Discussion

1. The first question in epilepsy to be considered is, importantly, can we help this patient? Obviously there is a high tolerance for many tests and surgeries if there is a chance of seizure freedom. Once we determine the patient has a focal onset epilepsy, if there is suspected overlap with cortical eloquent function, one should consider cortical grids and strip intracranial monitoring. However in most cases now confirming the hypothesis of epilepsy onset, sEEG is becoming more prominent due to the lower risks and better patient tolerability [1–5].
2. Outcome is always better with preoperative lesions such as cortical dysplasia, mesial temporal sclerosis, and cavernomas or tumors. However, most commonly one is presented with a normal MR of the brain. In these circumstances concordance of data such as semiology, SISCOM, MEG, etc. will lead to a better outcome. If one has significant discordance of data, preoperatively performing an intracranial implant would be inappropriate here as this puts the patient at risk without a very good chance of localizing seizure onest to find a surgical solution to their uncontrolled epilepsy.
3. Intracranial leads are used to confirm a hypothesis of the reason for the patient's epilepsy. If a good hypothesis is not formed to depict the network involved in epilepsy, it is not time to implant.
4. Intracranial EEG monitoring to map and define the seizure onset zone (Phase II monitoring) is a critical component of epilepsy treatment. It cannot be emphasized enough that teamwork, collaboration, and data must be integrated prior to surgery to create a viable seizure hypothesis for testing with the intracranial

monitoring. Random implantation of electrodes without a hypothesis (otherwise known as a fishing expedition), does a disservice to the patient and should be avoided. At our center we have transitioned over time to incorporate stereotactic EEG (sEEG) into our practice, which has become extremely valuable, however has by no means supplanted cortical application of electrodes for functional brain mapping via subdural grid monitoring.

5. The likelihood of seizure freedom has a lot to do with the structural findings on MRI. When a lesion is present on brain MRI, the likelihood of seizure freedom following resection may be as high as 80% when mesial temporal sclerosis is present. In those patients where the brain MR is unrvealing as seen in patients with extratemporal epilepsies, we have commonly seen that one of every ten evaluations will become seizure-free in the end.

Clinical Pearls

1. Selected patients with drug-resistant focal epilepsy may require intracranial EEG monitoring for surgical localization.
2. sEEG is an appropriate methodology for evaluation of patients with MRI-negative focal epilepsy, epilepsy with potentially more than 1 focus, or in patients with discordant imaging and scalp-recorded EEG recordings.
3. sEEG should be used in highly selected patients following a comprehensive presurgical evaluation when there is a clear hypothesis regarding the region of the seizure onset zone.
4. Continued reevaluation of patients as a multidisciplinary team may lead to favorable seizure outcomes, as in this patient with a long history of drug-resistant focal epilepsy.
5. Counseling patients regarding the potential risks and benefits associated with intracranial EEG is essential to provide quality care.

References

1. Guenot M, Isnard J, Ryvlin P, Fischer C, Ostrowsky K, Mauguiere F, Sindou M. Neurophysiological monitoring for epilepsy surgery: the Talairach SEEG method. Stereo Electro Encephalo Graphy. Indications, results, complications and therapeutic applications in a series of 100 consecutive cases. Stereotact Funct Neurosurg. 2001;77(1–4):29–32.
2. Gonzalez-Martinez J, Bulacio J, Alexopoulos A, Jehi L, Bingaman W, Najm I. Stereoelectroencephalography in the "difficult to localize" refractory focal epilepsy: early experience from a North American Epilepsy Center. Epilepsia. 2013;54(2):323–30.
3. Bulacio JC, Jehi L, Wong C, Gonzalez-Martinez J, Kotagal P, Nair D, Najm I, Bingaman W. Long-term seizure outcome after resective surgery in patients evaluated with intracranial electrodes. Epilepsia. 2012;53(10):1722–30.
4. Britton JW. Electrical stimulation mapping with stereo-EEG electrodes. J Clin Neurophysiol. 2018;35(2):110–4.
5. Bourdillon P, Ryvlin P, Isnard J, Montavont A, Catenoix H, Mauguière F, Rheims S, Ostrowsky-Coste K, Guénot M. Stereotactic electroencephalography is a safe procedure, including for insular implantations. World Neurosurg. 2017;99:353–61.

Seizures in the Operating Room

Anthony Ritaccio

Case

A 74-year-old right-handed man was evaluated urgently after having a witnessed generalized tonic-clonic seizure. Subsequent MRI imaging disclosed a 2 × 3 cm mass lesion with associated edema and distortion of gyral anatomy in the left inferior frontal gyrus. His expressive language skills were found to be intact on detailed neurologic exam. A decision was made for surgical resection of the lesion during an awake craniotomy with ESM for functional brain mapping of language function. After surgical exposure of the cortex and prior to surgical resection, a customized 22-channel circular subdural grid electrode array was placed circumferentially around the area of presumed resection and intended electrical stimulation (Fig. 43.1a). In the course of applying electrical stimulation to the cortical surface and during administering of visual naming tasks, an after-discharge (AD) was evoked at contacts numbered 5–7 of the circular grid (Fig. 43.2a). Over the next 5–10 s, the AD increased in amplitude and frequencies became admixed with faster frequencies to indicate an impending seizure (Fig. 43.2b). The neurophysiologist supervising the ECoG immediately called for cessation of ESM and iced Ringer's lactate solution was applied over the cortical surface which aborted the after discharge in less than 5 s (Fig. 43.2b). Within several minutes, the patient continued with the awake ESM. Functional localization of linguistic cortex was then resumed and a functional brain map achieved (Fig. 43.1b).

A. Ritaccio (✉)
Mayo Clinic, Department of Neurology, Jacksonville, FL, USA
e-mail: ritaccio.anthony@mayo.edu

© Springer Nature Switzerland AG 2021
W. O. Tatum et al. (eds.), *Epilepsy Case Studies*,
https://doi.org/10.1007/978-3-030-59078-9_43

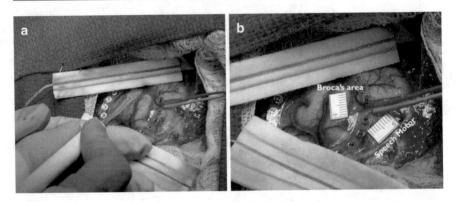

Fig. 43.1 (**a**) Surgeon's probe seen applying stimulation within circular electrode array. (**b**) Completed mapping exercise with sterile tickets placed over areas mark where electrical stimulation provoked language disruption

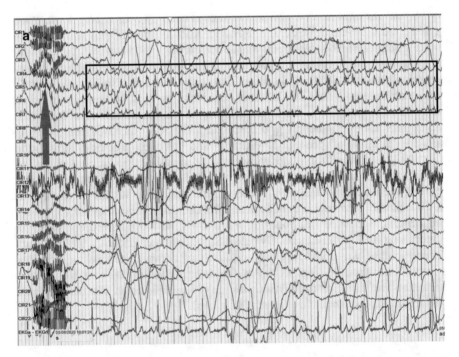

Fig. 43.2 (**a**) ECoG as recorded from 22-channel circular grid. *Red arrow* demonstrates electrical artifact generated during electrical stimulation by surgeon. *Black rectangle* encloses rhythmic pathologic afterdischarges in contacts 5–7. (**b**) Afterdischarges are rapidly aborted within seconds after topical administration of iced Ringer's solution

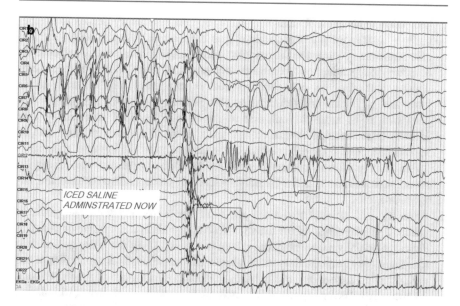

Fig. 43.2 (continued)

Questions

1. What is the incidence of intraoperative seizures?
2. What are the potential morbidities associated with intraoperative seizures?
3. What is the value of intraoperative ECoG during ESM?
4. How are intraoperative seizures managed?
5. What is the role of intraoperative ECoG in epilepsy surgery?

1. The incidence of intraoperative seizures in the literature is variable and typically defined by small retrospective series from individual centers [1]. Published series assessing the incidence of seizures evolving spontaneously during cortical resections record rates no higher than 3%. Whereas the occurrence of spontaneous seizures during neurosurgical resections is rare, the incidence of seizures induced during the course of ESM for functional localization may be as high as 25%. Intraoperative seizure rates have correlated with surgical volume and expertise in performing awake craniotomies in one large multicenter survey.
2. Seizures impact patient safety in the OR theater. Subclinical electrographic ictal activity recorded from subdural electrodes placed on the cortical surface for ECoG can lead to a generalized tonic-clonic seizure if not recognized and aborted. Seizures that occur during awake craniotomies specifically offer unique dangers [2]. The patient is awake and rigidly positioned with no airway

protection. This presents risk for aspiration and respiratory depression, especially if aggressive pharmacologic rescue is required. The post-ictal state will also prematurely terminate the mapping exercise due to somnolence and encephalopathy, independent of the contributory somnolence induced by rescue medications that may be employed, typically benzodiazepines or short-acting barbiturates. The electrical depression of the cortex post-ictally may make mapping with ESM more difficult and results unreliable. ESM post-seizure may identify false areas of eloquence that are a result of the seizure itself and its spread, unrelated to the discrete area being stimulated by the surgeon. The inability to fully perform functional mapping has been correlated statistically to incomplete resections and a greater incidence of postoperative motoric and linguistic deficits.

3. Neurosurgical lesional resections are typically performed with two goals in mind: [1] optimization of the extent of resection and [2] minimizing or avoiding deficit, especially when eloquent cortex is at risk [3]. In the context of nontumoral epilepsy surgery, functional mapping informs maximum resection of the epileptogenic zone to achieve seizure freedom in the absence of functional loss. ADs are provoked epileptiform EEG activity in response to electrical stimulation that resemble spontaneous seizures or may evolve into them. Stimulation intensities for AD production are widely variable among stimulation site, different lobes, adjacent electrodes, or even the same electrode pair from one trial to another. Identification of ADs and, if necessary, their termination are critical to prevent their potential evolution to generalized seizure with their associated morbidities. ADs and electrical seizures may produce functional deficits (false positive) that are misconstrued to be the result of the surgeon's discrete stimulation. Overestimates of eloquent areas that may ensue may lead to incomplete resections due to an abundance of caution. The neurologist/neurophysiologist and the timely identification of prolonged ADs and focal electrographic seizures in the real-time ECoG are one of the primary concerns when performing ESM to ensure functional brain mapping and subsequent resections are uninterrupted by intercurrent ictal events.

4. Intravenous administration of loading doses of conventional antiseizure medication (ASM) preoperatively has been shown to decrease the odds of triggering seizures by 45% even if the patient was maintained on ASM prior to surgery [4]. After the identification of a sustained AD or electrographic focal seizure, the most commonly utilized immediate therapy is not a pharmacologic one. Direct application of iced Ringer's solution applied to the cortical surface at the site of the AD/seizure is a potentially effective approach. As a mechanism of focal cerebral hypothermia, this therapy is extremely reliable in reducing spread of electrical activity, usually within 5–10 s. Cold water irrigation does not inhibit the surgeon from proceeding in mapping tasks and avoids the potential interruption and induced cognitive deficits of conventional ASDs and anesthetics.

5. ECoG is also used to define the irritative zone in a patient with seizures undergoing lesionectomy or epilepsy surgery [5]. Incomplete removal of epileptogenic tissue is one of the most common causes of failed temporal lobe surgery. Identification of irritative cortex to maximize the extent of resection may help

optimize seizure-free outcomes after surgery. Pre-resection spikes recorded by intraoperative ECoG in some patients with mesial temporal lobe has been correlated with good surgical outcome when eliminated by conventional temporal lobectomies and selective hippocampal resections. In MRI-negative temporal lobe onset seizures, patients with complete resection of tissue-generating interictal spikes recorded on intraoperative ECoG were less likely to have seizure recurrence compared to those with incomplete resection of spike producing cortex [6].

Pearls

1. Seizures may occur in an intraoperative setting and are most commonly observed during the ECoG that is recording during functional brain mapping using electrical stimulation.
2. Intraoperative seizures have unique morbidities in the OR setting.
3. Electrocorticography, recorded and interpreted in real time by the neurologist or neurophysiologist, is the principal means of identifying ADs and electrographic seizures.
4. Aborting nascent seizures can reduce intraoperative morbidity, allow for the potential to complete functional brain mapping. Overall, this leads to a more informed resection with greater probability of maximum resection without functional deficit.
5. Intraoperative pre-resection recording of interictal spikes by ECOG may result in more aggressive resections in both tumor surgeries and epilepsy surgeries and lead to higher long-term seizure-free rates.

References

1. Abecassis ZA, Ayer AB, Templer JW, Yerneni K, Murthy NK, Tate MC. Analysis of risk factors and clinical sequelae of direct electrical cortical stimulation-induced seizures and afterdischarges in patients undergoing awake mapping. J Neurosurg. 2020;22:1–8.
2. Spena G, Roca E, Guerrini F, Panciani PP, Stanzani L, Salmaggi A, Luzzi S, Fontanella M. Risk factors for intraoperative stimulation-related seizures during awake surgery: an analysis of 109 consecutive patients. J Neuro-Oncol. 2019;145(2):295–300.
3. Ritaccio AL, Brunner P, Schalk G. Intraoperative mapping of expressive language cortex using passive real-time electrocorticography. J Clin Neurophysiol. 2018;35(2):86–97.
4. Dineen J, Maus DC, Muzyka I, See RB, Cahill DP, Carter BS, Curry WT, Jones PS, Nahed BV, Peterfreund RA, Simon MV. Factors that modify the risk of intraoperative seizures triggered by electrical stimulation during supratentorial functional mapping. Clin Neurophysiol. 2019;130(6):1058–65.
5. Yao PS, Zheng SF, Wang F, Kang DZ, Lin YX. Surgery guided with intraoperative electrocorticography in patients with low-grade glioma and refractory seizures. J Neurosurg. 2018;128(3):840–5.
6. Grewal SS, Alvi MA, Perkins WJ, Cascino GD, Britton JW, Burkholder DB, So E, Shin C, Marsh RW, Meyer FB, Worrell GA, Van Gompel JJ. Reassessing the impact of intraoperative electrocorticography on postoperative outcome of patients undergoing standard temporal lobectomy for MRI-negative temporal lobe epilepsy. J Neurosurg. 2019;132(2):605–14.

Minimally Invasive Surgery

44

Sanjeet S. Grewal, Diogo M. Garcia, Erik H. Middlebrooks, and Robert E. Wharen

Case Presentation

A 17-year-old female presents with a history of gelastic and convulsive seizures. Exclusively nocturnal gelastic seizures (GS), lasting less than 30 s, were witnessed as early as at 9 months of age.

Currently, the patient was experiencing on average one seizure a day, lasting less than a minute, with preserved awareness. The patient did not report automatisms or amnestic episodes. At the termination of each event, the patient will yawn or stretch and does not have any postictal features. These events may cluster where she may have more than one seizure in a day. The best seizure-free interval for this type of event has been several weeks. The patient has proved to be drug-resistant to multiple antiseizure medications and is currently on levetiracetam 500 mg twice a day.

Separately, she has experienced nocturnal convulsive seizures, with multiple convulsions occurring monthly.

The general examination was unremarkable. The patient was awake, alert, oriented in time, place, and person, with normal speech and articulation, grossly intact cranial nerve function, normal motor function and deep tendon reflexes, preserved sensation to light touch and pinprick in all extremities, normal coordination, and normal gait.

S. S. Grewal (✉) · D. M. Garcia · R. E. Wharen
Mayo Clinic, Department of Neurosurgery, Jacksonville, FL, USA
e-mail: Grewal.sanjeet@mayo.edu; garcia.diogo@mayo.edu; Wharen.Robert@mayo.edu

E. H. Middlebrooks
Mayo Clinic, Division of Neuroradiology, Department of Radiology, Jacksonville, FL, USA
e-mail: Middlebrooks.Erik@mayo.edu

Clinical Questions

1. What is the classical epileptogenic lesion described for patients with gelastic seizures?
2. What are the two subtypes of hypothalamic hamartomas that are recognized?
3. What does her neuroimaging and EEG demonstrate?
4. What is the differential diagnosis for midline structural lesions?
5. How should she be managed?

Discussion

1. GS are the hallmark of seizures arising from the hypothalamus, with the most common etiology being a hypothalamic hamartoma (HH). In the setting of the aforementioned pathology, seizures typically have a childhood onset and are drug-resistant.
2. There are two types of HH:
   (a) Pedunculated, these hamartomas extend from the tuber cinereum between the mammillary body and the pituitary stalk and are commonly associated with precocious puberty [1]
   (b) Sessile hamartomas are often located along the roof of the tuber cinereum, asymmetrically lateralized, and more commonly associated with gelastic seizures [1]
3. The brain MRI (Fig. 44.1) shows a nonenhancing intra-axial, sharply defined, nodular lesion, arising from the left lateral wall of the hypothalamus and bulging into the left aspect of the third ventricle. The close relationship with the mammillary bodies can also be observed (Fig. 44.1).

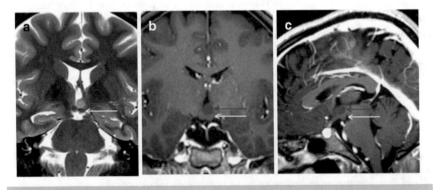

⟶ Hypothalamic Hamartoma
⟶ Mammillary Body

Fig. 44.1 The hypothalamic hamartoma (*red arrow*) and its close relationship with the mammillary body (*white arrow*) can be observed in the coronal T2 image of brain (**a**), post-contrast T1 coronal image of the brain (**b**), and post-contrast T1 sagittal image (**c**)

A 21-channel standard EEG recording with time-locked video and single-channel EKG was performed. The EEG background included sparse alpha activity of approximately 8 hertz over both posterior head regions. Intermittent short bursts of rhythmic theta or mixed frequency activity with a frontal central maximum, lasting for 0.5–1 s, were observed.

4. The differential diagnosis for hypothalamic lesions includes craniopharyngiomas, germinomas, hamartomas, lipomas, dermoid and epidermoid cysts, Rathke cleft cysts, colloid cysts, hypothalamic-chiasmatic gliomas, gangliogliomas, choristomas, hemangioblastomas, cavernomas, and systemic diseases with hypothalamic involvement. The patient's age, presentation with GS, imaging findings including near isointensity relative to the adjacent gray matter on all sequences, without associated abnormal restricted diffusion, and lack of enhancement support HH as the most likely diagnosis [2].

5. Drug-resistant HH-related epilepsy is best treated with surgery, which should be done as early as possible, regardless of the technique [3].

Open microsurgical resection has been largely abandoned due to its high rate of complications, up to 30%. Only Delande's type I purely cisternal peduncular forms remain a practical indication for an open pterional approach [4].

Stereotactic laser ablation and radiofrequency thermocoagulation procedures are an alternative to open microsurgical techniques as they can reduce approach-related morbidity. Both stereotactic radiofrequency thermocoagulation and fMRI targeted laser interstitial thermotherapy (LITT) allow a rate of seizure control of approximately 80–90%, while keeping the rate of complications at 0–2% [5, 6]. One advantage of LITT when compared to stereotactic radiofrequency thermocoagulation is the ability to image the ablation in real time and minimize heat spread to surrounding eloquent structures (Figs. 44.2 and 44.3). An important complication reported with interventions near the hypothalamic region is memory impairment. This has been largely prevented by recent advances, which allow the selective ablation of the epileptogenic focus [6].

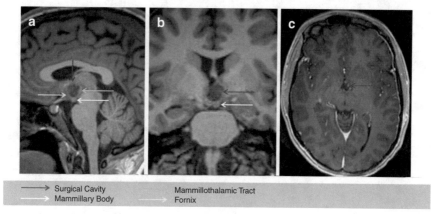

Surgical Cavity   Mammillothalamic Tract
Mammillary Body   Fornix

Fig. 44.2 The postoperative relationship between the surgical cavity (*red arrow*), mammillothalamic tract (*green arrow*), mammillary body (*white arrow*), and fornix (*yellow arrow*) can be observed in the sagittal T1 image of the brain (**a**), coronal T1 (**b**), and post-contrast T1 axial cut (**c**)

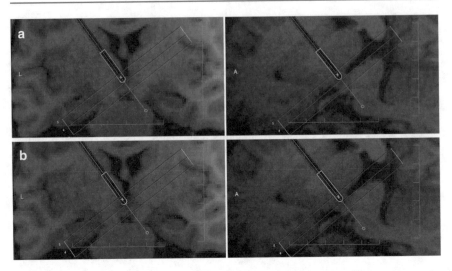

Fig. 44.3 The positioning of the laser fiber and anatomical relationship with the target can be observed (**a**), as well as the heat map of the ablation (**b**)

Pearls of Wisdom
- GS are characterized by laughter-like vocalizations, frequently accompanied by facial contraction in the form of a smile. Classically, GS have been associated with HH, which are rare congenital gray matter heterotopias associated with a triad of GS, precocious puberty, and developmental delay.
- Pedunculated HH are commonly associated with precocious puberty, while sessile HH are more commonly associated with GS.
- Standard EEG has a limited yield in the study of GS associated with HH. In the early stages of HH, the EEG is usually normal in the interictal period. Although GS are usually the first type of seizure presented by these patients, their clinical course may also include focal and focal to bilateral tonic-clonc seizures. Generalized convulsions/tonic-clonic seizures have been described in up to 70% of patients with GS associated with HH.
- GS in the setting of HH are often drug-resistant to antiseizure medication, and the progressive nature of the epileptogenic process eventually leads to cognitive and behavioral deterioration. As such, surgery offers the best chance at seizure control and should be considered as early as possible.
- Open microsurgical resection has largely been replaced by stereotactic radiofrequency thermocoagulation and is highly successful with MRI-guided LITT.

References

1. Mittal S, Mittal M, Montes JL, Farmer JP, Andermann F. Hypothalamic hamartomas. Part 1. Clinical, neuroimaging, and neurophysiological characteristics. Neurosurg Focus. 2013;34(6):E6.
2. Saleem SN, Said AH, Lee DH. Lesions of the hypothalamus: MR imaging diagnostic features. Radiographics. 2007;27(4):1087–108.
3. Ferrand-Sorbets S, Fohlen M, Delalande O, et al. Seizure outcome and prognostic factors for surgical management of hypothalamic hamartomas in children. Seizure. 2020;75:28–33.
4. Mittal S, Mittal M, Montes JL, Farmer JP, Andermann F. Hypothalamic hamartomas. Part 2. Surgical considerations and outcome. Neurosurg Focus. 2013;34(6):E7.
5. Boerwinkle VL, Foldes ST, Torrisi SJ, et al. Subcentimeter epilepsy surgery targets by resting state functional magnetic resonance imaging can improve outcomes in hypothalamic hamartoma. Epilepsia. 2018;59(12):2284–95.
6. Xu DS, Chen T, Hlubek RJ, et al. Magnetic resonance imaging-guided laser interstitial thermal therapy for the treatment of hypothalamic hamartomas: a retrospective review. Neurosurgery. 2018;83(6):1183–92.

Disconnection Surgery

45

Kai J. Miller and Elaine Wirrell

Case Presentation

A 15-year-old boy presented with a long-standing history of drug-resistant epilepsy. He was the product of a healthy term vaginal delivery to a 27-year-old G2P1 mother, and his birth weight was 3450 g. He enjoyed normal growth and development until 14 months of age when he was diagnosed with acute lymphoblastic leukemia. He received both chemotherapy with intrathecal methotrexate as well as whole brain radiation but unfortunately developed a toxic leukoencephalopathy which left him with moderate developmental disability.

His seizures began in his second year of life and included atonic seizures, atypical absences, myoclonic seizures, generalized tonic-clonic seizures, and tonic seizures. He was actively taking felbamate, valproate, clobazam, and lamotrigine but continued to have multiple drop seizures per week which had resulted in multiple head and dental injuries. With some of these he would lose tone, and with others would have generalized stiffness. His parents were concerned that medications made him dopey and less interactive. He had previously

K. J. Miller (✉)
Mayo Clinic, Department of Neurosurgery, Rochester, MN, USA
e-mail: miller.kai@mayo.edu

E. Wirrell
Mayo Clinic, Department of Child and Adolescent Neurology and Epilepsy,
Rochester, MN, USA
e-mail: Wirrell.elaine@mayo.edu

© Springer Nature Switzerland AG 2021
W. O. Tatum et al. (eds.), *Epilepsy Case Studies*,
https://doi.org/10.1007/978-3-030-59078-9_45

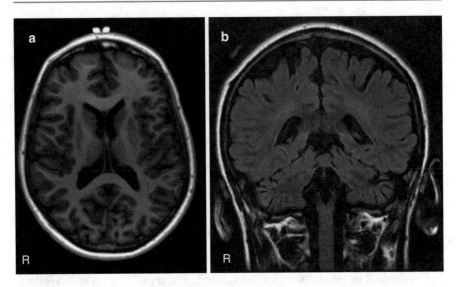

Fig. 45.1 Imaging. (a) Axial MPRAGE sequence. (b) Coronal T2 FLAIR sequence

been on multiple medications including levetiracetam, ethosuximide, rufinamide, and topiramate and had also tried therapy with the ketogenic diet without sustained benefit.

The general examination was unremarkable. His weight and height were at the 50th percentile, but head circumference was fifth percentile for age. He had approximately a 15-word vocabulary but could not combine words. He could follow some one-step commands. His optic discs were pale bilaterally, but otherwise cranial nerves were unremarkable. He had symmetric and appropriate strength in his arms and legs. His reflexes were slightly brisk bilaterally but with downgoing toes to plantar stimulation. He had slight bilateral hip contractures. He was able to walk independently although his gait was clumsy and somewhat stooped.

An MRI was obtained (Fig. 45.1).

He underwent video-EEG monitoring. The background EEG is shown (Fig. 45.2a, awake; Fig. 45.2b, sleep).

He was found to have atypical absence seizures, 2–4 times per day, lasting up to 2–3 min, as well as occasional myoclonic jerks. He had his typical drop seizures recorded during which his tone was increased (tonic seizure) (Fig. 45.3).

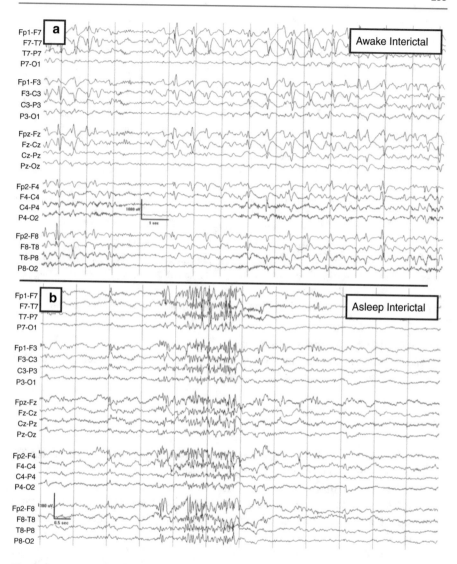

Fig. 45.2 Interictal EEG. (**a**) Awake. (**b**) Asleep. EEG sensitivity 10 uv/mm, filter settings 1–70 Hz, display speed 60 mm/s

Clinical Questions

1. What does his MRI show?
2. What does his interictal EEG show?
3. What does his ictal EEG show?

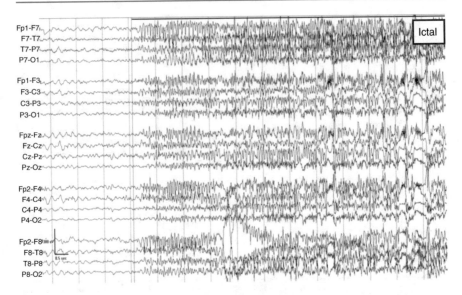

Fig. 45.3 Ictal EEG. EEG Sensitivity 10 uv/mm, filter settings 1–70 Hz, display speed 60 mm/s

4. What epilepsy syndrome does he have?
5. What treatment options might you suggest for his major seizure type? How likely are they to reduce his drop seizures?

Discussion

1. His MRI shows diffuse cerebral and cerebellar atrophy with hyperintense T2 changes in the white matter. His corpus callosum is intact.
2. The awake interictal EEG shows diffuse background slowing with high-amplitude, frontally predominant slow spike-and-wave (Fig. 45.2a). During sleep, there were frequent bursts of generalized paroxysmal fast activity (Fig. 45.2b).
3. The ictal recording shows abrupt onset of generalized polyspike discharge, which was clinically correlated with generalized tonic stiffening of his body, with a fall (Fig. 45.3).
4. He is presenting with Lennox-Gastaut syndrome. Lennox-Gastaut syndrome is a severe, lifelong epilepsy syndrome associated with multiple seizure types, most prominently drop attacks (atonic and tonic), in association with characteristic EEG changes (slow spike-and-wave and generalized paroxysmal fast activity) and intellectual disability. It is due to a broad range of diverse etiologies, including genetic (i.e., CDKL5, Trisomy 21, SCN8A), structural (developmental brain malformations, acquired diffuse brain injury), metabolic (i.e., mitochondrial disorders), and infectious causes (TORCH infection, prior meningitis). Approximately one quarter of cases are of unknown cause.

5. The goals of treatment in Lennox-Gastaut syndrome are to (1) reduce seizure frequency, particularly those seizure types that lead to injury, such as drop seizures, (2) minimize adverse effects of polypharmacy, and (3) maximize quality of life. Complete seizure freedom is not attainable. Medications which have been most helpful for seizures associated with this syndrome include valproic acid, lamotrigine, topiramate, clobazam, rufinamide, felbamate, and, most recently, pharma-grade cannabidiol [1]. The ketogenic diet also shows significant seizure reduction in approximately half of cases [2]. Rarely, cases with focal brain lesions are identified to benefit from resective surgery [3]; however, for most persons with Lennox-Gastaut syndrome, resective surgery is not an option.

Palliative surgical options are important therapeutic considerations in persons with Lennox-Gastaut syndrome, particularly with drug-resistant drop attacks. Corpus callosotomy is more efficacious at significantly reducing drop seizure frequency compared to vagus nerve stimulation with nearly half achieving freedom from drop seizures [4]. There is little evidence for disconnection syndrome in persons with Lennox-Gastaut syndrome who undergo callosotomy [5].

Follow-Up

He underwent complete corpus callosotomy with marked improvement in drop seizures. He can walk independently and has had no major falls or injury since surgery. He had no deterioration in his language skills nor any evidence to suggest disconnection syndrome. He has occasional clusters of minor head nods, which are often triggered by illness or fatigue, but these do not lead to falls. His atypical absence seizures and myoclonic seizures persist, with only minor reduction in frequency since surgery. He has been successfully able to wean off valproic acid and lamotrigine and continued felbamate with low-dose clobazam. His parents report a marked benefit in quality of life and feel that he is brighter and that his personality has re-emerged.

Pearls of Wisdom
1. Drop attacks are epileptic seizures that have significant impact on quality of life, can independently limit physical activities and cognitive development, often lead to recurrent injury, and generate unique challenges for the caregiver.
2. Callosotomy can be a highly successful surgical option for such cases as a palliative procedure.
3. Given the highly drug-resistant nature of seizures in Lennox-Gastaut syndrome, nonpharmacological therapies such as ketogenic diet and surgical options should be considered early in the course of management and not reserved only for patients who fail multiple antiseizure medications.

4. Persons with drug-resistant seizures are often treated with high doses of multiple antiseizure medications. It is essential to evaluate which medications are not significantly contributing to seizure control and wean and discontinue what medication is not working. Palliative surgical procedures may offer the benefit of reducing seizure burden but also the number and dosage of co-existing antiseizure medications.
5. Disconnection syndrome is rare following complete callosotomy in persons with Lennox-Gastaut syndrome.

References

1. Cross JH, Auvin S, Falip M, Striano P, Arzimanoglou A. Expert opinion on the Management of Lennox-Gastaut Syndrome: treatment algorithms and practical considerations. Front Neurol. 2017;8:505.
2. Lemmon ME, Terao NN, Ng YT, Reisig W, Rubenstein JE, Kossoff EH. Efficacy of the ketogenic diet in Lennox-Gastaut syndrome: a retrospective review of one institution's experience and summary of the literature. Dev Med Child Neurol. 2012;54(5):464–8.
3. Wyllie E, Lachhwani DK, Gupta A, Chirla A, Cosmo G, et al. Successful surgery for epilepsy due to early brain lesions despite generalized EEG findings. Neurology. 2007;69(4):389–97.
4. Lancman G, Virk M, Shao H, Mazumdar M, Greenfield JP, Weinstein S, Schwartz TH. Vagus nerve stimulation vs. corpus callosotomy in the treatment of Lennox-Gastaut syndrome: a meta-analysis. Seizure. 2013;22(1):3–8.
5. Graham G, Tisdall MM, Gill D. Corpus Callosotomy Outcomes in Pediatric Patients: A Systematic Review. Epilepsia. 2016; Jul;57(7):1053–68.

VNS and Epilepsy

46

Brian N. Lundstrom and William O. Tatum

Case Presentation

A 25-year-old right-handed woman with drug-resistant epilepsy presents to clinic with generalized tonic-clonic seizures since 12 years of age. Her ASM includes levetiracetam 1500 mg three times daily, lamotrigine 400 mg in the morning, 200 mg midday, and 400 mg nightly, and clobazam 20 mg twice daily. Two prior instances of inpatient scalp video-EEG monitoring recorded generalized polyspike-wave discharges as well as multiple diffuse onset seizures with varying focal features in the semiology. Seven years ago she had a left-sided vagus nerve stimulator (VNS) implanted for treatment of her seizures leading to an approximate 70% reduction in seizure frequency. Prior to VNS implant she reported approximately three generalized tonic-clonic seizures per month, and following VNS placement, she reports approximately one convulsive seizure every month. Her VNS battery is reaching end of service and needs to be replaced. Her settings are 1.5 mA, 20 Hz, 250 usec pulse width, and 25% duty cycle (30 s on and 1.8 min off). Symptoms of coughing and vomiting have precluded previous increases in VNS current.

Initially, her VNS settings were changed by increasing current to 1.75 mA and duty cycle to 35% while decreasing the pulse width to 130 usec, which improved tolerability. At 3-month follow-up, she reported only one convulsion in the past 3 months. Her VNS device was replaced with a newer model that included heart-rate-sensing autostimulation (Aspire SR, model 106; Liva Nova, Houston TX USA). Her new device was programmed to a lower current of 0.625 mA amplitude, as she

B. N. Lundstrom (✉)
Mayo Clinic, Department of Neurology, Rochester, MN, USA
e-mail: Lundstrom.Brian@mayo.edu

W. O. Tatum
Mayo Clinic, Department of Neurology, Jacksonville, FL, USA
e-mail: tatum.william@mayo.edu

© Springer Nature Switzerland AG 2021
W. O. Tatum et al. (eds.), *Epilepsy Case Studies*,
https://doi.org/10.1007/978-3-030-59078-9_46

could not tolerate higher levels due to stimulation-induced cough and hoarseness. At 9-month follow-up, she reported two convulsions over the previous 6 months, similar to just before her device replacement. However, she reported side effects of coughing during exercise. Normal mode current intensity was increased to 0.75 mA with autostimulation amplitude increased to 0.875 mA. Her autostimulation threshold was increased to 50% given the reported side effects during exercise. By 1 year she reported experiencing 1 seizure in the past 3 months with 24 autostimulations per day and was clinically tolerating her settings. Normal mode current intensity was increased to 0.875 mA. Autostimulation amplitude was increased to 1 mA, and the threshold was now decreased from 50% to 30%. At her 15-month follow-up, she continued to have approximately 1 seizure every 2–3 months with 76 autostimulations per day. Her amplitude was increased to 1.25 mA. As of her most recent follow-up, she had been seizure-free for 9 months.

Clinical Questions

1. How effective are VNS devices for controlling seizures?
2. Which patients are appropriate candidates for consideration of VNS therapy?
3. What is the patient's relative risk of sudden unexplained death in epilepsy (SUDEP)?
4. Are newer VNS devices more effective than older devices?
5. How long should one try to optimize stimulation parameters for implanted devices?

Discussion

1. The reported efficacy of VNS improves over time as with other forms of neuromodulation such as deep brain stimulation and responsive neurostimulation. Early trials suggested a 30% responder rate (greater than 50% seizure reduction) at 3 months and a 40% responder rate by 2 years. Overall long-term studies suggest that approximately 5–10% of patients experience seizure freedom for significant intervals of time after demonstrating drug resistance [1]. Many clinicians consider VNS to be somewhat less effective than other approved forms of neuromodulation for epilepsy.
2. VNS is approved as adjunctive therapy for the treatment of focal epilepsy in patients 4 years of age and older. Considerable experience suggests VNS is effective for treating generalized epilepsy as well [2]. VNS may be preferred to other forms of neuromodulation as it does not involve intracranial surgery. Since VNS is considered a palliative therapy, resective surgery that offers the potential for seizure freedom should still be considered if appropriate.
3. The relative risk of SUDEP occurs predominately in young people between 20 and 40 years of age who experience convulsions during unattended sleep at night. Substance abuse, cognitive disabilities, and low levels of ASM are also

risk factors for SUDEP. Long-term risk of SUDEP is decreased in those receiving VNS therapy [3].

4. Newer VNS models are at least as effective as the older models; heart rate sensing and different modes and frequencies of stimulation as high as 300 Hz (VNS Microburst®) may increase efficacy over older models. For example, the majority of focal seizure patients have tachycardia even before clinical manifestations of seizures, and heart rate sensing may allow for a "pre-emptive strike" that may be helpful in aborting seizures before they manifest clinically [4].

5. Evaluation of parameters using VNS have not demonstrated a single set of optimal parameter settings. There are many permutations of current intensity, pulse frequency, pulse duration, and duty cycles (i.e., on-off times). Further, autostimulation paradigms increase possible stimulation settings further emphasizing the need to individualize patient parameters. In general 3–6 months should be allotted before giving up on a particular approach and 2 years before determining that no benefit has occurred.

Pearls of Wisdom

1. VNS is one of the FDA-approved forms of neuromodulation for epilepsy. Responsive neurostimulation (RNS) and deep brain stimulation of the anterior nucleus of the thalamus (DBS-ANT) are other forms (Fig. 46.1). In general, the effects of neurostimulation appear to improve over time. Multiple mechanisms are proposed to explain this though it appears evident in all forms of neuromodulation. Related to this, the beneficial effect of neuromodulation may improve over time even without changes to the device. In contrast to clinical changes over days or a couple weeks typically expected with the addition of antiseizure medications (ASMs), the effects of neuromodulation should be measured in months and years.

2. Patients as young as 4 years of age with focal seizures, generalized seizures, and multifocal seizures may be candidates for VNS therapy. Because it does not require intracranial surgery, it is less invasive than other forms of stimulation such as responsive neurostimulation and deep brain stimulation. Patients with generalized tonic-clonic seizures are at risk for SUDEP. Evidence suggests patients with VNS show decreased rates of SUDEP.

3. More than 100,000 patients have been implanted with VNS device worldwide. Many clinicians are now familiar with this "pacemaker for the brain." However, newer developments including autostimulation and high-frequency stimulation are emerging, which may reflect improvements. The field of neurostimulation for epilepsy is rapidly advancing.

4. The side effect profile of VNS differs from typical ASMs. Typical side effects for VNS include hoarseness, pain or tingling at the electrode site, and shortness of breath [5]. Often these side effects can be ameliorated with appropriate programming changes. Typical side effects for ASMs

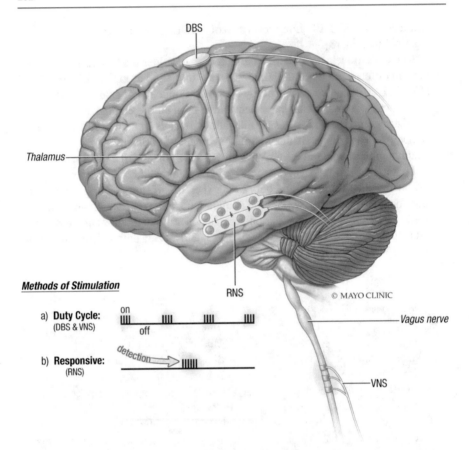

Fig. 46.1 FDA-approved approaches for brain stimulation for epilepsy include vagus nerve stimulation (VNS), responsive neurostimulation (RNS), and deep brain stimulation of the anterior nucleus of the thalamus (DBS-ANT). (**a**) DBS and VNS do not sense brain activity but rather stimulate periodically all the time. (**b**) In contrast, RNS is delivered in response to detected brain activity. Another difference is that DBS and VNS stimulate in the same analogous location for every patient, whereas RNS stimulates near the patient-specific seizure onset zone (Used with permission of Mayo Foundation for Medical Education and Research, all rights reserved)

include somnolence, dizziness, increased teratogenicity related to childbirth, and idiosyncratic life-threatening risks related to rash and organ function. These differences in side effects and predictability in VNS side effects make VNS therapy an attractive approach for adjunctive treatment.

5. It is important to realize that VNS is not a "cure" and is palliative in nature. The responder rates are similar to those experienced with ASM, perhaps somewhat better over time. While seizure reduction is important, disabilities related to the presence of seizures, such as driving restrictions, typically remain. ASMs may be reduced, but patients typically remain on ASMs. Typically, the possibility of epilepsy surgery should be excluded before VNS is considered. Nonetheless, quality of life improves with VNS therapy, and the unique side effect profile of VNS coupled with the possibility of reducing ASMs makes VNS an attractive option for patients with drug-resistant epilepsy.

References

1. Englot DJ, Rolston JD, Wright CW, Hassnain KH, Chang EF. Rates and predictors of seizure freedom with vagus nerve stimulation for intractable epilepsy. Neurosurgery. 2016;79(3):345–53.
2. Morris GL III, Gloss D, Buchhalter J, Mack KJ, Nickels K, Harden C. Evidence-based guideline update: vagus nerve stimulation for the treatment of epilepsy: report of the guideline development subcommittee of the American Academy of Neurology. Epilepsy Curr. 2013;13(6):297–303.
3. Ryvlin P, So EL, Gordon CM, Hesdorffer DC, Sperling MR, Devinsky O, et al. Long-term surveillance of SUDEP in drug-resistant epilepsy patients treated with VNS therapy. Epilepsia. 2018;59(3):562–72.
4. Hamilton P, Soryal I, Dhahri P, Wimalachandra W, Leat A, Hughes D, et al. Clinical outcomes of VNS therapy with AspireSR(®) (including cardiac-based seizure detection) at a large complex epilepsy and surgery centre. Seizure. 2018;58:120–6.
5. Révész D, Rydenhag B, Ben-Menachem E. Complications and safety of vagus nerve stimulation: 25 years of experience at a single center. J Neurosurg Pediatr. 2016;18:97–104.

Intracranial Stimulation and Epilepsy

47

Brian N. Lundstrom, Sanjeet S. Grewal,
and Robert E. Wharen

Case Presentation

An 18-year-old right-handed man presents with focal seizures with impaired awareness for the past 2 years. His imaging is consistent with a left posterior temporal ependymoma, and inpatient video-assisted scalp EEG recorded seizures arising from this region. Despite adequate trials of multiple antiseizure medications, his seizures were not controlled. The ependymoma was resected, and he was seizure-free for 1 year without any reported neurological deficits. Unfortunately, he had recurrence of seizures despite continued medical management. Repeat imaging revealed no signs of tumor recurrence. Intracranial EEG monitoring with subdural grids revealed seizure onset from the posterior lateral temporal cortex in the same region as eloquent speech areas, as determined by extra-operative speech mapping. A responsive neurostimulation system (NeuroPace, Inc., Mountain View, CA) was implanted with two 4-contact 1-cm spaced subdural leads placed on the inferior and superior lateral temporal cortex (Fig. 47.1). Three months after initiation of stimulation, he reported no clinical seizures. Stimulation parameters included eight negative contacts (device case was positive) at 8 mA (2.5 microcoulombs/cm^2 per contact) with pulse width 200 microseconds and 100-msec bursts at 200 Hz.

Twenty seven months after implantation, the patient reported a clinical seizure consistent with his prior seizures. Upon interrogation, the device battery was

B. N. Lundstrom (✉)
Mayo Clinic, Department of Neurology, Rochester, MN, USA
e-mail: Lundstrom.Brian@mayo.edu

S. S. Grewal · R. E. Wharen
Mayo Clinic, Department of Neurosurgery, Jacksonville, FL, USA
e-mail: grewal.sanjeet@mayo.edu; Wharen.Robert@mayo.edu

© Springer Nature Switzerland AG 2021
W. O. Tatum et al. (eds.), *Epilepsy Case Studies*,
https://doi.org/10.1007/978-3-030-59078-9_47

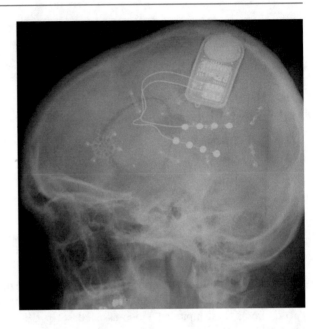

Fig. 47.1 Lateral skull X-ray revealing placement of two paddle electrodes over the left lateral temporal lobe connected to a left-sided RNS device

depleted and was no longer providing stimulation. After replacement he experienced prolonged seizure freedom with stimulation amplitude lowered to 4 mA (1.3 microcoulombs/cm^2 per contact). His neurostimulator was replaced two further times due to battery depletion at approximately 3-year intervals. During this time no clinical seizures were reported.

However, as he was nearing the time for his fourth battery replacement, it was noted that the skin overlying the stimulator location was thinning. Twice he underwent revision of his incision with plastic surgery in order to prevent dehiscence. However, there remained a small area that did not heal, and after a third revision of his incision with plastic surgery, the decision was made to explant the neurostimulator. At this point the patient had been seizure-free for 16 years. In an attempt to maintain the efficacy of neuromodulation, off-label use of FDA-approved hardware was used under an IRB protocol. The patient was implanted with two 2.8 mm spaced 1 × 8 contact subdural leads connected to an infraclavicular battery (Boston Scientific Spectra WaveWriter) for chronic subthreshold cortical stimulation (Fig. 47.2). The device was programmed such that all electrodes were negative and the device case was positive with a frequency of 100 Hz, pulse width of 200 microseconds, and device output of 2 mA (0.4 microcoulombs/cm^2 per contact). He has remained seizure-free with stimulation as of last follow-up 3 months following device programming.

Fig. 47.2 Lateral skull X-ray revealing placement of two paddle electrodes over the left lateral temporal lobe connected to a left-sided deep brain stimulating device. Only one row of each paddle was used for active stimulation

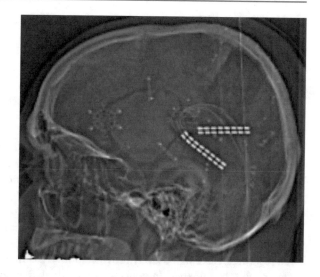

Clinical Questions

1. What are the intracranial stimulation options for this patient? Why might one option be chosen over another?
2. How efficacious are these stimulation options? What kinds of seizures do they treat?
3. What are typical risks and side effects associated with intracranial stimulation?
4. When should intracranial stimulation be considered?
5. How does intracranial stimulation affect risk for sudden unexplained death in epilepsy?

Discussion

1. Responsive neurostimulation (RNS) and deep brain stimulation (DBS) of the anterior nucleus of the thalamus are both FDA-approved intracranial stimulation options for patients with focal drug-resistant epilepsy [1–3]. The efficacy of each approach is similar, but each approach has different characteristics. RNS involves placement of a skull-based device, requires localizing the seizure onset zone for appropriate placement of stimulating electrodes, and has the advantage of recording intracranial brain signals [4]. DBS involves a chest-based device, does not require localization of the seizure onset zone, and is relatively more straightforward to program. Chronic subthreshold cortical stimulation is a form of continuous, open-loop stimulation provided near or at the site of seizure onset that is an investigational approach [5].

2. Both RNS and DBS typically lead to an approximate 50% seizure reduction after 1 year that improves to an approximate 70% reduction after 5 years. Treatment is considered to be palliative, and long periods of seizure freedom are rare, less than 15%. Both RNS and DBS are approved for the treatment of focal onset seizures.
3. Overall risks for the two approaches are similar with a risk of infection of 4–5% per procedure. Battery life depends on details of programming but is often reported as 4–8 years for non-rechargeable batteries. For RNS, battery replacement involves a skull-based procedure that may include complications with repeated replacements. For DBS, depressed mood and memory impairment have been reported but appear to be ameliorated by programming changes.
4. When antiseizure medications (ASMs) fail to completely control seizures, patients are typically considered for resective surgery, which can lead to seizure freedom. If resective surgery is deemed unlikely to lead to seizure freedom, neurostimulation approaches are considered. Occasionally, neurostimulation is considered earlier in the process. For example, the diagnostic capability of RNS in recording EEG signals may prove helpful in cases of apparent bilateral mesial temporal lobe epilepsy. In general, neurostimulation approaches are considered reversible, whereas resective surgery is irreversible.
5. Evidence suggests that both RNS and DBS significantly reduce the rate of SUDEP in treated patients.

Pearls of Wisdom
1. Neurostimulation for epilepsy is a rapidly changing field. FDA-approved approaches currently include vagus nerve stimulation as well as DBS and RNS. Many clinicians consider vagus nerve stimulation to be less effective but less risky than DBS and RNS. DBS and RNS are considered to be similar in efficacy.
2. Neurostimulation approaches are potentially less risky and reversible in comparison to resective surgery, which often requires a longer evaluation process, more inherent risk, and involves an irreversible procedure. However, neurostimulation approaches rarely lead to seizure freedom, although they can allow in some cases for ASMs to be reduced.
3. One significant difference between RNS and DBS is the need to adequately localize the seizure onset zone. For RNS, electrodes are placed near the estimated seizure onset zone. More recent evidence suggests that regional areas of seizure onset may beneft from being bracketed by the RNS electrodes to control seizures [6]. For DBS the seizure onset zone need not be localized because the electrodes target the anterior nucleus of the thalamus to involve widespread subcortical-cortical networks in patients treated for focal seizures.
4. Side effects to ongoing electrical stimulation by RNS and DBS are mild or not clinically relevant.
5. Future intracranial neurostimulation approaches will offer increasing options related to rechargeable batteries, sensing capabilities, and a greater number of implanted electrodes.

References

1. Salanova V, Witt T, Worth R, Henry TR, Gross RE, Nazzaro JM, et al. SANTE study group. Long-term efficacy and safety of thalamic stimulation for drug-resistant partial epilepsy. Neurology. 2015;84(10):1017–25.
2. Geller EB, Skarpaas TL, Gross RE, Goodman RR, Barkley GL, Bazil CW, et al. Brain-responsive neurostimulation in patients with medically intractable mesial temporal lobe epilepsy. Epilepsia. 2017;58(6):994–1004.
3. Jobst BC, Kapur R, Barkley GL, Bazil CW, Berg MJ, Bergey GK, et al. Brain-responsive neurostimulation in patients with medically intractable seizures arising from eloquent and other neocortical areas. Epilepsia. 2017;58(6):1005–14.
4. King-Stephens D, Mirro E, Weber PB, Laxer KD, Van Ness PC, Salanova V, et al. Lateralization of mesial temporal lobe epilepsy with chronic ambulatory electrocorticography. Epilepsia. 2015;56(6):959–67.
5. Lundstrom BN, Gompel JV, Khadjevand F, Worrell G, Stead M. Chronic subthreshold cortical stimulation and stimulation-related EEG biomarkers for focal epilepsy. Brain Commun. 2019;1(1):fcz010.
6. Ma BB, Fields MC, Knowlton RC, Chang EF, Szaflarski JP, Marcuse LV, Rao VR. Responsive neurostimulation for regional neocortical epilepsy. Epilepsia. 2020;61(1):96–106.

Ketogenic Diet

48

Rubina Bakerywala

Case History

A 3-year-old-girl was referred for evaluation of a drug-resistant epileptic encephalopathy manifest as recurrent convulsive and nonconvulsive seizures. In addition there were comorbid abnormal eye movements present. Her history was significant for global developmental delays thought to be developmental and worsened by her recurrent epileptic seizures. Her seizure types included generalized tonic-clonic seizures and staring spells that were previously uncharacterized. She was reported to have up to ten witnessed nonconvulsive seizures daily where she would abruptly stop and manifest a brief stare with a lapse of awareness. The generalized tonic-clonic seizures occurred two to three times within a month. She had experienced staring spells since infancy and failed high doses of phenobarbital, valproate, levetiracetam, topiramate, zonisamide, lamotrigine and was currently taking clobazam, rufinamide, and perampanel.

Her birth history included a full-term normal vaginal delivery with a birth weight of 7 pounds and 9 oz. She experienced initial problems shortly after birth that included developmental delay, initial feeding difficulty, hypotonia, and abnormal eye movements. A family history was unrevealing for a similar condition.

On physical examination, her weight was 15 kg, height was at the 45th percentile, and her head circumference was microcephalic at less than the 2nd percentile. A general examination revealed a baby that was small for her age. There were no abnormal signs visible to suggest a neurocutaneous syndrome. Her overall higher neurocognitive function was delayed. She was able to speak in two word responses. The cranial nerve examination was within normal limits. Her motor examination

R. Bakerywala (✉)
Nemours Children's Specialty Care, Department of Neurology, Jacksonville, FL, USA
e-mail: rubina.bakerywala@nemours.org

© Springer Nature Switzerland AG 2021
W. O. Tatum et al. (eds.), *Epilepsy Case Studies*,
https://doi.org/10.1007/978-3-030-59078-9_48

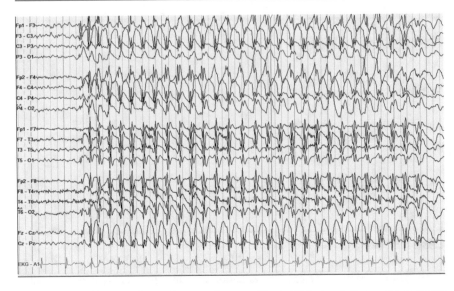

Fig. 48.1 EEG demonstrating an absence seizure manifest as 10.5-s burst of generalized anterior predominant 3-Hz spike-and-waves. Sensitivity 10 uV/mm, filter settings 1–70 Hz, display speed 30 mm/s

demonstrated diffuse hypotonia though there was good muscle strength throughout. The deep tendon reflexes were symmetrical in all four extremities, and the planter reflexes were downgoing. Her gait was wide-based.

Diagnostic Evaluation:

1. 3 T MRI brain done at 6 months and 28 months was normal.
2. Routine and special metabolic testing included a complete blood count, complete metabolic profile, serum amino acids, urine organic acids, and serum ammonia. All laboratory studies were within normal limits.
3. Lumbar puncture results included a normal cell count and protein, but the glucose in the cerebrospinal fluid was low at 24 mg/dl. A corresponding plasma glucose done at the same time was 80 mg/dl.
4. A sample of her EEG is depicted in the Fig. 48.1.

Clinical Questions

1. What type of seizures is she having and what is her diagnosis?
2. What is the best management option for this patient?
3. What are some of the side effects of treatment?
4. What are other indications and contraindications for this treatment?
5. What are other types of dietary options available for treating seizures?

Discussion

1. The EEG demonstrates 3 Hz spike- and polyspike-and-waves. When captured during a staring spell, this is diagnostic of an absence seizure. Given the history of early-onset drug-resistant absence epilepsy, development delays, hypotonia, and microcephaly, the history is concerning for metabolic or genetic form of epilepsy. Further genetic testing revealed a de novo mutation in SLC2A1 gene. The hypoglycorrhachia and genetic mutation reflects a diagnosis of GLUT1 deficiency syndrome (Glut-1). This is also known as GLUT1-DS or De Vivo disease [1], and Glucose transporter type 1 deficiency syndrome and represents a rare autosomal dominant genetic metabolic disorder associated with a deficiency of a glucose transport protein that transports glucose across the blood-brain barrier. This defect impairs glucose transport into the brain to maintain normal cellular function. The ratio of low spinal fluid glucose level compared to plasma is a crucial metric for diagnosis [2]. A spinal fluid to blood glucose ratio at or below the 25th percentile is the diagnostic hallmark of this entity. Approximately 80–90% of patients carry a mutation in the SLC2A1 gene. The phenotypic spectrum of Glut-1 is a continuum of epilepsy and movement disorders including the classic phenotype with absence seizures and paroxysmal dyskinesia, though spasticity, dystonia, choreoathetosis, and other movements may occur [3].
2. The ketogenic diet has become a first-line treatment involving epilepsy syndromes associated with gene mutations responsible for GLUT-1. The ketogenic diet initially was developed in the 1921 in response to the observation that fasting had antiseizure properties. During fasting, the body metabolizes fat stores and produces fatty acids which undergo beta-oxidation and produces ketones like acetoacetate, β-hydroxybutyrate, and acetone. The cell can then use these as precursors to generate adenosine triphosphate (ATP). The ketogenic diet is thought to simulate the metabolic effects of starvation by forcing the body to use fat as the primary fuel source. The diet fell out of favor with the development of new antiseizure medication in the late 1930s, but it has experienced a resurgence in use over the past 20 years, particularly in the treatment of patients with drug-resistant epilepsy. The classic ketogenic diet has a ratio of 3:1 or 4:1 of fat to carbohydrate and protein. The fat content in the classic ketogenic diet is composed of long-chain fatty acids; however, medium-chain triglycerides can be substituted. Several mechanisms have been proposed to explain efficacy of the diet, including changes in ATP production making neurons more resilient in the face of greater metabolic demands required during seizures, altered brain pH affecting neuronal excitability, direct inhibitory effects of ketone bodies, antiseizure effect of fatty acids on ion channels, and shifts in amino acid metabolism to favor the synthesis of the inhibitory neurotransmitter GABA [4, 5]. Approximately 50–60% of children experience seizure reduction of at least 50%, one-third have their seizures reduced by >90%, and about 10% become seizure-free.
3. Prior to initiating the ketogenic diet, a baseline laboratory evaluation is performed. Children are hospitalized for 24–48 h and undergo fasting. During this time, they are allowed limited amounts of sugar-free liquids and gelatin. Meal

plans are calculated from a ratio of grams of fat to grams of protein plus carbo-hydrate in a 3 to 1 or 4 to 1 ratio which means 3 or 4 g of fat to 1 g of protein and limited carbohydrate. Children may be kept on the diet for 1 to 2 years or longer when it is beneficial. Side effects may occur and, in general, are tolerable. The diet is tapered over several months by lowering the ratio of fat to protein plus carbohydrate and then slowly relaxing restrictions on the relative weighting of food intake while titrating the amount of carbohydrate intake.

4. Side effects of the ketogenic diet are listed below in the table. There is also the potential for hyperlipidemia caused by maintaining a diet that is very high in fat content. Lack of additional nutrients and minerals can result in compromised bone health. Rarely side effects may include damage to solid organs [6].

   Common side effects

- Weight loss/poor weight gain
- Dehydration
- Constipation (or less frequently diarrhea)
- Nausea
- Vomiting
- Renal calculi
- Poor weight gain
- Growth retardation
- Hypoglycemia
- Osteopenia and osteoporosis
- *Less common side effects*
- Kidney stones
- Hyperlipidemia
- *Rare side effects*
- Cardiomyopathy
- Prolonged QT syndrome
- Pancreatitis

5. The indication for using the ketogenic diet includes patients with drug-resistant epilepsy. Those patients with glucose transporter defect type-1(Glut-1 deficiency) and pyruvate dehydrogenase deficiency should have the ketogenic diet considered as an initial line of therapy. The diet works very well for these patients compared with traditional antiseizure drugs. Generating ketone bodies provides the brain with an alternative source of energy in conditions where metabolic functions are impaired. On the other hand, fasting or implementing the ketogenic diet in patients with inborn errors of metabolism that involves transport or oxidation of long-chain fatty acids is contraindicated and can lead to devastating catabolic crises due to the additional fat load that could perturb an already compromised system. Conditions where the ketogenic diet should be avoided include the following [6]:

- Primary carnitine deficiency
- Carnitine translocase deficiency

- Fatty acid beta-oxidation defects
- Pyruvate carboxylase deficiency
- Porphyria

6. Some alternatives to the ketogenic diet that are available for use in patients with drug-resistant epilepsy include the modified Atkins diet, low-glycemic diet, and medium-chain triglyceride diet. These are detailed below.

Low-Glycemic Index Treatment

This is a less restrictive diet which restricts carbohydrates to 40–60 g per day, does not restrict fluids or protein, and loosely monitors fat and calories. It is started as an outpatient without a fasting period [7]. Food quantities are not weighed out, but are based on portion sizes because of which, patients are able to live a more flexible lifestyle that includes eating at restaurants. On the low-glycemic index diet, the percentage of calories from fat is approximately 60%, compared with up to 90% on the ketogenic diet. About one-third of patients experience a > 50% seizure reduction after 3 months of implementation. Increased efficacy has been correlated with lower serum glucose levels, but not with changes in beta-hydroxybutyrate or change in ketosis status. The most common side effects include weight loss, acidosis, lethargy, nausea, vomiting, and headache. Acidosis may occur while initiating the diet which can be successfully treated with supplementation of a bicarbonate solution without affecting treatment efficacy of the diet.

Medium-Chain Triglyceride Diet

This diet is an alternate form of the classic ketogenic diet, where medium-chain triglycerides (MCTs) provided in an oil supplement are utilized as a major fat source. These MCTs yield more ketones and are more efficiently absorbed; as a result, less total fat is needed in the diet, and more protein and carbohydrates can be allowed. Many centers will also add MCT oils to the classic ketogenic diet as a supplement. The traditional MCT diet derived 60% of the energy from MCT. In some children, this needs to be reduced to 30–50% in order to minimize gastrointestinal symptoms, with the resulting decrement in energy source to be made up from long-chain fats.

Modified Atkins Diet

This diet is an alternative to the ketogenic diet. It is designed to mimic some aspects of the classic ketogenic diet, but there are no fluid or calorie restrictions. The diet is initiated as an outpatient without a fast. Carbohydrates are initially restricted to 10 grams per day (15–20 g per day in adolescents and adults) with patients counseled to increase their use of high-fat foods while decreasing the intake at of protein. Foods are not weighed and measured, but carbohydrate counts are monitored by patients and/or parents. This diet is more liberal than the ketogenic diet, and food restrictions are less and therefore may be eaten more freely in restaurants and other areas outside the home. Studies published on this alternative dietary therapy have established benefit in children as well as adults. Overall, 45% of patients experience a >50% seizure reduction, and 28% >90% seizure reduction, which is similar relative to the seizure control obtained with the traditional ketogenic diet but is much more palatable. Therefore, compliance may be easier when used in adults to adhere to than the ketogenic diet [8].

Pearls of Wisdom
1. The EEG pattern seen in patients with Glut-1 DS demonstrates a typical 3-Hz generalized spike-and-wave pattern associated with absence seizures. A similar mechanism is believed to be operational to typical childhood absence epilepsy involving the reticular thalamic nucleus and T-type calcium channels.
2. The ketogenic diet is an effective treatment for patients with epilepsy with >50% seizure reduction by 6 months in approximately 55–60% of children. It should be considered early as a treatment in patients with Glut-1 DS.
3. Side effects from the diet may emerge during treatment including dehydration, weight loss, renal stones, and osteopenia among others. Alternative types of diets such as the low-glycemic index diet and modified Atkins diet are other less rigorous forms of low-glycemic diets that are more palatable options for older children as well as young adults.
4. The ketogenic diet is the treatment of choice in GLUT-1 and pyruvate dehydrogenase deficiency though other conditions associated with altered lipid metabolism should be avoided. When the ketogenic diet is started in Glut-1 DS early in infancy, it may prevent ongoing developmental delay, microcephaly, and other comorbidities.
5. The hallmark of GLUT-1 DS is a low spinal fluid glucose level relative to a serum glucose done after 4–6 h of fasting, or a spinal fluid glucose to blood glucose ratio at or below the 25th percentile. A definitive means of support is to identify the gene mutation SLC2A1 which is present in up to 90% of patients with the typical phenotype of Glut-1 DS.

References

1. De Vivo DC, Trifiletti RR, Jacobson RI, Ronen GM, Behmand RA, Harik SI. Defective glucose transport across the blood-brain barrier as a cause of persistent hypoglycorrhachia, seizures, and developmental delay. N Engl J Med. 1991;325:703–9.
2. Leen WG, Klepper J, Verbeek MM, et al. Glucose transporter-1 deficiency syndrome: the expanding clinical and genetic spectrum of a treatable disorder. Brain. 2010;133:655–70.
3. Pong AW, Geary BR, Engelstad KM, Natarajan A, Yang H, De Vivo DC. Glucose transporter type I deficiency syndrome: epilepsy phenotypes and outcomes. Epilepsia. 2012;53:1503–10.
4. Freeman J, Veggiotti P, Lanzi G, et al. The ketogenic diet: from molecular mechanisms to clinical effects. Epilepsy Res. 2006;68:145–80.
5. Bough KJ, Rho JM. Anticonvulsant mechanisms of the ketogenic diet. Epilepsia. 2007;48:43–58.
6. Optimal clinical management of children receiving dietary therapies for epilepsy: Updated recommendations of the International Ketogenic Diet Study Group, Kossoff EH, Zupec-Kania BA, Auvin S, Ballaban-Gil KR, Christina Bergqvist AG, Blackford R, Buchhalter JR, Caraballo RH, Cross JH, Dahlin MG, Donner EJ, Guzel O, Jehle RS, Klepper J, Kang HC, Lambrechts DA, YMC L, Nathan JK, Nordli DR Jr, Pfeifer HH, Rho JM, Scheffer IE, Sharma S, Stafstrom CE, Thiele EA, Turner Z, Vaccarezza MM, van der Louw EJTM, Veggiotti P, Wheless JW, Wirrell EC. Charlie Foundation, Matthew's friends, practice committee of the child neurology society. Epilepsia Open. 2018;3(2):175. Epub 2018 May 21
7. Muzykewicz DA, Lyczkowski DA, Memon N, et al. Efficacy, safety, and tolerability of the low glycemic index treatment in pediatric epilepsy. Epilepsia. 2009;50:1118.
8. Kossoff EH, Dorward JL. The modifoed Atkins diet. Epilepsia. 2008 Nov;49(Suppl 8):37–41. https://doi.org/10.1111/j.1528-1167.2008.01831.

Complications from Seizures During Video-EEG Monitoring

49

Joseph F. Drazkowski

Case A 35-year-old man with uncontrolled seizures was admitted to the epilepsy monitoring unit (EMU) for presurgical evaluation. Greater than 20-year history of seizures persisted presumably related to febrile seizures as a child. The patient has been on antiseizure medications since childhood, many being older "enzyme-inducing" drugs. None of the drugs tried provided adequate seizure control to allow driving. They also interfered with personal relationships and employment for the patient who experienced both uncontrolled seizures and side effects from medications. He was therefore referred for epilepsy surgery evaluation and subsequently admitted to the EMU. The patient was surprised and expressed concern when he was told his usual antiseizure medication required reduction to capture seizures. The patient's current disabling seizures were classified as focal impaired awareness seizures. He has a preceding aura of déjà vu. He had not suffered from a convulsion since he was a teenager. After admission, ASMs were tapered, and he had two typical focal seizures with altered awareness over a 10 h period and had returned to baseline after each seizure. That evening, he suffered a convulsion and was given rescue intravenous (IV) lorazepam. It was noted that he had a deep tongue laceration and experienced urinary incontinence. He was given local lidocaine gel for his painful tongue and a change of clothing and bedsheets following incontinence. Cognition returned to normal after 20 min, and the lorazepam allowed him to sleep that evening. After the seizures, his usual ASM were restarted. Early in the morning, he was awakened by pain in his muscles and in the midthoracic spine and low back. X-Rays of the spine showed several compression fractures in the thoracic spine (Fig. 49.1).

J. F. Drazkowski (✉)
Mayo Clinic, Department of Neurology, Phoenix, AZ, USA
e-mail: Drazkowski.Joseph@mayo.edu

© Springer Nature Switzerland AG 2021
W. O. Tatum et al. (eds.), *Epilepsy Case Studies*,
https://doi.org/10.1007/978-3-030-59078-9_49

Fig. 49.1 Multiple compression fractures of the thoracolumbar spine following a convulsion (Note the intramedullary and superior endplate edema)

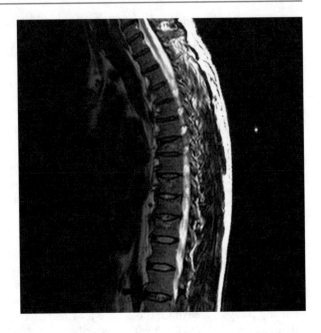

Clinical Questions

1. What are common complications associated with seizures in patients admitted to the EMU?
2. What are serious complications from seizures, and how often do they occur?
3. Can seizure associated complications be predicted and possibly avoided?
4. How should the complications of inpatient seizures be managed?
5. What should the patient be told about potential complications from seizure monitoring in the hospital?

Discussion

1. Most people with uncontrolled epilepsy, especially those who are admitted for continuous VEM, are aware of the more common complications of seizures as listed in Table 49.1. These complications may occur with any seizure, and most patients and families are often familiar with them, especially if seizures are drug-resistant and frequent [2]. These complications are often relatively minor and treated at home. Common seizure complications are typically effectively treated with minor first aid procedures. In the present case a local anesthetic was used to alleviate the pain due to a tongue laceration.
2. Thankfully the more serious complications listed in Table 49.2 are relatively rare compared with the common seizure complications listed above. These complications are a concern for physicians, nurses, and other allied healthcare

Table 49.1 Common seizure complications	Tongue laceration
	Bruises
	Myalgia
	Urinary/fecal incontinence
	Skin lacerations/abrasions
	Contusions

Table 49.2 Serious seizure complications	Status epilepticus
	Severe lacerations (especially head wounds)
	Concussion
	Ictal/post
	Ictal psychosis
	Fracture: vertebral/limb/facial
	Renal injury post convulsion (muscle breakdown)
	Cardiac asystole/arrhythmia/ischemia
	Flash pulmonary edema
	Deep vein thrombosis/pulmonary embolism
	Aspiration pneumonia
	Hypoxia

professionals. One cannot obviate all risk especially for unpredictable events such as seizures, but inhouse procedures, protocols, and training can help minimize the effects of such complications when they do occur. Being ready and having a plan to deal with these complications represents best practices and reduce suffering [3, 4]. Typically these serious complications occur rarely, less than 1–2% of admissions.

3. Being familiar with all complications can allow for institutional planning to both avoid and treat the complications of inpatient seizures. Simple first aid can be used for the more minor complications. Avoiding much of the minor complications can be anticipated especially in care procedures utilized in the monitoring unit. Classic examples include bed rail padding, fall precaution protocols, voluntary safety waist belt use for postictal confusion, intravenous (IV) access, postictal patient positioning, and cardiac telemetry/oximetry. These are in addition to careful behavioral monitoring of the patients with ongoing EEG surveillance to provide continuous observation of video-EEG. It has been noted that most VEM-associated falls occur on the way to or in the bathroom. We have adopted a safety vest system involving a ceiling-mounted track system that has prevented 99% of falls (even in the bathroom) during the admission mitigating injury to both patient and nursing personnel. Deep vein thrombosis prophylaxis in the form of regular mobilization/exercise and/or subcutaneous anticoagulation is also utilized.

4. Managing complications generally flows from protocols typically in place in anticipation of common and uncommon complications. One of the more common, meaningful, and effective treatments is judicious use of emergent antiseizure treatment with rescue medication to avoid status epilepticus. Use of a universal IV access policy for patients admitted to the EMU facilitates timely

administration of appropriate medications [1, 5]. Rapid IV access on the EMU can save minutes in an emergent situation. Clear orders placed for nurses to use rescue medication as part of a protocol, when needed to avoid having to obtain a verbal order from the covering physician, are efficient during seizure emergencies. Other forms of rescue medications may be also be utilized when there is no IV access. Nasal spray and rectal gels of benzodiazepine rescue medications are available. Shoulder dislocations and orthopedic injuries including compression fractures are fortunately uncommon but may occur following a convulsion. Having a plan in place in case of occurrence can help reduce patient's pain and suffering. Worrisome deterioration in vital sign issues associated with seizures include respiratory compromise and especially cardiac arrhythmia (Fig. 49.2). However, these can typically be managed with proper rescue protocols, rapid response teams, and appropriate subspecialty consultation to provide supportive care when necessary [6].

5. One cannot predict all complications that may occur in the EMU. Communicating common potential complications and having patient safety protocols in place alert the patient and family of potential safety concerns and are helpful to assuage fears and concerns about the hospitalization. Reviewing the details before or at admission has become a very useful practice at our program that patients, family, and nursing have come to appreciate.

Pearls of Wisdom

1. The nature of seizures is that they are associated with acute complications from minor to major severity. These indeed may occur in patients admitted to the EMU. Complications may be facilitated by the admission process when tapering ASMs takes place. Patients and families are often willing to risk the occurrence of potential complications due to seizure monitoring if it helps provide benefit in their overall treatment.

2. The occurrences of complications in the EMU are uncommon and are often treated effectively, especially when complications are anticipated and care protocols are in place.

3. Tapering ASMs in the EMU during VEM can lead to more frequent and more severe seizures. This should be anticipated when developing safety and rescue protocols.

4. Serious medical complications associated with seizures are significantly less common than minor complications but should be anticipated and able to be dealt with in the EMU.

5. Despite the possibility of complications, VEM remains the gold standard to diagnose patients with recurrent spells, classify those with epilepsy, and characterize person with epilepsy for possible surgery. Patients and families typically are willing to accept the risk of potential complications in the EMU especially when the process may lead to more effective treatment(s).

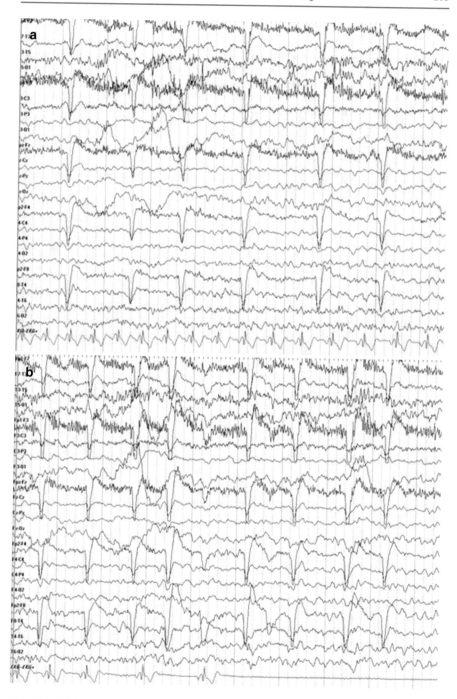

Fig. 49.2 (**a**) Ictal tachycardia during an ongoing seizure and (**b**) associated ictal asystole (Note the EKG with a dropped beat in second 5)

References

1. Noe K, Drazkowski J. Safety of the long-term video electroencephalographic monitoring for the evaluation epilepsy. Mayo Clin Proc. 2009;84(6):495–500.
2. Wirrell E. Epilepsy related injuries. Epilepsia. 2006;47(supp 1):79–86.
3. Rugg-Gunn F, Duncan J, et al. From unwitnessed fatality to witnessed rescue: nonpharmacologic interventions in sudden unexpected death in epilepsy. Epilepsia. 2016;57(supp 1):26–34.
4. Dobesberger J, Walser G, et al. Video-EEG monitoring: safety and adverse events in 507 consecutive patients. Epilepsia. 2011;52:443–52.
5. Dobesberger J, Hofler J, et al. Personalized safety measures reduce the adverse event rate of long term video EEG. Epilepsia open. 2017;2(4):400–14.
6. NAEC-Epilepsy.org National association of epilepsy centers; Updates and Resources; 2018 sample protocols. Accessed 31 May 2020.

Psychosocial Aspects and Stigma

50

Anthony L. Fine and William O. Tatum

Case

A 32-year-old right-handed single woman from the Middle East with anxiety-depression presented to epilepsy clinic for evaluation of a 7-year history of uncontrolled nighttime attacks. She was accompanied by her mother and younger sister who witnessed episodes of sudden arousal from sleep with violent thrashing of her arms and legs and screaming loudly jumping out of the bed. The duration was reported to be 2 to 3 min, and she would have no recall of the event, subsequently returning to sleep. The episodes reoccurred every night sometime 2–3 times per night. She was felt to be possessed by a demon by some of her distant family members. Anxiety and panic medications were unsuccessful in stopping the episodes. Brain MRI and several EEGs were normal. Seizures were considered, but carbamazepine and phenobarbital as well as several trials of alternative antiseizure medications (ASM) were unsuccessful.

Due to the nightly events, the patient was stigmatized by her paroxysmal bizarre behavior, age, and gender. She was isolated and even ostracized by others in her community due to religious underpinnings. She was unable to maintain outside personal or sexual relationships due to the episodes. She remained at home during the day to help around the house due to a periodic intercurrent postictal state and variable side effects from antiseizure medication limiting her ability to gain

A. L. Fine (✉)
Mayo Clinic, Department of Neurology, Division of Child and Adolescent Neurology, Rochester, MN, USA
e-mail: fine.anthony@mayo.edu

W. O. Tatum
Mayo Clinic, Department of Neurology, Jacksonville, FL, USA
e-mail: tatum.william@mayo.edu

© Springer Nature Switzerland AG 2021
W. O. Tatum et al. (eds.), *Epilepsy Case Studies*,
https://doi.org/10.1007/978-3-030-59078-9_50

employment. She came to the United States for treatment to be eligible for marriage like others who were younger than her and "have a normal life."

Questions

1. Is this epilepsy? What is the most likely epilepsy diagnosis?
2. What are some potential etiologies?
3. What factors need to be considered when developing a treatment plan?
4. What contributes to the stigma experienced by people with epilepsy, and what are some effects of stigma on quality of life in people with epilepsy?
5. What should be considered as next steps in the evaluation and treatment of this woman?

Discussion

1. Given the description of frequent, stereotyped events arising from sleep with hyperkinetic activity epileptic seizures merit principal consideration. Seizures arising from the orbitofrontal and mesial frontal lobes can be difficult to diagnose by semiology alone. Hyperkinetic seizures may also originate in the insula and temporal lobe and produce a semiology like those in frontal lobe epilepsy. Previously known as nocturnal frontal lobe epilepsy, sleep-related hypermotor epilepsy (SHE) can remain undiagnosed for years. It can be challenging to separate the semiology of nocturnal panic attacks from SHE, further accentuated by the limited ability for scalp EEG to detect epileptiform activity. Many people with hyperkinetic seizures are initially given a diagnosis of psychogenic non-epileptic attacks until they obtain a definitive diagnosis with video-EEG monitoring. Sleep disorders may also mimic SHE with sleep terrors, sleep walking, confusional arousals in NREM sleep and REM behavior disorder, and nightmares arising from REM sleep. Parasomnias including periodic limb movements of sleep, cataplexy, hallucinations, paralysis, hypnic jerks, and nocturnal enuresis may have semiologies that overlap with SHE, and while history is usually helpful to define seizures, video-EEG or video-polysomnography with an expanded EEG montage may be necessary to arrive at a diagnosis (Fig. 50.1).
2. Potential etiologies of SHE include genetic, structural, and unknown causes. Individuals with a family history of nocturnal hyperkinetic seizures and gene mutations that encode nicotinic acetylcholine receptor α and β subunits have autosomal dominant nocturnal frontal lobe epilepsy (ADNFLE), which has been shown to be caused by variants in the KCNT1 receptor. There are other genetic causes as well as gene variants which can cause structural changes resulting in an epileptogenic focus, such as variants in TSC1 or TSC2 genes in tuberous sclerosis complex and DEPDC5, which can be associated with focal cortical dysplasia and familial focal epilepsy with variable foci. Additional structural

Fig. 50.1 Signs during sleep may mimic frontal lobe epilepsy as well as psychogenic nonepileptic attacks. EEG electroencephalogram, FLE frontal lobe epilepsy, IEDs interictal epileptiform discharges, REM rapid eye movement sleep, NREM non-rapid eye movement sleep, SWS sleep wave sleep

Signs	Epilepsy	PNEA	REM	NREM
Recall	None except with FLE	Usually None	Bad Dream	None
Stereo-typed	Yes	No	No	No
EEG/PSG	IEDs or ictal discharges	Awake or drowsy	REM + EMG	SWS
Time	Anytime	Varies	Last ½ of night	1st one-third of night

considerations include malformations of cortical development, encephalomalacia from prior head injury, stroke, and brain tumors.

3. There are several factors which should be considered when counseling the patient regarding additional evaluations and treatment strategies. In our patient, there were cultural and personal beliefs which influenced her decision-making to pursue surgical help to allow her to marry. Being the subject of stigmatization due to epilepsy may lead to social isolation and psychosocial retardation, in addition to, culturally based practices which may further compromise the victim's quality of life. People with epilepsy have many social problems and may become socially withdrawn, become ostracized, and endure low self-esteem. The availability of certain ASM varies by country, and recommending medication alternatives should ensure the therapy is available in the patient's home country. When discussing medication options, the provider should be aware of any complications of treatment, particularly as they apply to women with epilepsy. These include the reduced effectiveness of oral contraceptives and increased chance of unplanned pregnancy, risk of reduced fertility, and teratogenic effects of antiseizure medication such as valproate or phenobarbital that carry the risk of major congenital malformations. Even if a woman is not currently planning on becoming pregnant or reports she is sexually inactive, counseling should be provided.

4. Despite large-scale global efforts in providing education to the public on epilepsy, there continues to be much misinformation and preconceived notions. In some cultures, people with epilepsy (PWE) are discriminated against or feel discrimination, particularly when it comes to employment and interpersonal relationships. A major reason for this stigmatization in PWE is a lack of public understanding of what epilepsy comprises [1]. Reasons found to contribute to a sense of perceived stigma include factors such as marital status (being single),

Table 50.1 Psychosocial issues affecting people with epilepsy

Stigma
Transportation
Education
Employment and Financial
Marriage and Children
Sexuality
Self-identity and social relationships
Quality of life

more severe epilepsy, having a high seizure burden, multiple ASM, and experiencing drug side effects, reduced medical literacy, and poor coping skills [2, 3]. The effects of stigmatization in PWE include impaired social interactions, higher rates of unemployment, and higher rates of anxiety and depression, which lead to overall reduction in one's quality of life [4]. In our patient, social and cultural barriers existed secondary to uncontrolled seizures resulting in stigmatization. Reduced quality of life was evident to our patient due to the inability to marry and have a family. This additionally led to isolation from others in her community. Increasing the individual's resilience and trying to change social attitudes requires targeting young school-aged people through education and social media (Table 50.1).

5. Patients with drug-resistant frontal lobe epilepsy and significant psychosocial impairment should have a comprehensive evaluation to identify them as a potential epilepsy surgery candidate. High-resolution brain MRI with an epilepsy protocol is the foundation of the evaluation for frontal lobe epilepsy given the limitation of discovering an abnormality on EEG. Video-EEG monitoring is the primary method for diagnosis and characterization of the electroclinical syndrome for patients with SHE. When anatomic brain MRI is "negative," additional functional neuroimaging studies such as PET-MRI or PET-CT may be helpful in localizing a hypometabolic focus or a region of cerebral hyperperfusion with ictal single-photon emission computed tomography. Magnetoencephalography may help as an adjunct to EEG to identify a cluster of electrical dipoles that localize the epileptogenic zone. When discordant information is found on the noninvasive evaluations and seizure localization is needed, phase 2 epilepsy monitoring with intracranial recording may be successful. In our patient, a malformation of cortical development was found (Taylor 2B focal cortical dysplasia); she underwent surgical resection following invasive EEG monitoring and has been seizure-free. She returned home and became involved in a romantic relationship with plans to marry.

Clinical Pearls

1. There is often significant stigma associated with a diagnosis of epilepsy. The level of perceived stigma can vary significantly. Stigma is based on many factors including one's level of education, social beliefs, cultural influence, and religious tendency.
2. The effects of stigmatization in people with epilepsy can be severe and lead to reduced or impaired psychosocial function from isolation, worsening anxiety and depression, and compromised general health and overall quality of life [5].
3. The sophistication of medical and surgical evaluations and treatments for the management of epilepsy varies in underdeveloped as well as developing countries. When treating an international patient, the clinician should take into consideration whether ASM is available in the patient's home country to continue maintenance medical therapy if initiated elsewhere.
4. In patients with drug-resistant frontal lobe epilepsy, nocturnal activation of recurrent seizures is often confused with psychiatric conditions or sleep disorders that stigmatize PWE.
5. When a definitive diagnosis of epilepsy is made with video-EEG monitoring and patients remain drug-resistant, an evaluation should be performed to see if the patient is an epilepsy surgery candidate.

References

1. Kroner BL, Fahimi M, Gaillard WD, Kenyon A, Thurman DJ. Epilepsy or seizure disorder? The effect of cultural and socioeconomic factors on self-reported prevalence. Epilepsy Behav. 2016;62:214–7.
2. Bautista RE, Shapovalov D, Shoraka AR. Factors associated with increased felt stigma among individuals with epilepsy. Seizure. 2015;30:106–12.
3. Shi Y, Wang S, Ying J, Zhang M, Liu P, Zhang H, et al. Correlates of perceived stigma for people living with epilepsy: a meta-analysis. Epilepsy Behav. 2017;70(Pt A):198–203.
4. Al-Khateeb JM, Al-Khateeb AJ. Research on psychosocial aspects of epilepsy in Arab countries: a review of literature. Epilepsy Behav. 2014;31:256–62.
5. de Boer HM, Mula M, Sander JW. The global burden and stigma of epilepsy. Epilepsy Behav. 2008;12:540–6.

Eloquent Cortex Resection in Rasmussen's Syndrome

51

Kai J. Miller, Cyrille Ferrier, Brian N. Lundstrom, and Peter van Rijen

Case Report

A 20-year-old pathologically left-handed woman presented with history of refractory epilepsia partialis pars continua and progressive loss of right-sided motor function. Serial MR imaging showed progressive atrophy of the left hemisphere. The clinical picture and MRI were compatible with diagnosis of Rasmussen's encephalitis.

Her epilepsy started at the age of 9 years with focal motor seizures involving clonic movements of the right arm, leg, and/or mouth. While initially intermittent, seizure activity progressed to a continuous state with waxing and waning severity of the clonic movements (epilepsia partialis continua). Language dysfunction fluctuated with seizure severity. She was noted to have a slight right-sided hemiparesis at age 14. Prolonged IVIG and steroid therapy were not helpful, and functional disability progressed such that her right arm motor ability was severely limited by age 20 [6]. She had been right-handed before onset of epilepsy at the age of 9, but

Kai J. Miller and Cyrille Ferrier contributed equally with all other contributors.

K. J. Miller (✉)
Mayo Clinic, Department of Neurosurgery, Rochester, MN, USA

University Medical Center Utrecht, Brain Center Rudolf Magnus, Department of Neurology and Neurosurgery, Utrecht, The Netherlands
e-mail: miller.kai@mayo.edu

C. Ferrier · P. van Rijen
University Medical Center Utrecht, Brain Center Rudolf Magnus, Department of Neurology and Neurosurgery, Utrecht, The Netherlands
e-mail: P.v.Rijen@umcutrecht.nl

B. N. Lundstrom
Mayo Clinic, Department of Neurology, Rochester, MN, USA
e-mail: Lundstrom.Brian@mayo.edu

transitioned fully to left-handedness by the age of 20. Visual fields were intact on neurological examination. Her neurological history is otherwise significant for meningococcal meningitis at age of 3.

The severity of her seizures, combined with her continued loss of right-sided motor function, is an indication to consider hemispherectomy, the definitive treatment for Rasmussen's syndrome. However, that would be expected to leave her with residual aphasia since she was left hemisphere dominant for language evident from her fluctuating aphasia during her focal seizures. Further language workup was not fruitful – an fMRI performed in 2009 was inconclusive for language dominance due to poor patient cooperation. Functional transcranial Doppler sonography for language lateralization was not possible because of an insufficient acoustic temporal bone window.

Surgery was initially deferred for 2 years in the interest of preserving language function and right-sided motor abilities. However, as the disease progressed to include severe right-sided hemiparesis, surgery was reconsidered by a multidisciplinary epilepsy team. The recommendation was to pursue a modified surgical approach sparing language function. We believed that a complete left sensorimotor (rolandic) resection for palliation would stop motor aspects of disease while preserving language, cognitive, and visual function with the understanding that language-related disruptions might continue and progress. The patient was also counseled for worsening of motor abilities with her right-sided extremities.

Surgical Intervention

The complete sensorimotor resection was performed in the following steps:

- The outward projection of the pre- and postcentral gyri was identified using stereotactic navigation (Stealth Navigation system, Medtronic, Minneapolis, MN). A question mark-shaped incision was made in the scalp, extending across the midline. The cranial and dural openings were then made, incorporating the pre- and postcentral gyri with generous margin (Fig. 51.1).
- Median nerve somatosensory evoked potential identified postcentral gyrus using a 5x4 electrode grid overlying the central cortex. Thereafter, electrocorticography was performed in several stages over central and adjacent frontal and parietal cortex. It demonstrated multifocal ictal activity over the frontal lobe and pre- and postcentral gyri (Fig. 51.1).
- The pre- and postcentral gyri were confirmed based upon anatomical landmarks and confirmed with navigation. Subpial resection was performed with ultrasonic aspiration, following gray matter to the base of the precentral sulcus anteriorly, the postcentral sulcus posteriorly, and around all the gray matter lining the central sulcus, preserving the white matter beneath. Some minimal injury to the extreme capsule was assumed involving U-fibers connecting the pre- and

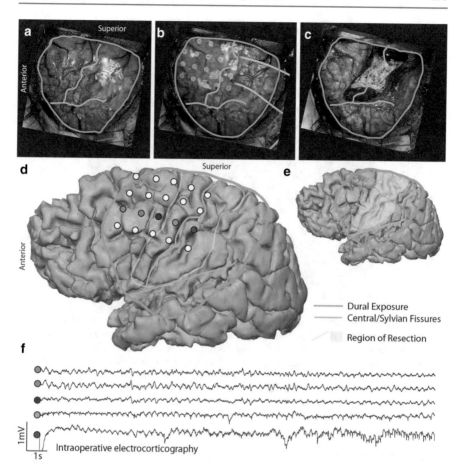

Fig. 51.1 Total primary sensorimotor cortex resection. (**a**) A left hemispheric craniotomy was performed. (**b**) Intraoperative electrocorticography (ECoG) was measured. (**c**) The pre- and postcentral gyri were removed in entirety. (**d**) A left-hemispheric brain surface reconstruction from preoperative MRI shows the extent of craniotomy, placement of ECoG array, and extent of resection. Note the relative occipital sparing in cortical atrophy that is characteristic of Rasmussen's syndrome. (**e**) Region of resection shown independently on left-hemisphere reconstruction. (**f**) Intraoperative ECoG, colors correspond to locations noted in (**d**). Note epileptic activity in orange and red sites. Blue outline shows region of intraoperative dural exposure. Green line shows central/Sylvian fissures. Yellow trace (in **d**) and shading (in **e**) show the region of resection (**c**)

postcentral gyri (Fig. 51.2), extending ventrally to the Sylvian fissure and dorsally to the midline. This maintains the integrity of the internal capsule within which the arcuate fasciculus and inferior fronto-occipital fasciculus are contained, carrying important information between language association regions [7].
• Hemostasis and wound closure were performed in the standard fashion.

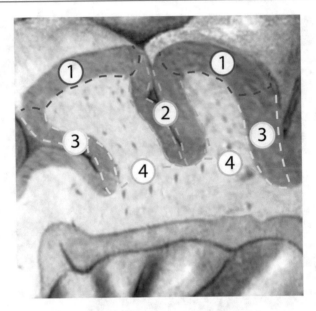

Fig. 51.2 Steps in the subpial resection: *1* (*red dashed line*), remove *gray* matter on the gyral caps of the pre- and postcentral gyri; *2* (*green dashed line*), remove *gray* matter lining the central sulcus, limiting the depth of the resection to the *gray-white* interface beneath the pial plane; *3* (*yellow dashed line*), removal of precentral and postcentral sulci *gray* matter to the *white-gray* junction at the base of the sulcal plane; *4* (*orange dashed line*), the *white* matter is taken down to a depth defined by the subpial section to avoid damages to the tracts beneath. (Case courtesy of Assoc Prof Frank Gaillard, Radiopaedia.org, rID: 58883, https://radiopaedia.org/cases/subcortical-u-fibres-and-juxtacortical-lesions-illustration)

Postoperative Function

In the immediate postoperative period, she was found to have preserved motor function on the right side of her body, with right-hand grip and sensation documented in the surgical recovery ward. She was found to have a right hemianopia. At her first postoperative clinic visit, she was noted to be able to walk without the use of a wheelchair, something she was unable to do preoperatively due to continuous seizure activity. She was able to ride a bike, which she had not been able to do preoperatively. Her family felt that she had an overall subjective improvement in function and cognition in her interpersonal interactions as well as activities of daily living. This level of function was maintained as of her most recent year follow-up visit 3 years later.

Questions

1. What are typical characteristics of Rasmussen's syndrome?
2. How does the disease usually progress?

3. What other types of neurological conditions can provoke epilepsia partials continua with motor symptoms but can be successfully treated surgically without a significant (or with minor) neurological deficit?
4. What is the end stage of Rasmussen's syndrome?
5. What is an emerging option for high-functioning patients with Rasmussen's syndrome, but no relocation of representation to the contralateral hemisphere?

Discussion Points

1. Rasmussen's syndrome (f.k.a. Rasmussen's encephalitis) is a progressive inflammatory childhood disease marked by hemispheric atrophy, focal seizures, and intellectual decline. For the vast majority of patients, focal seizures are the initial sign of the disease, typically occurring before age 10 years. Seizures are often resistant to antiseizure medication, and focal motor seizures such as epilepsia partialis continua (EPC) are typical.
2. Disease progression has been described by three stages. Seizures begin first. After several years, worsening hemiparesis, neurological decline, and intellectually decline follow. After another several years, disease stabilization is often noted, with cessation of further decline and some improvement in seizure activity.
3. In our experience, patients with a ganglioglioma, focal cortical dysplasia (type 2B), and dysembryoplastic neuroepithelial tumor (DNET) can provoke epilepsia partials continua with motor symptoms but can be successfully treated surgically without a significant (or with minor) neurological deficit, due to the relative sequestration from, rather than integration into, the functioning brain tissue.
4. Anecdotally, we have come across patients with Rasmussen's syndrome in which no surgery was performed, despite many years of seizures. Eventually, patients became seizure-free but had a significant hemiparesis (hand/arm more pronounced than leg) yet were able to walk.
5. Implanted cortical stimulation therapies in the form of responsive neurostimulation or constant subthreshold cortical stimulation represent a potential alternative to disconnection or resective surgery.

Pearls
1. Selective resection can treat epilepsia partialis pars continua in Rasmussen's syndrome while preserving language.
2. The primary features of Rasmussen's syndrome are progressive neurologic decline and drug-resistant focal epilepsy. Neurological deficits may fluctuate due to ongoing or frequent seizures.
3. Although focal motor seizures emerging from the perirolandic region are the most common, a variety of seizures with posturing, visual, auditory, or somatosensory manifestations can develop over time in patients with Rasmussen's syndrome; however, drop attacks rarely occur.

4. A detailed history can help to provide an understanding of cortical reorganization of eloquent function and transference from one hemisphere to the other.
5. Surgical resection can successfully treat patients with drug-resistant epilepsy including epilepsia partialis continua associated with Rasmussen's syndrome. When the disease progresses with recurrent focal seizures, a hemispherotomy can be safely performed without sustaining significant postoperative neurological deficits.

Acknowledgments We are grateful for ongoing communication with the patient and their family. KJM is supported by the Van Wagenen Fellowship and CTSA Grant Number KL2 TR002379 (NIH - NCATS).

References

1. Rasmussen T, Olszewski J, Lloydsmith D. Focal seizures due to chronic localized encephalitis. Neurology. 1958;8:435–45.
2. Varadkar S, Bien CG, Kruse CA, Jensen FE, Bauer J, Pardo CA, et al. Rasmussen's encephalitis: clinical features, pathobiology, and treatment advances. Lancet Neurol. 2014;13:195–205.
3. Hart YM, Cortez M, Andermann F, Hwang P, Fish DR, Dulac O, et al. Medical treatment of Rasmussen's syndrome (chronic encephalitis and epilepsy): effect of high-dose steroids or immunoglobulins in 19 patients. Neurology. 1994;44:1030.
4. Takahashi Y, Yamazaki E, Mine J, Kubota Y, Imai K, Mogami Y, et al. Immunomodulatory therapy versus surgery for Rasmussen syndrome in early childhood. Brain Dev. 2013;35:778–85.
5. Bien CG, Granata T, Antozzi C, Cross JH, Dulac O, Kurthen M, et al. Pathogenesis, diagnosis and treatment of Rasmussen encephalitis: a European consensus statement. Brain. 2005;128:454–71.
6. Matthews WB. Aids to the examination of the peripheral nervous system [internet]. J Neurol Sci. 1977;299. https://doi.org/10.1016/0022-510x(77)90205-2.
7. Almairac F, Herbet G, Moritz-Gasser S, de Champfleur NM, Duffau H. The left inferior fronto-occipital fasciculus subserves language semantics: a multilevel lesion study [internet]. Brain Struct Funct. 2015:1983–95. https://doi.org/10.1007/s00429-014-0773-1.

Epilogue

I wish to express gratitude to my colleagues at the Mayo Clinic in Florida, Arizona, and Minnesota for the privilege to work and learn from them. This multiauthored work from the Mayo Clinic enterprise is comprised of many outstanding epileptologists and amazing individuals who ontributed freely and generously of their time without prompting or hesitancy. It serves as a testimony to their dedication and reflects the strength of the Mayo Clinic to attract the best clinicians, educators, and researchers within the field of epileptology. Each author has contributed a case report of a patient represented in a vignette to illustrate a specific condition or situations that involved someone afflicted by epilepsy. It is the details of the situation that are encoded in their memory. These are based on the person and special characteristics that makes the memory of that particular situation last. To a large degree, all our experiences treating patients have been shaped by the unique qualities of a single person that makes us remember it when asked to recall a specific clinical condition or situation.

In the second edition of this book, 51 people had their lives suddenly change and take a different course after being affected by epilepsy. The stigma and painful lack of predictability they have endured, as have their families, is something that most of us will hopefully never know. Much of what we take for granted exists as an unknown for the patients in this book. I hope the readers of this book never know and experience the life-changing event that occurs following a seizure. Instead, it is hoped that from these stories, drawn from real-life experiences, that the breadth and individuality of epilepsy will stimulate compassion for those who suffer and endure the constant fear wondering if and when they will experience their next seizure.

WO Tatum

Index

© Springer Nature Switzerland AG 2021
W. O. Tatum et al. (eds.), *Epilepsy Case Studies*,
https://doi.org/10.1007/978-3-030-59078-9

Printed in the United States
by Baker & Taylor Publisher Services